Vulnerabilities, Impacts, and Responses to HIV/AIDS in Sub-Saharan Africa

Vulnerabilities, Impacts, and Responses to HIV/AIDS in Sub-Saharan Africa

Edited by

Getnet Tadele
Associate Professor, Addis Ababa University, Ethiopia

and

Helmut Kloos
Research Associate, University of California, USA

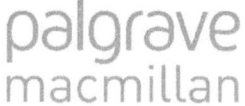

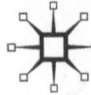

First published 2013 by
PALGRAVE MACMILLAN

Palgrave Macmillan in the UK is an imprint of Macmillan Publishers Limited,
registered in England, company number 785998, of Houndmills, Basingstoke,
Hampshire RG21 6XS.

Palgrave Macmillan in the US is a division of St Martin's Press LLC,
175 Fifth Avenue, New York, NY 10010.

Palgrave Macmillan is the global academic imprint of the above companies
and has companies and representatives throughout the world.

Palgrave® and Macmillan® are registered trademarks in the United States,
the United Kingdom, Europe and other countries.

ISBN 978–1–137–00994–4

This book is printed on paper suitable for recycling and made from fully
managed and sustained forest sources. Logging, pulping and manufacturing
processes are expected to conform to the environmental regulations of the
country of origin.

A catalogue record for this book is available from the British Library.

A catalog record for this book is available from the Library of Congress.

10   9   8   7   6   5   4   3   2   1
22 21 20 19 18 17 16 15 14 13

Contents

Part I Contextualizing HIV/AIDS

Part II Impacts and Responses to HIV/AIDS

Figures and Tables

Figures

Tables

Preface and Acknowledgments

The idea for this book was conceived after the completion of several research projects between 2003 and 2006 in many Sub-Saharan African countries that culminated in an international conference, 'The Social Sciences and HIV/AIDS in Africa: New Insights and Policy Perspectives', held in Addis Ababa in November 2006. After this conference, the Organization for Social Science Research in Eastern and Southern Africa (OSSREA) took further responsibility of supporting this book project. We hope that the fully revised and updated synthesis presented in this volume ensures that the main ideas we put forward will further influence students, practitioners, and health planners.

The social science perspective articulated in this volume can broaden understanding of the dynamics of the HIV/AIDS epidemic in infamously hyperendemic Sub-Saharan Africa and may help guide the development of comprehensive policies and appropriate, effective, and sustainable interventions. The chapters of this volume are written by several anthropologists and sociologists, an economist, a demographer, a social epidemiologist, and a health services specialist/physician, thus providing a wide interdisciplinary discourse. They go beyond the shortcomings of the biomedical approach to the HIV/AIDS problem described by earlier investigators. By embracing a more holistic approach, this book can contribute to further promoting and strengthening interdisciplinary studies involving the social and biomedical sciences. This promising approach offers considerable potential for an analytical contextualization of the pandemic and the development of equitable, culturally acceptable, and sustainable interventions within Sub-Saharan Africa. The identification of and elaboration on socioeconomic and cultural factors and contexts of HIV vulnerability, impacts, and responses are increasingly recognized as a prerequisite of an AIDS-free world and put this book at the center of efforts toward that end. We hope it will contribute to overcoming the persisting, albeit narrowing, divide between the biomedical and social sciences and promote a collective *harambee* spirit that is needed to mobilize all available resources to control the HIV/AIDS problem in the most affected and poorest region of the world.

We owe much gratitude to a number of people and organizations that contributed in various ways to the publication of this book. We are grateful to OSSREA, CODESRIA (Council for the Development of Social Science Research in Africa), SOMA-Net (Social Science and Medicine Africa Network), and UAPS (Union for African Population Studies) for initiating the project, deploying researchers, and giving inspiration for preparing this volume. Special thanks go to OSSREA for providing strong support throughout the project and hosting the international conference *The Social Sciences and HIV/AIDS in Africa: New Insights and Policy Perspectives* in Addis Ababa in 2006 that laid the groundwork. We are also indebted to SIDA/SARAC (Swedish International Development Agency) and Norad (Norwegian Agency for Development Cooperation) for providing financial assistance and unfailing encouragement during all phases of the project.

We also would like to express our appreciation to all the chapter contributors to this volume. We felt privileged to work with these committed researchers, who were responsive and patient during the preparation and editing of the manuscript. In making the extensive revisions, we are particularly grateful to the anonymous editors who forwarded many incisive comments. Asrat Ayalew provided technical assistance during the preparation of Chapter 1 and Benjamin Kloos during finalization of the manuscript. Paulos Chanie of OSSREA was particularly supportive throughout the process of writing. Ann Byers tirelessly and meticulously edited both revisions of the manuscript and worked with us far beyond the call of editorial duty. Aynalem Adugna kindly assisted in preparing the map and Worku Mulat prepared several graphs at short notice. At Palgrave, Senior Commissioning Editor Christina Brian provided valuable comments for the revision of the first draft and her assistant Amanda McGrath was a constant support. Anne Scott was kind enough to critically review the revised manuscript. Finally, our gratitude goes to all our families, for their support and inspiration throughout this book project.

Contributors

Woldekidan Amde is a PhD candidate and manager of an intercountry capacity development project covering South Africa, Mozambique, Ethiopia, and Rwanda at the School of Public Health, University of Western Cape, South Africa. His research interests include HIV/AIDS intervention, social determinants, health policy, systems analysis, and research and capacity development. He published (with Getnet Tadele) a chapter for the book *Adolescent Psychology around the World* (2012) and the monograph *Barriers to HIV Testing: Investigating HIV Testing Practices in a Rural District in Ethiopia* (2011).

Tekalign Ayalew is a lecturer in social anthropology in the Department of Social Anthropology of Addis Ababa University in Addis Ababa, Ethiopia. He has carried out research on gender-related issues in girls' education in southern Ethiopian communities and published the monograph *Risks, Resilience and Adaptations in Child Life: Success Stories of Resilient Children and Youth in Arba Minch Town* (2010).

Sebsib Belay is a lecturer in the School of Social Work, Indira Gandhi National Open University in Addis Ababa. He has extensive experience in social, anthropological, development, and public health research and in advising, monitoring, and evaluating community-based HIV/AIDS and social works projects in various Ethiopian communities. He has submitted research results to the HIV/AIDS Prevention and Control Office of the Ministry of Health, Addis Ababa, and various UN agencies (UNAIDS, WHO, and IOM) and contributed a chapter to the book *Grass-roots Justice in Ethiopia* (2010).

Ayalew Gebre is an assistant professor in the Department of Social Anthropology of Addis Ababa University. His current research interests include social aspects of HIV/AIDS and sexually transmitted infections (STIs), sexual abuse and exploitation of children, and child welfare. He published, among others, a chapter on care and support needs of HIV-infected young people and AIDS orphans in the CODESRIA Monograph Series (2009) and an article on community knowledge and perceptions of HIV/AIDS in *Northeast African Studies.*

Damen Haile Mariam is a medical doctor and professor in the School of Public Health, Addis Ababa University, and a consultant community health specialist in the Federal Ministry of Health in Addis Ababa. He has a wide range of interests and extensive research experience in Ethiopian public health, particularly in health services development, the *iddir* traditional social institution, and other HIV/AIDS-related issues. He has published numerous book chapters and articles in the *Ethiopian Journal of Health Development, Journal of Public Health Policy, AIDS Patient Care and STDs, Ethiopian Medical Journal, Journal of Health Services Research & Policy, BMC Health Services Research,* and *Social Science and Medicine* and edited (with Yemane Berhane and Helmut Kloos) the book *The Epidemiology and Ecology of Health and Disease in Ethiopia* (2006).

Charles Hongoro is the director of the Health Systems Research Unit of the South African Medical Research Council and a professor at Tshwane University of Technology. His work is currently focused on the provision of primary health care services, particularly scaling and improving the quality and cost-effectiveness of HIV services. He has published articles on equity of access to hospital services in *BMC Health Services Research,* cost analysis of hospital palliative care (*Journal of Pain and Symptoms Management*), and on human resources in health services in southern Africa in the *Lancet* and other journals.

Anne A. Khasakhala is a senior lecturer at the Population and Research Institute at the University of Nairobi in Kenya. Her research interests are in the areas of child health and development; maternal health; family planning; adolescent reproductive health; and social aspects of HIV/AIDS, fertility, morbidity, and mortality in Kenya. She has published articles in the *Journal of Biosocial Science, African Population Studies, Demography India, BMC Pregnancy and Birth,* and several book chapters. Dr. Khasakhala is the coauthor of the book *Urban Integration in Africa: A Socio-demographic Survey of Nairobi* (CODESRIA Monograph Series).

Helmut Kloos is an associate professor retired from Addis Ababa University and currently a research associate in the Department of Epidemiology and Biostatistics of the University of California, San Francisco, USA. He has a wide range of interests in public health and in strengthening interdisciplinary research involving the social and biomedical sciences in developing countries. He has carried out field research on access to health services, traditional medicine, and the transmission and control of neglected tropical diseases in Ethiopia, Kenya, Egypt, and Brazil. His current research interests include epidemiological, socioeconomic, and cultural aspects of HIV/AIDS. He has published articles on HIV/AIDS and STIs in the journals *Geospatial Health, BMC Health Services Research, Human Ecology Review, Ethiopian Medical Journal,* and the *Ethiopian Journal of Health Development* and co-edited with Zein Ahmed Zein, Yemane Berhane, and Damen Haile Mariam three editions of the book *The Ecology of Health and Disease in Ethiopia* (1988, 1993, and 2006).

Getnet Tadele is an associate professor in the Department of Sociology, Addis Ababa University, Ethiopia. His research interests are in child and adolescent issues, sexuality, HIV/AIDS, and other health problems. He has carried out several consultancy projects and evaluations for a number of nongovernmental organizations (NGOs) in the field of health science and recently conducted field research on livelihoods, economic strengthening and HIV/AIDS, prevention of mother-to-child transmission (PMTCT), and private sector involvement in sexual and reproductive health services delivery in Ethiopia. He published a book entitled *Bleak Prospects: Young Men, Sexuality and HIV/AIDS in an Ethiopian Town* (2006) and numerous articles in *Culture, Health & Sexuality, Journal of HIV/AIDS and Social Services, Northeast African Studies, CODESRIA and IDS Bulletin* and *Medische Anthropologie (Medical Anthropology)*.

Damtew Yirgu is a freelance anthropologist research consultant working in community development, poverty alleviation, and related areas and was a lecturer in an institute of the Ministry of Agriculture in Arsi Region, Ethiopia. He carried out research on maternal and child health-seeking behavior for Save the Children, UK, and conducted a longitudinal study of poverty, inequality, and well-being in rural communities in Oromia and Amhara regions in Ethiopia. His study results have been submitted in reports to these organizations.

Acronyms and Abbreviations

ACU	AIDS Control Unit
ART	antiretroviral therapy
ARV	antiretroviral
CODESRIA	Council for the Development of Social Science Research in Africa
DHS	Demographic and Health Survey
GAMET	Global Monitoring and Evaluation Team
HID	Human Development Index
HIV/AIDS	Human Immune Deficiency Virus/Acquired Immune Deficiency Syndrome
HPC	high-prevalence country
LSE	life skills education
M&E	monitoring and evaluation
MARPs	most-at-risk populations
MDGs	Millennium Development Goals
MSM	men who have sex with men
NACC	National AIDS Control Council
NGO	nongovernment organization
NSF	National Strategic Framework
OSSREA	Organization for Social Science Research in Eastern and Southern Africa
OVC	orphans and other vulnerable children
PEPFAR	President's Emergency Plan for AIDS Relief
PLWHA	people living with HIV/AIDS
PMTCT	prevention of mother-to-child transmission
PRSP	Poverty Reduction Prevention Plan
PSABH	Primary School Action for Better Health
RECs	research ethics committees
SIDA/SAREC	Swedish International Development Cooperation Agency
SOMA-NET	Social Science and Medicine Africa Network
STIs	sexually transmitted infections
UNAIDS	United Nations Joint Program for HIV/AIDS
UNDP	United Nations Development Program
UNESCO	United Nations Educational, Scientific, and Cultural Organization

UNGASS	United Nations General Assembly Special Session on HIV/AIDS
UNICEF	United Nations Children's Fund
USAID	United States Agency for International Development
VCT	Voluntary HIV counseling and testing
WHO	World Health Organization

Part I
Contextualizing HIV/AIDS

1
Introduction

Getnet Tadele

We are now approaching four decades since AIDS was first reported from Africa and yet, notwithstanding tremendous progress during the last decade, we are far from containing the pandemic caused by the human immuno-deficiency virus (HIV). In 2010, an estimated 68% of all people living with HIV/AIDS (PLWHA) and 70% of all new infections were in Sub-Saharan Africa (UNAIDS 2011, p. 7). Even though 22 countries in this region reported declines in HIV incidence of 25% or more and 20% fewer people died in 2009 than in 2001, the total number of PLWHA in Sub-Saharan Africa increased by 2.2 million during that period, 1.5 million of which lived in southern Africa, the most highly affected region. South Africa, the country with the largest epidemic worldwide, reported 220,000 AIDS-related deaths in 2001 and 310,000 in 2009; 15 other countries in Sub-Saharan Africa reported smaller increases in mortality although a downward trend appeared in the region after 2004 as a result of intensified interventions (UNAIDS 2010, pp. 16, 180, 185). AIDS continues to severely impact households, communities, businesses, public services, and national economies in the Sub-Saharan African region and local, national, and international stakeholders searching for new, effective, and sustainable ways to contain the epidemic.

Recognizing that HIV/AIDS is a social, behavioral, and biomedical problem requires that socioeconomic, cultural, and political factors be carefully examined toward unraveling this complex phenomenon in Africa. Our understanding of the historical, social, economic, cultural, and political contexts of the disease and of human sexuality, which accounts more than any other factor for the transmission of the virus in Sub-Saharan Africa, is paramount to the development of effective prevention and control programs (Kalipeni et al. 2004). Toward achieving that understanding, this book examines how the web of socioeconomic factors and cultural norms surrounding sexuality and stigma influences the trajectory of HIV and AIDS and identifies both persisting and emerging challenges and opportunities for HIV prevention and control and care and support for AIDS patients in Sub-Saharan Africa. From a social science perspective, it extensively frames how broader

3

structural issues such as religion, culture, gender, food insecurity, masculinity, and other socioeconomic factors influence transmission, prevention, care, and treatment of HIV/AIDS. This book strongly argues that placing HIV/AIDS within the broader social, cultural, economic, and political context of the region goes a long way toward an appropriate understanding of the dynamics of the epidemic and the development of effective, contextual, and multisectoral strategies and programs aimed at not only halting and ultimately reducing the spread of the epidemic, but also devising ways of addressing its enormous social, economic, demographic, and institutional consequences.

Mapping the context: the epidemic in historical and spatial perspectives

Historical perspective

Emerging in the late 1970s and reaching epidemic proportions in the early 1980s, HIV could not have come at a worse time to Africa. Much of Sub-Saharan Africa was in crisis either because of war, famine, bad governance, and coups or structural adjustment programs that forced governments to cut spending on social services. Of the 19 major famines in the world between 1975 and 1990, 18 occurred in Africa, and more than half of all African countries experienced military conflicts from the 1980s on, leading to the displacement of more than 10 million people and sharp declines in food production (Caraël 2006). The economies of those countries were, as a result, ill prepared to deal with the HIV/AIDS epidemic. Adding to the problem, the structural adjustment programs of the 1970s and 1980s had devastating effects on social sectors such as education and health, leaving them unable to respond to the emerging epidemic (Caraël 2006; Farmer 1999; Nattrass 2004; Seckinelgin 2008).

Conflicts, famines, and economic crises were not, however, the only reasons the epidemic spread rapidly over the continent in its early stages. In much of Africa, leaders were often reluctant to acknowledge the very presence of HIV/AIDS or the danger it caused during its initial phase (1984–1988). A disease that was associated in the affluent countries of the West with homosexual behavior, prostitution, and intravenous drug usage seemed, at the time, impossible in Africa. Even when its presence was acknowledged, AIDS was seen as a foreign disease spread on the continent by white homosexuals, or as an elaborate conspiracy by the West aimed at bringing down the birth rate of Africans by imposing the use of condoms, or as an attack against African traditions such as polygamy (Caraël 2006; Farmer 1993, cited in Seckinelgin 2008). In some countries of the region, such thinking led to the denial of the disease at the highest political levels. President Mobutu of Zaire (now the Democratic Republic of the Congo), for example, banned the subject of HIV/AIDS from the press between 1983 and 1987. Government warnings in the 1980s and early 1990s that AIDS kills and that it is incurable intensified the confusion, discrimination, and blaming that surrounded the condition (Iliffe 2006, pp. 81–86). The situation was worsened by the apparent (although short-lived) hesitation of the industrialized countries to accept the seriousness of HIV/AIDS. This was perhaps best epitomized by the now infamous 1985 comment of the then Director General of WHO that tropical diseases such as malaria were in danger of being neglected because of HIV/AIDS (Iliffe 2006, p. 68).

As world leaders began to realize that HIV/AIDS could not be simply denied as a mythical construct or an elaborate conspiracy of the West or dismissed as less important than other challenges facing African nations, prevention campaigns slowly swung into action in many Sub-Saharan African countries. But these were largely ineffective in curtailing the spread of the epidemic. The international community was yet to take decisive action, and many national government programs were underfunded, corrupt, or otherwise ill equipped to deal with the escalating crisis. It took the world until 1996 to establish UNAIDS (The United Nations Joint Programme on HIV/AIDS) as the responsible body for coordinating actions worldwide against the pandemic. But by then the seriousness of the epidemic was blatantly clear to even the most hardened skeptics and some countries, including Kenya, had already declared AIDS a national disaster (AFP 1999).

At the turn of the new millennium, the international effort to fight HIV/AIDS gained momentum. The Global Fund to Fight AIDS, Tuberculosis, and Malaria was created in 2001 following a special meeting of the UN General Assembly called to discuss HIV/AIDS. United States President George W. Bush announced the establishment of the President's Emergency Plan for AIDS Relief (PEPFAR) two years later. Overall global funding for HIV/AIDS increased threefold between 2002 and 2007, when it reached $10 billion (Figure 1.1). Funding rose to $15.9 billion in 2009 but fell to $15 billion in 2010 (Sidibe 2011).

Sub-Saharan Africa has received about half of all international AIDS spending in recent years and 54.2% from the Global Fund to Fight AIDS, Tuberculosis and Malaria in 2009, the major distributor of HIV/AIDS funds (Salaam-Blyther 2010). This fact, together with the actions of governments to strengthen health services, issue guidelines, and launch initiatives facilitating treatment activities, especially in rural areas, yielded positive results almost immediately. Between 2003 and 2009, the number of people receiving antiretroviral treatment (ART) for HIV/AIDS in eastern and southern Africa increased from fewer than 100,000 to 3.1 million. Treatment coverage was particularly high in these two regions, where national rates between 55% and 67% were reported for females and rates between 31% and 45% for males in 2009 (UNAIDS 2010, p. 256). Although the full impact of the stepped-up intervention remains to be determined, HIV prevalence has declined in

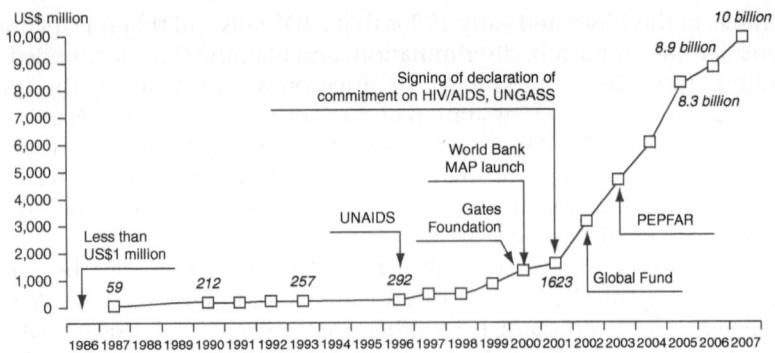

Figure 1.1 Total annual funds made available for HIV/AIDS programs, 1986–2007
Notes: [1] 1986–2000 figures are for international funds only
[2] Domestic funds are included from 2001 onwards
[i] 1996–2005 data: Extracted from 2006 Reported on the Global AIDS Epidemic (UNAIDS 2006)
[ii] 1986–1993 data: Mann & Tarantola (1996)
Source: UNAIDS (2008, p. 188).

Sub-Saharan African countries since the late 1990s, when the number of new HIV infections peaked in much of the region (UNAIDS 2010, p. 27).

But the increasing involvement of international actors brought a new complication to HIV/AIDS governance in Africa. There is now a well-established global governance of HIV/AIDS, which, while providing the much needed resource base for interventions, does not adequately reflect the way local people perceive, experience, and respond to the disease within their sociocultural and economic contexts. As a result, researchers have questioned the appropriateness of international governance of HIV/AIDS to deal with the prevailing issues in a multiplicity of contexts across Africa (Seckinelgin 2008; see also Tamale 2011a). There is also a danger in relying on HIV/AIDS-related funding to bring about the multifaceted socio-economic structural transformations (such as universal education, economic opportunities for women, social protection systems, and support for the agricultural sector) that are required to bring about and sustain a meaningful and viable local capacity to challenge the threat posed by HIV/AIDS (UNAIDS 2008).

The Global Fund jeopardized the progress made in preventing HIV/AIDS and increasing the number of people on ART when it cancelled Round 11 of funding in 2011 because of dwindling resources. Most HIV/AIDS and tuberculosis (TB) programs in Africa are financed by the Global Fund, and reduced funding may endanger the gains made in the fight against HIV/AIDS so far. Though this new development is worrisome for Africa, it may provide an opportunity for African governments to mobilize domestic resources and take ownership of the HIV/AIDS response. Moreover, the mobilization of activists and health care consumers has pressured global and national leaders toward a stronger sense of accountability and urgency, and a number of innovative preventive and health services approaches, as well as greater participation of the private sector in Sub-Saharan Africa promise to render HIV/AIDS programs more cost-effective and sustainable (Berhe 2011; Idoko and Bequele 2011; Traore 2011).

Spatial aspects

The increased testing of general populations and improvements in the reliability of HIV prevalence data have enabled planners to better understand the geographic distribution of HIV infections. The pattern that is emerging from recent national sample surveys in Sub-Saharan Africa indicates that several countries have concentrated epidemics, usually in urban areas that are characterized by sharply higher prevalence of infection in vulnerable groups than in the general population. The heterogeneous distribution of HIV infection in all countries, not only in those with concentrated epidemics affecting mostly high-risk groups but also those with generalized epidemics, demands that interventions be well designed and adequate resources allocated to highly infected high-risk groups (Forsythe et al. 2009). Furthermore, the uneven HIV distributions can give only a general indication of the real prevalence and total number of people infected in individual countries (Forsythe et al. 2009) but not of regional differences.

Nine of the ten countries in continental Southern Africa had HIV prevalence rates among 15- to 49-year-olds between 11% and 25.9%, the highest worldwide, and five countries in eastern Africa (Uganda, Tanzania, Kenya, Burundi, and Rwanda) and eleven countries in Central and West Africa (Cameroon, Equatorial Guinea, Central African Republic, Gabon, Nigeria, Togo, Guinea Bissau, Côte d'Ivoire, Congo, Chad, and Gambia) reported rates between 2% and 5.3% (Figure 1.2 and Table 1.1). Swaziland, with an estimated HIV prevalence rate of 25.9% among adults aged 15–49 in 2009, had the highest infection rate in the world, and South Africa had the largest population living with HIV, about 5.6 million. The most populous countries in eastern Africa (Ethiopia, Tanzania, and Kenya) had larger HIV-infected populations than Nigeria and all but three countries in southern Africa (South Africa, Mozambique, and Zimbabwe) in spite of relatively low HIV prevalence rates (Table 1.1). HIV rate in Madagascar was only 0.2% in 2009, the lowest in Sub-Saharan Africa, apparently due to the island's geographic and political isolation, but lack of data for high-risk groups and recent social instability render available data questionable. Little information is also available for Somalia and the newly independent South Sudan, both of which were brutalized by civil war, although rates are thought to be low (Ahmed 2011). This information is consistent with the relatively low HIV prevalence reported from Angola (2%), another war-ravaged country. These figures contradict the common assumption at the turn of the millennium that armed

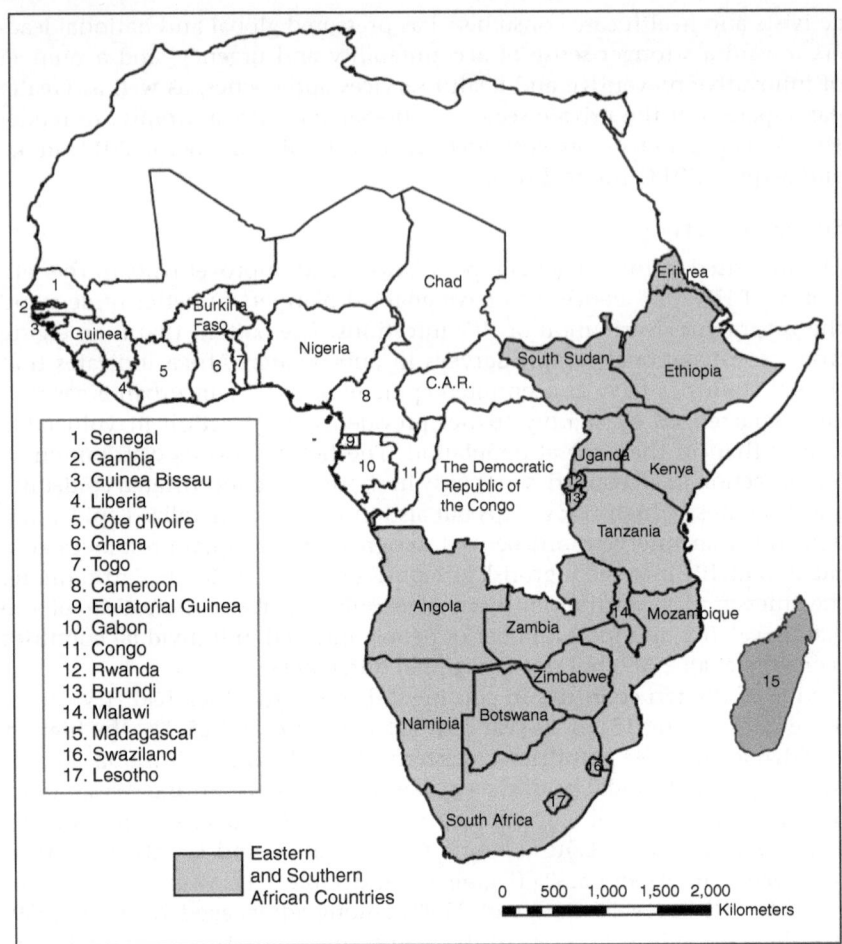

Figure 1.2 Sub-Saharan Africa, eastern and southern subregions (shaded) and the countries in Central and West Africa referenced in the text (white), with names and numbers

conflict significantly fuelled the epidemic; this assumption diverted attention from the major driving forces of the epidemic, identified by de Waal (2010) and Kalipeni et al. (2004) as gender and socioeconomic inequities, stigma, and discrimination.

Although we examine studies and data from nearly all Sub-Saharan African countries (Figure 1.2), the focus is on the eastern and southern subregions mainly because they are impacted most severely by the epidemic and are the focus of most research on HIV/AIDS published in the English language.

Table 1.1 HIV prevalence (%) among children and adults and the number of infected adults (15- to 49-year-olds) in Sub-Saharan African countries with rates of 2% and higher in 2009

Country	Prev.(no.)[a]	Country	Prev.(no.)	Country	Prev.(no.)
Swaziland	25.9(1.8)	Uganda	6.5(8.4)	Côte d'Ivoire	3.4(5.7)
Botswana	24.8(3.2)	Kenya	6.3(15.0)	Chad	3.4(2.1)
Lesotho	23.6(2.9)	Tanzania	5.6(14.0)	Burundi	3.3(1.8)
South Africa	17.8(56.0)	Cameroon	5.3(6.1)	Togo	3.2(1.2)
Zimbabwe	14.3(12.0)	Gabon	5.2(0.5)	Rwanda	2.9(1.7)
Zambia	13.5(9.8)	Equat. Guinea	5.0(0.2)	Guinea Bissau	2.5(0.2)
Namibia	13.1(1.8)	C.A.R.[b]	4.7(1.3)	Ethiopia[c]	2.2(11.0)
Mozambique	11.5(14.0)	Nigeria	3.6(33.0)	Gambia	2.0(0.2)
Malawi	11.0(9.2)	Congo	3.4(0.6)	Angola	2.0(2.0)

[a] in 100,000s.
[b] Central African Republic.
[c] The data for Ethiopia are for 2007.
Sources: Based on UNAIDS (2010, pp. 180, 181) and Federal Democratic Republic of Ethiopia (FDRE) (2010).

These regions have additional importance as high HIV impact areas because of the regional distribution of the two strains of HIV.

Whereas HIV1, more easily transmitted and more virulent than HIV2, is the only strain in eastern and southern Africa, both strains are endemic in Central and West Africa (Levy 2007, p. 7), possibly accounting for the lower HIV and AIDS rates in the latter two regions (Oppong and Agyei-Mensah 2004). Differences in HIV infection and risk behavior, as well as increasing ART and other interventions reported from eastern and southern Africa as well as Central Western Africa must be better understood (WHO/UNAIDS/UNICEF 2011). This volume contributes to a better understanding of the vulnerabilities, impacts, and interventions at the regional level within the context of the multitude of contexts in which HIV occurs in Sub-Saharan Africa. Our focus on the eastern and southern subregions allows for pertinent discussions of the management and governance of the epidemic in the most affected areas.

Counting the toll of the epidemic

As pointed out above, the most devastating impact of the HIV/AIDS epidemic has been in eastern and southern Africa. In some Southern African countries, infection rates increased from 4% to 20% or more in adult populations in the 1990s. Moreover, although the cumulative number of AIDS patients has been decreasing in the last five years, the social and economic impacts of the epidemic remains at high levels and may even increase in some populations (see Chapters 5 and 6).

Demographic impact

While HIV prevalence declined in most countries between 2001 and 2009 and the rapid scale-up of ART since 2002 lowered mortality from AIDS in several eastern and southern African countries, infection rates among 15- to 49-year-olds continued to increase during that eight-year period in South Africa, Swaziland, and Mozambique. The majority of people infected with HIV are adults in their most productive years (age 15–49) (UNAIDS 2010, p. 181). In Botswana, South Africa, Swaziland, Zambia, and Zimbabwe, mean life expectancy plummeted by more than 20 years between 1970–1975 and 2005–2010 as a result of AIDS (UNAIDS 2006). In addition to being an immediate public health challenge, HIV/AIDS has impacted countries in more systemic ways as it has affected the most productive element of African economies: prime-aged adults. High mortality in middle-aged people has greatly affected the labor force and household demographics, as detailed in Chapter 6.

Socioeconomic impacts

While its demographic impacts are relatively easy to anticipate, the economic impact of HIV/AIDS has always proved difficult to fully comprehend. A number of studies conducted in the 1990s, using classical economic models, predicted that HIV/AIDS would have only a minor effect (between 0.3% and 1.0% decline) on the macroeconomic performance of countries as measured by mean annual gross domestic product (GDP) per capita. More recent models have attempted to capture the multiple dynamics of the pandemic, incorporating a number of new variables. Although these models estimated that the aggregate impacts will remain fairly low for now (about 1.5%), impacts are likely to increase in the long run (Greener 2004). As the lead time between HIV infection and the onset of AIDS is relatively long, no African country has yet experienced the full implications of the pandemic.

The structural implications of HIV-related mortality on public services are also projected to be substantial. Morbidity from HIV-related opportunistic infections, usually occurring over a number of years, is often associated with increased absenteeism and decreased productivity at home and at the workplace. Thus the toll on public services includes the costs of absenteeism, replacing lost staff, and operating with fewer staff (ECA 2010).

The burden is likely to be felt most in the health sector, which, in addition to coping with the loss of its own personnel, has to find ways to meet the increasing demands for AIDS treatment as well as care and treatment of opportunistic infections. The increased burden on the health sector is reflected in the fact that more than half of all hospital beds were occupied by AIDS patients in the 1990s and early 2000s (UNAIDS 2006). The situation perhaps must have improved as fewer PLWHA are getting ill and occupying hospital beds with increased accessibility of antiretroviral drugs (ARVs).

The increased demand for medical services comes in the face of high losses of staff in the health sector due to AIDS and migration of labor to better paying positions in non-governmental organizations and in industrialized countries. Labor force losses have reached 30% in Zambia and several other countries (Tawfik and Kinoti 2006).

The education sector is also feeling the brunt of the epidemic as a huge number of teachers are affected by HIV/AIDS. In South Africa, 21% of teachers aged 25–34 are estimated to be HIV-infected (UNAIDS 2006). On the other hand, the epidemic has created a new job market as the United Nations, bilateral donors, and NGOs are recruiting staff specifically for HIV-related interventions. While the implications for the public sector have not been studied comprehensively, the diversion of trained health workers appears to have weakened this sector in many African countries and made it a popular 'poaching ground' upon which a multitude of bilateral and multilateral Western development agencies rely for recruitment of local staff (ECA 2010).

Impacts on communities

It is at the family and community levels, however, where the impact of the HIV epidemic is most severely felt, particularly among poor households. In Africa's predominantly subsistence and extractive economies, the most vulnerable people are often also the most productive economically. As these people die, their families struggle to cope both emotionally and economically. As limited savings dwindle, families fragment economically. One consequence of this fragmentation of families is the rising number of orphaned children in Sub-Saharan Africa, which reached 14.8 million in 2009 (UNAIDS 2010, p. 186). Many of these and other vulnerable children have to quit school to help families cope and are exploited or sexually violated.

HIV/AIDS exacerbates household poverty in other ways. It changes household characteristics and negatively affects human and physical capital endowments in a reciprocal relationship with poverty. Households affected by HIV/AIDS are more likely to be poor and show a greater risk of drifting into and remaining in chronic poverty than non-affected households (Marzo 2004). Poorer households and individuals, especially females, are at a greater risk of becoming infected in a down-spiraling reciprocal relationship (Nattrass 2004).

Interventions

The dramatic 20-fold increase in ART between 2001 and 2010 in low- and middle-income countries has given rise to euphoric expectations that HIV/AIDS can be controlled in the foreseeable future. However, enthusiasm over the remarkable progress made to date has been tempered by recent funding shortfalls and concerns that the projected target of increasing the number of people on ART from 6.6 million in 2010 to 15 million in 2015 cannot be met (Sidibe 2011). The socioeconomic and cultural barriers continuing to impede progress toward this and other prevention and control goals as well as patient care and support are less frequently mentioned. We identify many causal pathways leading to various types of risk that must be considered by planners and administrators of anti-HIV/AIDS programs in Sub-Saharan African countries. We also present in this book considerable evidence that gender equity, raised living standards, and sharing of wealth and power may reduce the social and economic drivers of HIV risk and vulnerability.

Evolving social science research on HIV/AIDS in Sub-Saharan Africa

In this section we review historical developments in researching HIV/AIDS in Africa from a social science perspective in order to understand the past, the present, the continuities, and the changes. Since the mid-1990s, awareness that the social, cultural, and political aspects of the HIV epidemic need to be understood and that the virus is spreading in Africa primarily through heterosexual sex prompted research on the social and cultural aspects of sexual behavior. As the mode of transmission became better known, the biomedical researchers turned to social scientists for help. The epidemic in Sub-Saharan Africa appeared to take a totally different route from what was witnessed in Europe and North America. Why was transmission of AIDS in Africa different from that in the industrialized countries? Why were as many women infected in Africa as men? And was there something unique in African sexuality that caused the disease to spread so rapidly in such a short time? Social scientists were expected to provide the answers to these questions (Schoepf 1995). But these questions were answered, at least at first, through ethnographic analysis of past studies of African sexuality which portrayed exotic sexual traditions and cultures, and, not surprisingly, these traditions and cultures were held to blame (Tamale 2011a).

The public health community was generally content with old ethnographic accounts of 'African' sexual behavior to make sense of an epidemic that actually demanded up-to-date epidemiological data. Information on how such behavior may have changed over a generation or more and the implications of the enormous social, economic, and political transformations of the 1980s and 1990s on the validity of the explanations and insights such data 'offered' were conveniently ignored (Stele 1999; Tamale 2011a). Even worse, Africans were being blamed for all sorts of 'apparent' facts, ranging from the evolution of the simian to human transmission of the virus to the spread of HIV in cities that were considered places of open sexual promiscuity for inhabitants who supposedly had lost touch with their traditional sexual morality. Africans were criticized for a number of high-risk cultural practices, such as polygamy, wife inheritance, weak marriage ties, and even the exclusive role of the mother in the education of children (Iliffe 2006; Tamale 2011a).

Fortunately, contextualized studies of gender, sexuality, and power relations revealed that females adhered to traditional norms in HIV prevention. For example, female university students used traditional discourse about virginity and premarital sex to resist sexual requests, and wives were able to negotiate condom use with their husbands indirectly under the guise of family planning (Schoepf 1995). These studies showed that culture, and African culture in particular, which many epidemiologists often viewed as part of the problem or even the problem, presented opportunities for change rather than constituting an impediment (Nyanzi et al. 2008; see also Chapter 2). In other words, culture is a 'double-edged sword' (Tamale 2011a) that can be used to prevent the spread of HIV/AIDS. But identifying and utilizing the opportunities does, above all else, require an understanding of the nature of sexual behavior as manifested within the broader cultural hemisphere.

Social science research into HIV/AIDS in Sub-Saharan Africa faced other stumbling blocks as well. Even when epidemiologists understood that dated colonial ethnographic accounts did not shed any light on the epidemic and the need for up-to-date and rigorous studies became acute, the epidemiological thinking that dominated HIV/AIDS research for far too long continued to creep into social science research. KAP (knowledge, attitude, and practice) studies that kept the individual's sexual history at the center became the norm. The sociocultural contexts and the power and gender relations that influenced, dictated, and at times even determined individual behavior were pushed aside while sexual behaviors of individuals and risk groups were portrayed in ever greater detail (Schoepf 1995; Tamale 2011a). But, perhaps unsurprisingly, the countless KAP surveys and the intervention strategies derived from them did little to achieve their aim.

In the 1990s, scientists called for an urgent redirection of social science research to insure adequate contextualization of the disease. Prominent authorities in social science (Schoepf 1995) and interdisciplinary research (Farmer 1999) on HIV/AIDS were very critical of the output of KAP studies that obstructed the proper understanding of the epidemic and the framing of effective interventions. Rather than understanding the complexity of human sexual behavior in its entirety and within the social, cultural, and political environment, research aims prevailing at that time were much more epidemiologically defined – often limited to counting frequencies of certain forms of sexual expression at the individual level and identifying risk factors and groups. While documenting the frequency of certain forms of sexual expression is undoubtedly important for monitoring changing risk behavior in a population, understanding the subjective as well as the sociocultural meanings attached to these forms of expression is just as important (Parker 1995). The role social forces such as gender inequality, poverty, and denial played in HIV risk was neglected in biomedical, epidemiological, and even social science research (Farmer 1999, p. 149; Parker 1995; Tamale 2011a).

Therefore a growing number of social scientists started questioning the individualistic nature of research into HIV/AIDS. Schoepf (1995) argued that the semiology and biochemistry of AIDS are equally important and Parker (1995) lamented the absence of well-informed and extensive studies on the social and cultural aspects of sexuality and its implication for understanding the spread of HIV/AIDS. Questioning sometimes even extended to the appropriateness of social science methods (the entrenched relativism of anthropology in particular) for studying HIV/AIDS (Bolton 1995), and some asserted that AIDS research in developing countries must include an element of social justice (Farmer 1999). These and other objections against the dire state of social science research into the relationship between sex and sexuality and HIV/AIDS argued that those who used the individualistic model of the medical approach in their studies had utterly failed to capture the complexity of human sexuality. They focused on the individual expressions of sexual behavior in the hope of identifying risk factors and risky behaviors. Sexual research appeared literally obsessed with the 'risk' of sex and painting a morbid picture of sex as a dangerous endeavor, often ignoring the pleasures of sex (arguably the very reason people have sex) as well as the richness and complexity it has in its varied forms of expression and in its meaning (Bolton 1995).

But why was such a decontextualized, individualized, and fragmented account of HIV/AIDS so widespread? Parker (1995) argued that the abysmal state of research into sexual behavior in the context of AIDS should not come as a surprise as such research has almost never been driven by a theoretical framework but by the expectation that large amounts of quantitative and descriptive data would provide theoretical insight. The lack of a comprehensive theoretical and conceptual framework has been compounded by changing priorities in the research agenda. Funding for social science studies of the epidemic was dependent on asking the appropriate questions, which often were determined by the health units of Western development agencies (Parker 1995; Schoepf 1995). Rather than shaping the research agenda based on the most pressing and relevant problems at hand, social scientists often followed the diverse interests of funding agencies and the fashionable questions of the day as posed by those agencies. These organizations do not – and cannot – reasonably be expected to have a coherent and consistent research agenda that can incrementally lead to a complete and meaningful portrayal of human sexual behavior in all its complexity (Parker 1995; see also Tamale 2011a).

There has been an encouraging growth of social science literature on HIV/AIDS in Sub-Saharan Africa since the mid-1990s. This includes the proceedings of the 1996 *AIDS and Social Sciences in Africa* conference, published following the conference at Champaign-Urbana (United States), and a growing number of books such as *The African AIDS Epidemic: A History* by John Iliffe (2006), *Human Sexuality in Africa: Beyond Reproduction* by Eleanor Maticka-Tyndale et al. (2007), *A Tapestry of Human Sexuality in Africa* by Oka Obono (2010), *HIV/AIDS in Africa: Beyond Epidemiology* by Ezekiel Kalipeni et al. (2004), *The Socioeconomic Dimensions of HIV/AIDS in Africa* by David A. Sahn (2010), *'Letting Them Die': Why HIV/AIDS Prevention Programmes Fail* by Catherine Campbell (2003), *African Sexualities: A Reader* by Sylvia Tamale (2011b), *28 Stories of AIDS in Africa* by Stephanie Nolen (2007), *Working with Spirit: Experiencing Sangoma in Contemporary South Africa* by Joanne Wreford (2008), and *Witchcraft, Violence and Democracy in South Africa* by Adam Ashforth (2005). What is interesting about some of the recent publications is that they describe the vulnerabilities and coping behaviors of PLWHA from the point of view of Africans themselves. For instance, Tamale (2011a) provided new insights into sexuality by incorporating 51 contributions from all over the continent; Nolen (2007) presented the stories of 28 PLWHA cast in their socioeconomic, cultural, and political settings; Wreford (2009) described health-seeking behaviors of South Africans in the context of indigenous healing systems and advocated closer collaboration between biomedicine and traditional practice in South Africa. Both an *isangoma* healer and a social anthropologist, she suggested that biomedicine may be empowered and health outcomes improved through serious engagement with African healing and spirit evocation. Similarly, Ashforth (2005), working in Soweto, South Africa, identified questions infected people face in everyday life pertaining to spiritual insecurity and their coping behaviors. He emphasized that health workers in local contexts need to understand the questions lay people ponder about issues such as the action of ARVs and the complexity of stigma in order to ward off unintended consequences of treatment and prevention efforts, including poor treatment adherence and lack of follow-up. Concerned that prevailing knowledge, behaviors, and attitudes be properly examined, Obono (2010) called for a responsible and broad-minded view of sexual practices in Sub-Saharan Africa, a plea that needs to be extended to include all populations affected by HIV/AIDS, as we demonstrate in this volume.

Researchers need to do more to uncover and understand the social, political, and cultural history that underlies AIDS rather than accept a decontextualized presentation of AIDS that limits itself to a description of sexual practices of potential carriers of the virus or to the identification of the cultural phenomena promoting the spread of HIV (Denis 2006). Seckinelgin (2008, citing Farmer 1999) noted that we know little about the disease in context even though we know its biomedical features. Seckinelgin (2008,

p. 124) and Parker (1995) emphasized that conceptually sound policies and practices require a good understanding of the social, cultural, economic, and political aspects of sexuality. Due to increasing recognition that HIV is predominantly a social disease, biomedical researchers are stepping up demands for more holistic research with the full participation of social scientists, as illustrated in the publication of a special issue in the *Journal of the International AIDS Society* in 2011 (Kippax et al. 2011).

While the picture today has significantly improved, in part due to the contributions of social scientists and greater recognition among biomedical scientists of the need to more fully understand the drivers of the epidemic and the barriers to successful prevention and control, most research into HIV/AIDS is still focused on biomedical aspects (Kippax et al. 2011). Social science research continues to be relegated to civil society interventions and conducted primarily to inform policy implementations. MacQueen (2011) noted that because of many challenges facing the integration of social, behavioral, and biomedical perspectives and lack of close collaboration in trial design and implementation, social scientists feel forced to either adapt to the priorities of biomedicine and public health or maintain their autonomous HIV social science agenda. MacQueen considered the latter insufficient for social scientists to optimally contribute to HIV/AIDS research. In the absence of a strong social science presence, narrowly focused biomedical researchers often fail to ask if they have the right ideas and approaches and, in the urgency to stem the epidemic, they seem preoccupied with particularities and rarely go beyond the question of whether a particular initiative has worked somewhere or not. The medicalization of HIV/AIDS, defined by Seckinelgin (2008) as a process by which non-medical problems get defined and treated as medical conditions, regrettably continues to dominate the intellectual discourse surrounding HIV/AIDS in Africa. On the other hand, the importance of HIV coming to the forefront as a major development hurdle for the continent continues to be periodically called into question.

This volume builds on earlier studies on the vulnerability to HIV/AIDS, on impacts on different levels of society, and on evolving interventions in the socioeconomic and cultural context of Sub-Saharan Africa. We expand earlier discussions of HIV prevention and AIDS treatment and patient care by addressing the challenges posed by persisting stigma and inequalities. New topics treated here include the intricacies of youth sexuality and vulnerabilities in the social and cultural context of Sub-Saharan Africa, mainstreaming HIV prevention into educational systems, monitoring and evaluating HIV/AIDS prevention programs, and HIV/AIDS impacts on businesses in Southern Africa. The overarching theme is that all areas of HIV risk, its burden on society, and efforts to prevent, mitigate, and control the epidemic must consider the central role of socioeconomic and cultural factors.

Sources, structure, and content

Against the background summarized above, the Swedish International Development Cooperation Agency (SIDA/SARAC) provided funding for four African organizations to support social science research on the HIV/AIDS pandemic: the Organization for Social Science Research in Eastern and Southern Africa (OSSREA), the Council for the Development of Social Science Research in Africa (CODESRIA), the Social Science and Medicine Africa Network (SOMA-NET), and the Union for African Population Studies (UAPS). Between 2003 and 2006, these four research organizations carried out several research projects in African countries that culminated in the international conference held in Addis Ababa in November 2006. The organizations' programs were: (1) A Political Economy of Patient Welfare and Rights in Relation to HIV/AIDS (CODESRIA); (2) The HIV/AIDS Challenge in Africa: The Socioeconomic Impact of HIV/AIDS and Responses (OSSREA); (3) Reversing the HIV/AIDS Pandemic among Youth through Participatory Action Research in Kenya and Uganda (SOMA-NET); and (4) The Demographic, Social and Economic Determinants and Consequences of the HIV/AIDS Pandemic in Africa (UAPS). SIDA/SARAC supported these programs to achieve the following objectives: enhance capacity for HIV and AIDS research among African scholars, come up with new research findings, and produce applied results that could feed into policy and practice. And, 15 research projects were supported by CODESRIA, 16 by OSSREA, and 12 projects were carried out by multidisciplinary teams working within the SOMA-NET project. CODESRIA took over stewardship for the UAPS research in 2005, supporting nine projects. Some in-house publications focusing on social science aspects of HIV/AIDS were produced by the organizations, particularly by OSSREA. Most results of the studies have not appeared in the social science or medical literature, so we present them in this volume.

This book examines the concepts, issues, and information presented by these different research projects. Additional resources showing the current state of knowledge about the region were identified through online searches of the social science and epidemiological literature, particularly in Internet archives and journal articles.

The four chapters in Part I place HIV/AIDS in its socioeconomic and cultural contexts in Sub-Saharan Africa, and the seven chapters in Part II describe the impacts of HIV/AIDS and interventions. Some overlap of issues across chapters is the result of interacting factors that influence HIV/AIDS transmission, prevention, and treatment; the overlap provides an opportunity to consider different aspects of the same issue or problem.

In Chapter 2, Getnet Tadele and Woldekidan Amde examine the literature linking HIV/AIDS with tradition, religion, and culture in Sub-Saharan Africa, where these inadequately understood forces are pivotal in shaping views and conceptions relating to sex and sexuality and thus the risk of infection and people's response to HIV/AIDS. The authors review evidence of the negative impacts of the culture of silence, gender norms, and the broader social environment on girls and young women, sexual relations, stigma and discrimination, and non-disclosure of HIV status. They examine the economic dependence of women on men, inheritance laws, and other traditional, religious, and cultural practices that lead to vulnerability to HIV infection and impede behavioral change. Tadele and Amde briefly review the still sparse literature on men who have sex with men (MSM), including studies on the role of religious morality in stigma and the denial and lack of legal protection of MSM. They show that the same moral judgments that attach stigma to HIV-infected people have discouraged the use of condoms. The authors address the rapid decline of traditional means of socialization in youth sexuality and their replacement by modern education, identifying both positive and negative outcomes. But they found strong, persisting demand for traditional healers, some of whom have started to contribute to HIV prevention efforts. The chapter ends by addressing some of the unwarranted accusations against African culture.

Chapter 3 explores the linkages between gender norms, values, and beliefs regarding sexuality and vulnerability to HIV infection in an effort to explain the significantly higher infection rates in women than men. Ayalew Gebre et al. examine gendered decision-making power in sexual relationships, the traditional role of sex in socialization, women's lower socioeconomic position, societal myths and misconceptions regarding HIV/AIDS, harmful traditional practices, and role of women's physiology in HIV risk. They give due attention to the meaning and role of various notions of masculinity and femininity and their effect on the sexuality and HIV risk of young men and women in the context of Sub-Saharan African social realities. This includes a detailed examination of how differing social expectations of sexuality among adolescent men and women, as well as cultural ideals of manhood and womanhood, put young women at risk of infection.

Getnet Tadele and Woldekidan Amde examine a number of still poorly understood and understudied aspects of cultural notions of masculinity and femininity regarding HIV risk in Chapter 4. Case studies of the vulnerability of married adolescents, sexuality of in-school and out-of-school youth, competing concerns of pregnancy and HIV infection, homosexuality, and sexual violence vividly illustrate the vulnerability of youth in general and females in particular. But the discussion also provides a balanced picture of gendered vulnerabilities by considering male HIV risk associated with masculinity and male sexual behaviors. The authors discuss lesser-known aspects of sexuality and their health consequences, including the clandestine sexual activities of unmarried girls who fear pregnancy more than HIV because of the social rejection and disrepute pregnancy would bring to their families. The authors also discuss briefly the well-known epidemic of sexual violence against females, and they present recent evidence of sexual violence against boys, another culturally denied and understudied HIV transmission route. Amde and Tadele emphasize the need for innovative, youth-friendly approaches to increase knowledge about HIV and safe sex and to overcome negative perceptions of condom use.

In Chapter 5, Ayalew Gebre et al. examine the strong relationship between food insecurity and poverty and HIV/AIDS. They describe the impacts of HIV/AIDS on agricultural labor and food production; coping strategies, including distress sale of household assets and commercial sex work by females; and the role of malnutrition in the progression of HIV infection to AIDS. The information on gender inequality and poverty in Chapters 3 and 6 supplements the arguments of this chapter. Less documented information on recurrent medical expenses and recent sharp increases in food prices in Africa and the plight of orphan-headed households provide additional insights into the nexus of poverty, food insecurity, and vulnerability to HIV/AIDS. The authors note the great variability in the relationship between poverty and HIV/AIDS vulnerability, especially across rural/urban lines. Moreover, they show that increasing levels of education and consequent social mobility are associated with higher HIV infection rates in urban areas in eastern and southern Africa. Gebre and colleagues conclude that the mutually reinforcing and converging dynamics of the epidemic must be proactively addressed through more effective AIDS-responsive and context-sensitive food policy and poverty reduction programs.

Ayalew Gebre et al. examine the literature dealing with social, economic, cultural, and political impacts of HIV/AIDS and responses of individuals, households, communities, and governments in Chapter 6. They describe the coping strategies of HIV-positive individuals who must face stigma and discrimination. They investigate how the social and economic pressures on HIV/AIDS-affected households have disrupted the nuclear and extended families, impacting household size and composition. The increase in child- and grandparent-headed families illustrates this trend. The authors discuss impacts at the workplace, still poorly understood, including reduced productivity and profitability, declining quality of the dwindling labor force, and weakened relationships among workers due to actual and perceived stigma and discrimination. The authors call for studies of stigmatization and discrimination and for policy makers to address the persisting problems of widespread non-disclosure of HIV infections, low utilization of voluntary counseling and testing services, and default from ART. They also point out the potential of using traditional institutions such as the *iddir*, a community-based self-help program in Ethiopia, to provide prevention, care, and support services.

Chapter 7 gives insights into the still poorly known vulnerabilities, impacts, and responses to HIV/AIDS in the mining and commercial agricultural sectors in southern Africa. Charles Hongoro et al. provide evidence that the socioeconomic and cultural environment of the mines and farms is highly conducive to HIV transmission, especially among migrant workers and females. The authors describe various impacts of HIV/AIDS on mining companies and agricultural enterprises. They document a trend among enterprises, particularly in the mining sector, to expand HIV/AIDS services to protect their businesses and demonstrate corporate social responsibility. The authors identify several areas needing further research, including the need for case studies documenting the vulnerability of companies' workforces and their workforces' access to health services.

In Chapter 8, Getnet Tadele et al. discuss the rapid upscaling of ART and HIV prevention and patient care and support services within the context of the changing funding environment, persisting socioeconomic challenges, and several new prevention approaches. The authors discuss the potential contribution of recently developed ART-based prevention approaches, including prevention of mother-to-child transmission (PMTCT) and preexposure prophylaxis. The chapter presents much needed information on structural approaches, community capacity enhancement, strengthening of the evolving community-based health services, and other decentralized approaches to service delivery. The authors point out persisting impediments to ART coverage and adherence among pregnant women and high-risk groups. They conclude that the current shift from hospital-based services to community-based interventions may result in greater coverage and cost-effectiveness and that the integration of prevention and treatment strategies can improve services, particularly where collaboration between government agencies and community groups can be achieved.

Woldekidan Amde and Getnet Tadele explore the widely contested issue of care for the growing AIDS orphan population in Chapter 9. They note the ongoing debates among researchers and service providers over how best to provide for the care, support, and nurturing of these orphans. After providing definitions for the often-misused term 'orphan', the authors describe the psychological damage, social exclusion, and sexual and economic exploitation and abuse of affected children. They reference studies of the differential effect of fathers and mothers dying of AIDS on the welfare and coping behavior of surviving children and on the survivability of affected families. A comparison of orphan care provided by extended families and orphanages illuminates the worrisome trend of children being enrolled in often-deficient orphanages because families lack the means to support them. Amde and Tadele recommend the development of alternative approaches to orphan care, particularly community-based care.

In Chapter 10, Anne Khasakhala reviews efforts to mainstream HIV/AIDS interventions in education programs in order to integrate prevention and mitigation efforts in education policies, programs, and projects in hyper-endemic countries. Khasakhala examines the effects of the HIV/AIDS epidemic on educational systems and shows how interventions can be mainstreamed within the infrastructure of Sub-Saharan African institutions of learning. She explores discrepancies between governments' use of good practices for mainstreaming HIV/AIDS in the education sector, particularly attempts to implement prevention programs and curriculum changes, and persisting bureaucratic, cultural, and religious barriers that impede the scaling-up and effectiveness of the programs. Although some countries have made progress in integrating prevention and mitigation programs, the author concludes that most ministries of education have failed to take decisive steps necessary to protect schools from HIV. Khasakhala calls for further studies to address these and other difficulties encountered in streamlining efforts.

Chapter 11 examines the needs and recent progress in monitoring and evaluating HIV/AIDS programs to gauge the dynamics of the epidemic, identify impacts and responses, and insure that available resources are used effectively and efficiently. Although considerable progress has been made in developing monitoring and evaluation (M&E) policies, essential documentation, and implementation of programs, some aspects of M&E remain underdeveloped in most HIV prevention programs. Summaries of 2010 national HIV/AIDS progress reports reveal impediments to the effectiveness and efficiency of M&E programs: non-adherence to reporting requirements; failure to link different databases and track resources for HIV/AIDS; limited data use for decision making; lack of timely and accurate data; limited capacity at sub-national, district, and regional levels; and widespread failure to report on high-risk populations. Anne Khasakhala and Helmut Kloos end the chapter by emphasizing that M&E programs are at the center of sound governance and necessary for evidence-based policy making, budget decisions, management, and accountability in Sub-Saharan Africa's HIV/AIDS prevention programs.

In Chapter 12, Anne Khasakhala and Helmut Kloos review pertinent ethical issues in HIV/AIDS biomedical research in the areas of informed consent; research collaboration between Sub-Saharan African countries and industrialized countries; and the effectiveness, functionality, and shortcomings of ethics committees in the region's challenging political environment. The authors find the combination of corporate greed and regulatory weakness in Sub-Saharan African countries a fertile ground for exploitive and culturally insensitive biomedical research that may not be in the best interest of host countries. In particular, poor and under-educated local people enrolling in vaccine and drug trials are poorly informed about their objectives, risks, and benefits due to the absence of prior counseling, and many research projects are not adequately screened by ethics committees for their relevance in host countries. Ethical irregularities persist in spite of national and international guidelines, standards, and protocols. The author concludes that national and international guidelines, standards, and protocols need to be enforced, corporate research protocols modified, and transactions and interactions between corporations and local communities overseen to control ethical irregularities.

In the final chapter, Damen Haile Mariam and Helmut Kloos conclude that contextualizing HIV/AIDS in the socioeconomic and cultural settings of Sub-Saharan Africa can provide valuable insights into the vulnerabilities and coping behaviors of affected populations and institutions during the current stepped-up interventions. There is much evidence that the ever-increasing complexity and cost of interventions – both the massive ART programs and the less successful programs focused on orphans, children, females, and other high-risk populations – can benefit from more interdisciplinary research involving social scientists. A number of still poorly understood problems and possible solutions highlighted in Part II of this volume need to be more fully addressed. They include the potential of community-based approaches to providing more people-friendly – and thus more accessible and more sustainable – treatment, care, and support programs; sectoral mainstreaming of HIV/AIDS in education; further upgrading of monitoring and evaluation programs; the ethics of biomedical research; and the impact of HIV/AIDS on individual companies and the responses of those companies. The authors end the chapter by identifying needs and opportunities for interdisciplinary research projects predicated on the intransigence of HIV transmission and spread, a continuing increase in the number of AIDS patients, and increasing communication and collaboration between biomedical and social scientists.

References

AFP. 1999. Kenya-AIDS: AIDS as a national disaster but condoms not the answer: Kenya's Moi. Agence France Press news article, 26 November. http://www.aegis.com/news/afp/1999/AF991135.html

Ahmed, S. 2011. HIV/AIDS: A window of opportunity for South Sudan, 8 July 2011. http://health.gbiportal.net/2011/07/08/hivaids-a-window-of-opportunity-for-south-sudan/

Ashforth, A. 2005. *Witchcraft, Violence and Democracy in South Africa*. Chicago and London: University of Chicago Press.

Berhe, C. 2011. Special Session: Ministerial Panel-Health and Social Affairs: Making Health Systems Work to Effective HIV Response. *Program of the 16th International Conference on AIDS and STIs in Africa*. Addis Ababa, 4–8 December, Abstract TUSS05.

Bolton, R. 1995. Rethinking anthropology. In Brummelhuis, H. ten and Herdt, G. (eds.), *Culture and Sexual Risk: Anthropological Perspectives on AIDS*, pp. 285–314. New York: Gordon and Breach.

Campbell, C. (ed.). 2003. *'Letting Them Die': Why HIV/AIDS Prevention Programmes Fail*. Oxford: The International African Institute in association with James Currey.

Caraël, M. 2006. Twenty years of intervention and controversy. In Denise, P. and Becker, C. (eds.), *The HIV/AIDS Epidemic in Sub-Saharan Africa in a Historical Perspective*, online edition. http://rds.refer.sn/IMG/pdf/AIDSHISTORYALL.pdf

Denis, P. 2006. Towards a social history of HIV/AIDS in Sub-Saharan Africa. In Denise, P. and Becker, C. (eds.), *The HIV/AIDS Epidemic in Sub-Saharan Africa in a Historical Perspective*, online edition. http://rds.refer.sn/IMG/pdf/AIDSHISTORYALL.pdf

de Waal, A. 2010. Governing a world with HIV and AIDS: An unfinished business. In Shan, D.E. (ed.), *The Socioeconomic Dimensions of HIV/AIDS in Africa*, pp. 42–73. Ithaca, NY: Cornell University Press.

ECA (Economic Commission for Africa). 2010. *Africa: The Socio-Economic Impact of HIV/AIDS*. Commission on HIV/AIDS and Governance in Africa. http://www.aec. msu.edu/fs2/adult_death/SOCIO_ECO_IMPACT.pdf

Farmer, P. 1999. *Infections and Inequalities: The Modern Plagues*. Berkeley, Los Angeles and London: University of California Press.

FDRE (Federal Democratic Republic of Ethiopia). 2010. *Report on Progress towards Implementation of the UN Declaration of Commitment on HIV/AIDS 2010*. Addis Ababa: Federal HIVAIDS Prevention and Control Office.

Forsythe, S., Stover, J. and Bollinger, L. 2009. The past, present and future of HIV, AIDS and resource allocation. *BMC Public Health* 9(Suppl 1):S4.

Greener, R. 2004. The impact of HIV/AIDS on poverty and inequality. In Haaker, M. (ed.), *The Macroeconomics of HIV/AIDS*, pp. 167–181. Washington, DC: International Monetary Fund.

Idoko, J. and Bequele, A. 2011. Special Session: Value for Money: Sustaining HIV Response. *Program of the 16th International Conference on AIDS and STIs in Africa*. Addis Ababa, 4–8 December, Abstract MOSS02.

Iliffe, J. 2006. *The African AIDS Epidemic: A History*. Oxford: James Curry and Athens, Ohio: Ohio University Press.

Kalipeni, E., Craddock, S., Oppong, J.R. and Ghosh, J. (eds.), 2004. *HIV/AIDS in Africa: Beyond Epidemiology*. Oxford: Blackwell.

Kippax, S.C., Holt, M. and Friedman, S.R. 2011. Bridging the social and biomedical: Engaging the social sciences and political sciences in HIV research. *Journal of the International AIDS Society* 14(Suppl. 2):S1.

Levy, J.A. 2007. *The Pathogenesis of AIDS*. 3rd edn. Washington, DC: ASM Press.

MacQueen, K.M. 2011. Framing the social in biomedical HIV prevention trials: A 20-year retrospective. *Journal of the International AIDS Society* 14(Suppl. 2):S3.

Marzo, F. 2004. *The Impact of HIV/AIDS on Chronic and Transient Poverty*. http://www. csae.ox.ac.uk/conferences/2004-GPRAHDIA/papers/1h-Marzo-CSAE2004.pdf

Maticka-Tyndale, E., Tiemoko, R. and Makinwa-Adebusoye, P. (eds.), 2007. *Human Sexuality in Africa: Beyond Reproduction*. Johannesburg: Action Health Incorporated.

Nattrass, N. 2004. *The Moral Economy of AIDS in South Africa*. Cambridge: Cambridge University Press.

Nolen, S. 2007. *28 Stories of AIDS in Africa*. New York: Walker & Company.

Nyanzi, S., Nassimbwa, J., Kayizzi, V. and Kabanda, S. 2008. 'African sex is dangerous!': Renegotiating 'ritual sex' in contemporary Masaka District. *Africa* 78:518–539.

Obono, O. (ed.). 2010. *A Tapestry of Human Sexuality in Africa*. Johannesburg: Fanele.

Oppong, J.R. and Agyei-Mensah, S. 2004. HIV/AIDS in West Africa: The case of Senegal, Ghana, and Nigeria. In Kalipeni, E., Craddock, S., Oppong, J.R. and Ghosh, Y. (eds.), *HIV/AIDS in Africa: Beyond Epidemiology*, pp. 71–82. Oxford: Blackwell.

Parker, R.G. 1995. The social and cultural construction of sexual risk, or how to have (sex) research in an epidemic. In Brummelhuis, H. ten and Herdt, G. (eds.), *Culture and Sexual Risk: Anthropological Perspectives on AIDS*, pp. 257–270. New York: Gordon and Breach.

Sahn, D.A. (ed.). 2010. *The Socioeconomic Dimensions of HIV/AIDS in Africa: Challenges, Opportunities, and Misconceptions*. London: Cornell University Press in cooperation with United Nations University.

Salaam-Blyther, T. 2010. *The Global Fund to Fight AIDS, Tuberculosis, and Malaria: U.S. Contributions and Issues for Congress*. Congressional Research Service. htpp://healthlegislation.blogspot.com/2010/08/globalfund-to-fight-aids-tuberculosis.html

Schoepf, B.G. 1995. Culture, sex research and AIDS prevention in Africa. In Brummelhuis, H. ten and Herdt, G. (eds.), *Culture and Sexual Risk: Anthropological Perspectives on AIDS*, pp. 29–51. New York: Gordon and Breach.

Seckinelgin, H. 2008. *International Politics of HIV/AIDS: Global Disease – Local Pain*. London and New York: Routledge.

Sidibe, M. 2011. Antiretrovirals for prevention: Realizing the potential. Closing commentary by the Executive Director of UNAIDS. *Current HIV Research* 9:470–472.

Stele, P.W. 1999. *A Plague of Paradoxes: AIDS, Culture, and Demography in Northern Tanzania*. Chicago and London: University of Chicago Press.

Tamale, S. 2011a. Researching and theorizing sexualities in Africa. In Tamale, S. (ed.), *African Sexualities: A Reader*, pp. 11–36. Capetown, Nairobi and Oxford: Pambazuka Press.

Tamale, S. (ed.). 2011b. *African Sexualities: A Reader*. Capetown, Nairobi and Oxford: Pambazuka Press.

Tawfik, L. and Kinoti, S.N. 2006. *The Impact of HIV/AIDS on the Health Workforce in Developing Countries*. Background Paper Prepared for the World Health Report 2006 – Working Together for Health. www.who.int/hrh/documents/Impact_of_HIV.pdf

Traore, N. 2011. Workshop: Quality Improvement: A Strategy to Promote Ownership, Sustainability and Scale-up. *Program of the 16th International Conference on AIDS and STIs in Africa*. Addis Ababa, 4–8 December, Abstract TULSBW17.

UNAIDS. 2006. *Report on The Global AIDS Epidemic*. Geneva: UNAIDS.

UNAIDS. 2008. *Report on The Global AIDS Epidemic*. Geneva: UNAIDS.

UNAIDS. 2010. *Report on the Global AIDS Epidemic*. Geneva: UNAIDS.

UNAIDS. 2011. *UNAIDS World AIDS Day Report 2011*. Geneva UNAIDS.

USAID. 2010. *Madagascar: HIV/AIDS Health Profile*. Washington, DC: USAID.

WHO/UNAIDS/UNICEF. 2011. *Global HIV/AIDS Response: Epidemic Update and Health Sector Progress towards Universal Access*, Progress Report 2011. Geneva: WHO, UNAIDS and UNICEF.

Wreford, J. 2008. *Working with Spirit: Experiencing Sangoma in Contemporary South Africa*. Oxford and New York: Berghahn Books.

Wreford, J. 2009. The pragmatics of knowledge transfer: An HIV/AIDS intervention with traditional health practitioners in Southern Africa. *Anthropology Southern Africa* 32:37–47.

Books, papers, websites, and other resources for further reading

Africa Regional Sexuality Resource Centre (ARSRC). www.arsrc.org

Dilger, H. and Luig, U. (eds.), 2010. *Morality, Hope and Grief: Anthropologies of AIDS in Africa*. New York and Oxford: Berghahn Books.

Ouédraogo, J.B. and Cardoso. A. (eds.), 2011. *Readings in Methodology: African Perspectives*. Dakar: CODESRIA.

PubMed's biomedical, health services and social science resource site: http://ncb.nlm.nih.gov/pubmed

United Nations. 2011. *The Millennium Development Goals Report 2011*. New York: UNAIDS.

2
Contextualizing HIV/AIDS in Sub-Saharan Africa: The Link with Tradition, Religion, and Culture

Getnet Tadele and Woldekidan Amde

Introduction

Tradition, religion, and culture are interrelated and overlapping concepts. Social scientists in general and anthropologists in particular have given numerous definitions of culture. Of all the definitions offered by different scholars, Edward Tylor's is among the most widely accepted. Tylor defined culture as that broader reality that comprises a gamut of belief systems, perception of righteousness, competencies, and long-established practices that are passed across generations in society (Tylor 1987, in Helman 2007, p. 2). This definition suggests that tradition and religion are part of the culture of any society. The overlap between culture, tradition, and religion must be considered in evaluating their roles in prevention or spread of HIV/AIDS. Distinctions between aspects of culture that have religious origin or backing of religious texts and those that are simply the result of age-old tradition are relevant for analytical studies, although the two are joined seamlessly in many instances. Patriarchy, for instance, is a cultural practice having the backing of religion.

This chapter examines the role of tradition, religion, and culture in sexuality, illness behavior, and condom use in Sub-Saharan Africa, relationships between which need to be further clarified. Although gender and HIV/AIDS are explored in detail in Chapter 3, gender issues have been broached in this chapter as well in order to consider additional specific perspectives on tradition, religion, and culture. Gender relations are also included in the discussions of the influence of religion on sexual initiation, homosexuality, condom use, and the link between sexuality and culture.

Clearly, religion, tradition, and culture play significant roles in the lives of many people all over the world. Consciously or subconsciously, people explain significant or minor life events with reference to tradition, religion, and culture. Tradition, religion, and culture also disapprove or sanction countless activities human beings carry out every day, from mundane practices such as what and how one should eat or dress to serious issues such as when and with whom one should engage in sex. Throughout human history, sexuality in particular has been surrounded by social values and norms that emanate from tradition, religion, and culture. Premarital and extramarital sex, abortion, and homosexuality always remain a source of contention, and the basis for or against these behaviors is either religion or tradition, or both.

Thus, almost everywhere, culture, religion, health, illness, and sexuality intersect in the everyday lives of people. Despite this strong connection, the scientific discourse regarding HIV/AIDS is dominated by biomedical understanding and pertinent social and cultural aspects of the disease are often marginalized. According to McFadden (1992, in Ampofo et al. 2004), focusing on the biomedical dimensions of HIV/AIDS constrains appreciation of social and cultural dynamics that impact vulnerability to the virus and uptake of HIV-related services. A plethora of structural barriers having economic, cultural, and political dimensions undermine the agency of individuals to undergo appropriate behavioral change that would protect them from becoming victims of the AIDS epidemic. Regardless of the effectiveness of strategies for effecting behavioral change, if the context does not favor transformation, outcomes tend to be poor. Thus scholars reiterate the need for changing the social environment in a manner that would empower individuals to make the best of their knowledge and available HIV/AIDS prevention programs (Faigle and Koijane 2000). Some of the proposed structural changes include empowering women to be educated and economically independent and addressing inheritance laws and other traditional, religious, and cultural practices that may make people prone to HIV infection.

Although the social science literature describes the diversity in the social, cultural, and political contexts in Sub-Saharan Africa, conclusions from these numerous published and unpublished works regarding the relationship between HIV/AIDS and structural and behavioral factors are largely inconclusive. Some believe tradition, religion, and culture undermine the fight against HIV/AIDS by negatively portraying the disease and condom use or promoting behaviors that expose people to the virus. Others reject the unqualified attacks against African culture and tradition, insisting that culture goes through constant change and contains aspects that reduce HIV risk and facilitate care of the sick (Oppong and Kalipeni 2004).

Religion and HIV/AIDS

Sub-Saharan Africa has been described as one of the most religious regions in the world, based on the high proportion (69–98%) of the population that considers religion to be very important in their lives and the preference of both Christians and Moslems for the Bible or Sharia, respectively, as the official law of the land (Pew Forum 2010). The region's population now consists of nearly twice as many Christians as Moslems and a small proportion of adherents to numerous African religions. Although the traditional African religions have significantly declined since 1900 due to the growth of Christianity and Islam, many indigenous beliefs and practices that have a bearing on vulnerability to HIV survive today among followers of Christianity and Islam (Pew Forum 2010).

Studies of the association between religion and vulnerability to sexually transmitted infections (STIs) in Sub-Saharan Africa were undertaken as early as the beginning of the nineteenth century (Barton 1991). The Western paradigm of the generally positive effects of religion on health appears less applicable in developing countries, where considerable variation exists in AIDS-related behavior by religious affiliation (Trinitapoli and Regnerus 2006). Many studies in Sub-Saharan Africa have examined differences in risk behavior and HIV prevalence of the major religious groups – Moslems and Christians, particularly Protestants, Catholics, and members of African churches and indigenous African religions. A review of HIV prevalence in 38 countries using national data indicated that Moslems generally had lower infection rates than Christians (Trinitapoli and Regnerus 2006). These broad studies have been expanded in recent years by research into specific risk behaviors among different religious groups, including sexual initiation, homosexuality, and condom use.

Religion and sexual initiation

Using data from the Ghana Demographic and Health Survey of 1993, Addai (2000) found a relationship between religious affiliation and sexual initiation for married women aged 15–49 years but not for unmarried females of the same age. The relationship between religious affiliation and sexual initiation varied according to religious denomination and was closely associated with whether the women subscribed to a progressive or conservative religion; those in the latter group were less likely to engage in sexual activity prior to wedlock. The probability of sexual initiation prior to marriage was least likely among Moslem women, apparently due to their adherence to strict religious and traditional norms that assign high value to maintaining virginity until marriage (Addai 2000). Similarly, a study in Nigeria of 1,870 students from two universities examined the influence of religion on perceptions and sexual practices of youth. Results confirmed existing literature: Those affiliated with certain religions were more likely to have relatively conservative opinions regarding sex before marriage and abstain from sexual activity as opposed to their peers with little religious attachment. The study also associated difference in attitudes and behaviors with different levels of religiosity. Thus ardent followers, both males and females, who tended to practice their religion and invested time and effort in religious causes were more likely to abstain from sex (Odimegwu 2005).

Religion, together with marriage, is at the forefront of institutions that associate meaning with sexuality and its manifestations and offer benchmarks for appropriate behavior (Reddy 2004, in Makinwa-Adebusoye and Tiemoko 2007). Christianity and Islam discourage premarital and extramarital sex, activities that are contrary to the moral creeds of these religions. Devout followers normally adhere to these proscriptions (Lehrer 2004, in Odimegwu 2005). Christianity insists on attaching sexuality to the institution of marriage, whereby sex is acceptable only within wedlock, and provides teachings to that effect (Makinwa-Adebusoye and Tiemoko 2007). This has prompted scholars to emphasize the need for public health policies that promote the participation of religious leaders in HIV/AIDS programs for the purpose of changing prevailing perceptions and practices of fledgling followers. Odimegwu (2005) cited the significant progress in HIV prevention made in Uganda and Zambia via innovative projects with religious components such as 'True Love Waits' and 'Abstinence Lie Che' (Trafford 2002, in Odimegwu 2005).

There is some evidence that clergy may not be applying religious dicta to HIV/AIDS issues adequately. A recent survey among 3,303 Orthodox priests in Ethiopia, for instance, showed that only 14% did not know how to advocate against promiscuity, 96% wanted the practice of early marriage to continue, and fewer than one-third of them advised families to delay marriage of their daughters and abandon female genital cutting (Mekbib et al. 2011). This demonstrates the elevated status the institution of marriage enjoys, being entrenched in tradition and religion, and how it mediates perceptions toward sexual intercourse. Priests appear to be concerned far more about whether sex happens outside wedlock than its premature initiation or the implication early initiation may have on youngsters.

Although religion can have a positive influence on HIV prevention, its impact can also be negative. Smith (2004a) found that evangelical and Pentecostal religious traditions in two Nigerian cities undermined the consistent use of condoms and instilled a false sense of security among young rural and urban migrants. According to these religious perspectives, HIV/AIDS is God's punishment for those who have been immoral and sinful. This belief was promulgated through media outlets and church programs in these two cities. More than one-third of the youth in Kano and 26% of those in Aba considered AIDS to be God's wrath or a disease the cause of which only God knows; many others attributed the disease to decadent behavior. Ethiopian Orthodox priests expressed similar beliefs in an anti-AIDS leadership course (Surur and Kaba 2000). Such perceptions, Smith (2004a) argued, are problematic as they undermine bargaining of safe sex.

Thus religious interpretations of the disease and moral assessments of personal sexual behavior may create obstacles for young, sexually active people attempting to evaluate risk, both those in 'moral partnerships' and those participating in more stigmatized sexual relationships. By providing doctrinaire explanations for who is at risk and who is not, Christianity creates contexts in which individuals tend to ignore or deny their actual risk (Smith 2004a; see also Schmid 2007; Tadele 2006).

Schmid (2007) underlined the problem that ensues when religions promote faithfulness as the only prevention against HIV/AIDS: This line of reasoning leaves many faithful people unprotected from the harm their not-so-faithful partners can cause them. This dilemma is evident from the experience of many married women in Sub-Saharan Africa. Smith (2004a) observed the need to address the gap in existing interventions in Nigeria that fail to recognize the role religious morality plays in sexuality. Emphasis on abstinence and fidelity in religious morality introduces stigma into any discussion on condom use and leaves many either ignorant or relegated to unsafe sex. This is disconcerting in a situation where youth engage in risky sexual behavior before or in marriage.

Several other studies demonstrate that religion has little impact on the sexual behavior of individuals or on preventing the spread of the virus. Most young people surveyed in an Ethiopian town reported that religion did not have any effect on their sexual behavior (Tadele 2006). In Uganda, adolescent girls used religiosity to evade social control and maintain respectability in the eyes of the community (Romberg 2001). Garner (2000) found that among the great majority of South Africans he studied who were affiliated with various Christian denominations, sex before marriage and infidelity within matrimony were rampant. This study in a KwaZulu-Natal township noted the inability of religion to curb followers from engaging in sexual practices that are against the moral teachings of their respective churches. Differences in sexual behavior were associated with different churches, but only Pentecostal churches had significantly lower extra- and premarital sex among members. They achieved this by emphasizing indoctrination, religious experience, exclusion, and socialization (Garner 2000).

Garner (2000) described in some detail the difficulty of using the experience of the Pentecostal churches to guide interventions in other parts of South Africa. For one, adopting some of the nuances of the Pentecostal church – such as requiring members to avoid sex before marriage but allowing affairs once married – is generally frowned upon. The factors that brought success in a religious environment cannot be simply injected into a secular setting. Indoctrination that is not religious, but is limited to the facts of HIV transmission and prevention, does not have the same strength as it is devoid of emotional content. The exclusiveness of a religious sect, which motivates adherence to the sect's norms, is lost when the distinctives of the sect are offered to a wider group. And socialization without religious fervor and exclusivity is not sufficient to effect behavior change.

Religion and homosexuality

Much of the discourse on homosexuality in Sub-Saharan Africa is dominated by religious morality that considers it a decadent Western practice to be fought and suppressed, and many deny the very existence of this practice in their respective countries (Maticka-Tyndale 2007; Tadele 2008). Between 79% and 98% of representative populations in 18 Sub-Saharan countries, including 9 countries in eastern and southern Africa, consider homosexual behavior to be morally wrong, with minor differences between Christians and Moslems (Pew Forum 2010). The denial and stigma surrounding men who have sex with men (MSM) emanates primarily from the perception that the behavior is contrary to the religion, tradition, and culture of the continent. Nevertheless, researchers have concluded that this behavior has existed in many African societies for long periods. Barton (1991) identified more than 150 studies on homosexuality for both genders in Sub-Saharan Africa. According to Murray and Roscoe (1998, in Niang et al. 2003), evidence of same-sex relationships has been found in approximately 50 African societies in numerous geographical areas with different family structures and kinship patterns.

Despite a body of literature underlining the high risk of HIV infection to which MSM are exposed, little HIV/AIDS-related programming is directed at them in most African countries. This is because homosexuality is criminalized, associated with violence against perpetrators, and shrouded by strong stigma, exacerbating the vulnerability of MSM (UNAIDS 2010). Religion accounts for much of the stigma and denial (Niang et al. 2003).

MSM are divided in regard to religious affiliation. Some reject religion, believing it has no space for them; others hold on to their religion and hope to find healing and become 'straight' believers (Tadele 2008). In Senegal, men often concede their homosexual orientation to be a sinful indulgence and claim they will abdicate it when they attain a certain age of maturity and fully embrace the ways of Islam (Niang et al. 2003).

Similarly, in Ethiopia there are MSM who recognize the contradictions between their behavior and the dictates of their religion but choose to affiliate themselves with the religion and are optimistic that they can renew their heterosexual orientation and reclaim their religious status. One study captures the complexity of the situation, acknowledging that religion creates distress among homosexuals who feel they have gone astray and experience social rejection, but at the same time recognizing that religion offers a path for cleansing, solace, and regaining a sense of belonging with fellow religious followers. Some MSM who are totally overwhelmed by the contradiction between their sexuality and their religion abandon the latter for the former. Some of these men adopt alternative belief systems that embrace their sexuality. In Ethiopia, where the major religions strongly denounce homosexuality, some MSM turn to certain traditional belief systems that tolerate and allegedly give meaning to their sexuality. These belief systems proclaim that MSM and their behaviors are dictated by powerful spirits that possess the men, a notion that separates the practice from the practitioner, possibly abdicating the latter from any sense of wrongdoing (Tadele 2008).

Religion and condom use

In a study in Nigeria, Smith (2004a) attempted to explain the recurrent research finding of a discrepancy between knowledge and practice of individuals in relation to HIV/AIDS. In a survey of 863 youth, Smith found that traditional gender norms, values, and perceptions toward having a child determined the choices youth made in relation to whether they would have unprotected sex or use contraception, similarly to the way such decisions are mediated by the perception of HIV/AIDS risk. However, the cultural expectations and leverage to make individual decisions involving choosing partners, having sex, and using condoms were different for men and women (Smith 2004a).

The dialogue on HIV/AIDS spearheaded by religious leaders and institutions tends to interpret the epidemic as God's punishment for people's sins. It suggests certain groups are responsible for AIDS, stigmatizing those living with the virus (Schmid 2007). A number of studies make evident that discourse about the use of condoms is marred by the same traditional and moral judgments that attach stigma to HIV/AIDS and people living with HIV/AIDS (PLWHA). Notwithstanding the role condom use plays in reducing transmission of the virus, it carries a great deal of stigma as it is associated with immorality and sexual indiscretions that are characteristics of the stigma attributed to the pandemic (Hillier et al. 1998, in Smith 2004a). For example, Smith (2004a) demonstrated that migrant youth in Nigeria have difficulty dealing with issues of sex prior to marriage, putting them at further HIV risk, as any attempt to address risk behavior or suggested use of protection provokes all the negative moral sentiments attached to the disease. Hence, the issue of having sex is intertwined with the fear of getting infected by HIV, prompting many young migrants to avoid engaging in such discussions (Smith 2004a).

In communities where Christian norms are highly influential and in a period of life when the idea of romance and going steady leading to marriage and children is in vogue, youth, particularly females, find the issue of having sex before marriage entangled with various religious and moral values. This dilemma makes contraceptive use difficult to negotiate. It is rather tragic that in the context of the AIDS pandemic condoms appear to be the most difficult form of contraception for young women to negotiate because their use requires the obvious cooperation of men and, ironically, condoms are stigmatized as a symbol of the epidemic they are meant to control (Smith 2004b). Despite being one of the most effective prevention strategies against HIV and pregnancy in Africa, the use of condoms has been sternly denounced or rejected by different belief systems, including Christianity,

Islam, and traditional belief systems; and there is much stigma attached to it, as it is considered synonymous with promiscuity or infidelity. Married couples look on condom use as signaling a lack of trust (Francis-Chizororo and Natshalaga 2003).

The relationship between religion and condom use continues to be very contentious. As a case in point, the Ethiopian Evangelical Church Mekane Yesus, in its training manual on HIV/AIDS/STI prevention and control, vividly described condom use as a futile measure against the disease because it gives a false sense of security and fosters indulgence in sexual indiscretions. The church prescribed refraining from sinful practices as the only sure way to fight the disease (EECMY 1999).

Dominant discourses in Sub-Saharan African societies on condom use, such as ones that proclaim the use of condoms as a violation of God's command or insinuate that it is unbecoming for anyone but sex workers, play a great part in undermining the acceptance of condoms by individuals, particularly by married couples (Kaler 2004). Similar notions of condoms that associate them with prostitution and infidelity undermine their use in Swaziland (Daly 2001).

To overcome moral and religious challenges related to using condoms, a number of researchers recommend promoting condoms as a means of contraception rather than as HIV/AIDS prevention. In Malawi, for instance, one researcher who found strong opposition to promoting condom use suggested that the idea of using condoms for contraception would be better accepted. She argued that the use of condoms is invariably mediated by the social context that informs perception toward it, which contains long existing societal notions of wellness, vulnerability, and risk. Thus any effort to curtail the spread of the virus by increasing condom use has the daunting task of altering existing social contexts that undermine condom use (Kaler 2004).

To get around the stigma attached to condoms and the opposition of men, married males in particular, toward their use, Francis-Chizororo and Natshalaga (2003) recommended promoting the product as a contraception mechanism rather than emphasizing its effectiveness in preventing disease. However, studies in Nigeria (Ezumah 2003) and the former Zaire (Schoepf 1997) proved this strategy by itself to be problematic. The researchers found that even when individuals considered condoms a means of preventing unwanted pregnancy, that fact may not be sufficient ground for many of them to use condoms because using them clashed with their religious beliefs. Among unmarried male youth members of the African Independent Church in three districts in rural Mozambique, however, religious affiliation had little effect on condom use and sexual activity (Noden et al. 2010). For women, their inferior social position in most parts of Africa means they have no voice in making decisions on having children or using condoms, even in situations where they feel they would be at high risk of becoming infected with

HIV, as in the case of those with unfaithful partners (Francis-Chizororo and Natshalaga 2003).

In spite of the limited effectiveness of religion in impacting sexual behavior, religious institutions have a unique potential for delivering HIV/AIDS messages to a large segment of the population. Therefore, their strength in addressing the problem of HIV/AIDS should not be underestimated (Tadele 2006).

Traditional medical systems

One of the areas demanding better understanding of its relationship to HIV/AIDS in Sub-Saharan Africa is the widespread practice of traditional medicine, particularly because it is intertwined with both culture and religion. According to World Health Organization (WHO), the region experiences a quarter of the world's disease burden but has at its disposal only 3% of the global health workforce, necessitating reliance on traditional healers and extensive lay healing knowledge in nearly all communities (UNAIDS 2006; WHO 2006). Against this backdrop, traditional medicine is widely practiced, with close to 80% of the users relying on it to treat, inter alia, sexually transmitted diseases, including HIV/AIDS. Traditional healers play a prominent role in dealing with the health needs of the people, and they are by far more accessible than any other form of health care in the region, with a ratio of one traditional healer to 500 people as opposed to one medical doctor to 40,000 people (Truter 2007). People esteem traditional medicine for it is entrenched in indigenous culture, is readily available, and provides a holistic approach to treating illnesses that not only considers the physical condition of the patient but also psychological, spiritual, and social conditions. Despite continuous efforts by Western missions and doctors since colonial times to eliminate cultural healing practices, traditional healing continues to be widely practiced in both rural and urban areas. Because of their influential role in setting and enforcing societal and spiritual norms and practices, including traditional medicine, many healers enjoy higher respect and acceptance than Western-trained doctors, and many PLWHA therefore seek their help (Truter 2007; UNAIDS 2000, 2006). Some governments in Africa have recognized the role of traditional medicine as complementary to modern practice. However, a study in Ethiopia reported that although the government of Ethiopia has fully recognized the presence and role of traditional medicine in health care, professional medical personnel have failed to integrate it into their practices (Villanucci 2010).

Diversity in the beliefs and practices of traditional healers in Africa reflects the diversity of culture and experience on the continent (Good 1987, in UNAIDS 2000). Studies investigating the knowledge, beliefs, and practices of traditional healers in the region generally conclude that despite difference in nomenclature and inability to provide descriptions matching biomedical understanding, many traditional healers are aware of the various sexually transmitted infections. There seems to be consensus among many traditional healers that AIDS is an ailment that is foreign to Africa (Green et al. 1993, in UNAIDS 2000).

Traditional healers have identified various HIV and STI prevention strategies, most of which are typical to traditional medicine. Traditional medicine considers HIV infection a state of impurity and thus traditional healers offer help to either maintain or reclaim purity, mostly through the use of herbs and cauterization. Traditional healers are increasingly recognizing the value of condom usage and promoting it as well as denouncing promiscuity as HIV prevention strategies (Green et al. 1993, in UNAIDS 2000; Schoepf 1992, in UNAIDS 2000); they may serve as effective information, education, and communication agents advocating condom use and other behavioral changes (Gbodossou et al. 2011).

As traditional healers are becoming increasingly aware of the benefits of condoms, they are able to give them meaning in the context of their existing beliefs. For more conservative healers, though, the idea of using condoms contradicts their belief regarding semen, and so some discourage their use. Traditional healers on the continent commonly perceive semen to be an invaluable nutrient that ensures well-being of pregnant mothers and unborn children. Notwithstanding this perception, many have accepted and even promoted condom use due to its far superior benefit: ensuring continuation of life and long established ways of communal living (Schoepf 1992, in UNAIDS 2000).

Health institutions and administrations in Sub-Saharan Africa have recognized the potential contribution traditional healers can make to HIV/AIDS prevention and control, and collaborative initiatives between traditional and biomedical practitioners have emerged in recent years. These initiatives have been beneficial to both HIV/AIDS programs and the wider community as they have assisted with the formulation and support of government policy on traditional medicine and patient counseling and treatment in their homes (UNAIDS 2006). Project HOPE in Western Cape Province in South Africa is an encouraging collaborative that mobilizes social health assets that were underused in that country's pluralistic medical system. This project emphasizes the need for biomedicine to consider folk knowledge of illness causation and perceptions of 'appropriate remedies' within the context of local belief systems (Wreford 2009).

Nevertheless, many hurdles remain in integrating relevant elements of traditional medicine into prevention and control programs. For example, a study in the Central African Republic found that traditional healers who had gone through a one-week training course on STIs and AIDS showed few signs of attitudinal change toward the use of condoms or practices that favored the spread of the virus. Persistent non-use of condoms emanated from the perception that they undermine fertility (Johnson 1996, in UNAIDS 2000), indicating that the belief systems and medical practices of traditional heal-ers are unlikely to change quickly, even after they are exposed to biomedical education and training.

Gender, sexuality, and culture

Most studies dealing with tradition, religion, and culture in relation to HIV/AIDS highlight the relative vulnerability of women to the virus due to a number of structural factors (Bankole et al. 2004; Makinwa-Adebusoye and Tiemoko 2007). Brown et al. (2005) stressed the need to investigate how notions of sexuality and gender mediate the behavior of individuals in the effort to curb the spread of HIV in Sub-Saharan Africa. Likewise, Wekwete and Madzingira (2008) expressed the need for a gendered approach to exam-ining women's vulnerability to HIV and AIDS in Zimbabwe, observing that women's vulnerability is closely related to the gendered nuances of their social milieu that operate to promote sexual subjugation of women and expose them to different forms of sexual violence.

The societal norms or traditions that relate to sexuality prescribe different behaviors for men and women that put both under pressure to act in cer-tain ways, and those ways tend to contribute to the spread of HIV (Ezumah 2003; Wekwete and Madzingira 2008). Bankole et al. (2004) also demon-strated that strong cultural norms and values pushed individuals to engage in risky sexual practices. Studies indicate that young men in Sub-Saharan Africa experience strong social pressures to prove their manhood by having sex, engaging in sexual intercourse with commercial sex workers, having sex with many partners, or having unprotected intercourse (Awusabo-Asare et al. 1999, in Bankole et al. 2004).

Several researchers have examined the link between masculinity and sex-uality. In Zambia, for example, young men consider sexual relationships an essential aspect of their sense of self and of their standing in society (Price and Hawkins 2002, in Brown et al. 2005). A boy's initiation of relationships with girls is a confirmation of his transition to manhood, according to stud-ies in Nigeria and in a Xhosa township in South Africa (Caldwell et al. 1997, in Otive-Igbuzor 2007; Wood and Jewkes 2001, in Brown et al. 2005). Such strong notions of masculinity undermine the efficacy of programs meant to bring about change in sexual practice among men. This has been shown in a study among mine workers in South Africa who embraced having sex-ual relationships with multiple partners, engaged in unprotected sex, and wished to bear several children (Campbell 1997, in Brown et al. 2005).

Another aspect of masculinity that is closely related to increased risk of HIV is high consumption of alcohol, which is closely linked to lack of con-dom use (Mbulaiteye et al. 2000). Brown et al. (2005) reasoned that in some contexts alcohol use might help explain linkages between masculin-ity and HIV infection in Sub-Saharan Africa. Describing the situation in contemporary Namibia, he seemed to suggest the need to develop alternative notions of masculinity in Ovambo society, notions that would challenge existing concepts whereby men are culturally pressured into having multiple sexual partners, indulging in excessive alcohol consumption, and bearing several children, all to live up to culturally prescribed notions of being a man (Brown et al. 2005).

There is a growing body of literature about how cultural notions of femininity and masculinity undermine the safety of women regarding HIV. Examples include the practices of polygamy and having multiple sexual relations within or outside marriage. Another example is that women generally receive inadequate care once they are infected. Despite knowledge about the infidelity of their sexual partners, women cannot decline sex or even negotiate safe sex with their partners. Their powerlessness in sexual relationships and thus their lack of control over their sexuality puts women at high risk of HIV/AIDS infection (Ampofo et al. 2004).

Due to the illness and the vulnerability associated with it, notions of sexuality in Africa bring to mind not ideas of excitement, but rather hurt and death (Reddy 2004, in Makinwa-Adebusoye and Tiemoko 2007). Women's experiences of sexuality, HIV/AIDS, and violence go hand in hand. Women experience violence not only from their partners, but also from the broader social context that sets and enforces gendered norms to police their sexuality (Makinwa-Adebusoye and Tiemoko 2007). Wekwete and Madzingira (2008) pointed out that gendered roles that favor men and patriarchal marital arrangements in Zimbabwe render women powerless in the society. For instance, following payment of the bride price, men tend to feel they own their wives and that ownership gives them free reign in sexual relations. Women thus have little say and are in no position to protect their sexual and reproductive rights.

Ezumah (2003) set out to understand the gender and sexuality-linked root causes of unsafe sex among the Igbo of Awka and Agulu in Anambra State in Nigeria. The study identified the high prevalence of certain cultural practices and values as major culprits. Because the society placed a high cultural value on parenthood, married women engaged in extramarital sex when they could not conceive from their husbands. Further, parents wanted to have a male child in the family, so they pressured their unmarried female children to have sex prior to marriage. Women in this patriarchal society have low socioeconomic status, so they succumb to these cultural pressures, exposing themselves to HIV. They cannot bargain protected sex; they might face wrath for even suggesting it. Hence, efforts to promote positive perceptions about sexuality and sexual practices have been undermined by the patriarchal status quo that stifles expression of sexuality, particularly among women (Ezumah 2003; Otive-Igbuzor 2007).

Other sociocultural practices that encourage sexual relationships involving young people, such as child marriage and rituals initiating boys and girls into adulthood, are still common in Sub-Saharan Africa. Some of these practices increase young people's, especially young women's, risk of HIV infection (Bankole et al. 2004; Mann 1997, in Otive-Igbuzor 2007). Younger women's risk of HIV/AIDS infection is heightened by the fact that they are often sought after by men who are much older than they because the men assume the younger women are less exposed to HIV/AIDS (Rajani and Kudrati 1996, in Ampofo et al. 2004) and because of a belief that sex with a virgin cures HIV/AIDS (Leclerc-Madlala 2002).

Early marriage for women is a common phenomenon in most parts of the region, especially in rural areas where traditional cultural norms and values are particularly strong. Women are expected to get married early to men who are far older. Life in wedlock puts women at further risk (Bankole et al. 2004). Many believe the age gap between husbands and wives creates a power imbalance between them that makes negotiation for safer sex unattainable for women (Maticka-Tyndale 2007).

Traditional practices exercised to control the sexuality of women in the region exacerbate the situation. One such practice is the prenuptial tradition of virginity testing in KwaZulu-Natal in South Africa, a highly celebrated and politically charged issue in the aftermath of Thabo Mbeki's pro-traditional political ideology (Wickström 2010). The practice, although banned by the government in South Africa, is gaining wider acceptance as a way of fighting the spread and impact of HIV/AIDS. Local people of KwaZulu-Natal see virginity testing as a way of using community pressure and symbolism to increase individual and collective responsibility for sexual relations (Wickström 2010). Leclerc-Madlala (2001) suggested that virginity testing is primarily a manifestation of the strong desire of a male-dominated society to maintain the existing gender status quo to the detriment of the rights and well-being of women.

Makinwa-Adebusoye and Tiemoko (2007) cautioned against the gendered response to HIV/AIDS whereby stringent moral rules on the sexuality of women are revamped throughout Sub-Saharan Africa with relatively little emphasis on the implication of the sexuality of men. For example, Seidel (1993, in Schmid 2007) reported that in response to the alarming spread of the virus, religious conservatism, which was on the rise in Africa, reinforced stringent norms on women that further alienated them from the public sphere and accentuated the importance given to maintaining virginity. Such ill-informed policy and programs against HIV/AIDS in Africa have inadvertently resulted in further entrenching men's control over women's sexuality and increased women's vulnerability to the virus (Makinwa-Adebusoye and Tiemoko 2007; Otive-Igbuzor 2007). This type of gendered response toward HIV/AIDS draws disproportionate attention to women and exempts men from any responsibility even though they are the most responsible for spreading the virus. Society exhibits a lot of tolerance toward men, even if they engage in risky sexual practices and put their women partners at high risk of infection. In a context in which men's reckless behavior is not tackled head on, addressing women only continues to undermine the fight against the epidemic (Leclerc-Madlala 2001).

The culture of silence surrounding sexuality

The culture of silence regarding issues of sexuality has put youth at risk of HIV/AIDS. Conversations in the Meru and Maasai communities revealed that youth lack awareness about their sexuality and ways they can avoid pregnancy and STIs, including HIV/AIDS (Mwangi 2006). In these and other East African societies, HIV/AIDS is perpetuated by a culture of silence between children and parents regarding issues of sexuality. Several misperceptions surround youth sexuality, including the beliefs that girls engaging in sexual intercourse can relieve menstrual cramps and that boys not engaging in sex can die from an erection.

The significance of traditional/local means of socialization about sexuality through social networks such as kinship, extended families, and clans has been challenged by modernization. In South Africa, for example, youth is no longer ruled by authoritative and hierarchical structures and the gulf between the generations is widening, affecting all areas of youth sexuality (Pelzer et al. 2006). The modern community lacks competence to address the issues by relying on traditional knowledge. However, widely prevalent public education on HIV/AIDS, which is increasingly replacing traditional education about sex, has its shortcomings. The public education disregards the significance of the social milieu on the choices individuals make and places correspondingly greater emphasis on the agency of individuals. Public education also fails to take into account local knowledge and resources and thereby creates dependence on exogenous support (Mwangi 2006). On the other hand, reliance on traditional social structures or networks for disseminating information on sexuality and HIV/AIDS may fail to reach women, who are often not present in meetings in patriarchal societies where such matters may be discussed. Men's dominance in family and clan settings means that the use of these social settings as platforms for raising awareness, notwithstanding their benefits, would fail to reach women, who are often marginalized in these structures (Mwangi 2006).

Policy makers increasingly recognize that families can play a significant part in educating youth about sexuality. As a result, many studies call for closer communication between parents and children and greater willingness of parents to offer information about sexuality to their children. This method of disseminating information to young people contrasts with existing public education campaigns that address youth and adults separately, but the need to engage both in working communication is undeniable. The underlying cause of poor communication between parents and their children is a lack of awareness regarding sexuality (Mwangi 2006).

The culture of silence is reinforced by fear of stigma and other social sanctions. Fear has been found to be the reason HIV-infected persons do not disclose their status. Studies (Ekanem and Gbadegesin 2004; Otive-Igbuzor 2007) have shown that women are inhibited from disclosing their positive sero-status for fear of backlash in the form of annulment of marriage or violence. As a result, researchers have called for incorporating disclosure as an important aspect of HIV/AIDS prevention (Olley et al. 2004). This would change situations such as the one in which only 12% of 141 AIDS widows interviewed at an HIV clinic in Sokoto, Nigeria, knew of their husbands' infection status while they were still alive (Ahmed et al. 2011).

Unqualified criticism of African culture and sexuality

Some scholars squarely blame African culture for the spread of HIV. Early in the epidemic, Caldwell and collaborating authors (1989) came up with an African sexuality thesis that held that African people are permissive and sexuality has never been at the center of their moral concern. In a Euro-centric tone and unrealistic way, these 'scholars' advocated that Africans should emulate the West's model of sexuality. Caldwell et al. made sweeping generalizations about sexuality in Africa, which they assumed was subject to little societal supervision, notwithstanding the presence of norms and values of modern religions such as Christianity. Hence, they anticipated that HIV/AIDS campaigns based on education would bear little fruit. Instead, they recommended using fear to induce behavioral changes, speculating that once behavior is changed, the continent would finally be ready to implement best practices from Europe and Asia that are rooted in religion (Ahlberg 1994; Tamale 2011).

Nyanzi et al. (2008) criticized such attacks against African culture as a major factor in the spread of the epidemic. Their criticism was directed at Caldwell et al. (1989) and allies, whom they dubbed 'Caldwellians', who categorically portrayed African culture as the cause of the HIV epidemic. Specifically, they criticized Caldwellians for lumping all African groups together under the banner of a single, rigid 'African' culture that determines their behavior. The Caldwellian view purports that an ethnic culture exerts tremendous influences on every facet of society – including sexuality, gender norms, and health – but that those social realities have no reciprocal impact on the larger culture (Nyanzi et al. 2008, p. 518; see also Tamale 2011).

Cultural practices pertinent to ritual sex are a good case in point refuting the Caldwellian stance. These practices are not static; they can be changed and adapted in response to the onslaught against them from religion, colonization, and lately from HIV/AIDS prevention campaigns (Nyanzi et al. 2008). Nyanzi et al. (2008) explained that when traditional ritual sex practices become unacceptable in a given community for any reason, members of that community can create symbolic replacements that serve the same purposes. The symbolism is more important in ritual sex than the actual sexual acts. The purpose of ritual sex is to mark certain significant life events, usually but not always between husband and wife. If the ritual is seen as dangerous – as, for example, it may expose one party to HIV/AIDS – the community may settle upon a different symbol that would convey the same meaning (Nyanzi et al. 2008). Changes in these practices illustrate the agency of the local community to adapt to threats and risks without the need for demeaning campaigns from outside that attempt to overhaul their way of life and 'sexual culture.'

Schoepf (1997) also vociferously criticized discourse that grossly put the blame for the upsurge of HIV/AIDS on African culture and tradition (see also Tamale 2011). She concluded, like a growing number of researchers, that Africans are not more promiscuous than other peoples, that behavior found today cannot be considered traditional, and that the major impediments to change did not originate in African cultural traditions. She further emphasized that the most intransigent obstacles to AIDS prevention in Africa – moralizing, stigma, denial, and blame casting – are essentially the same as in the United States. In the context of poverty and inequality, they create numerous risks for women and youth (Schoepf 1997).

Other studies tout the role of local agency and adaptation in reducing the risk of HIV/AIDS. An example comes from a study in Malawi in which Schatz (2005) examined 50 married women, vulnerable because of physiological and structural factors, who took measures to address their vulnerability. These women challenged the assumption that married African women have no agency against HIV/AIDS and can be empowered only by exogenous interventions. They also rejected the widely publicized HIV/AIDS prevention strategies of those exogenous groups that were completely unworkable in their rural setting. When they thought their husbands were engaging in risky practices, these women applied their own interventions, ranging from discussions with their spouses, with or without the mediation of a third party, to ending the relationship if their husbands failed to comply. Such novel indigenous practices need to be nurtured and should be incorporated into prevention programs that are adopted from outside to make them more relevant to particular contexts (Schatz 2005).

The relatively low incidence of infidelity in the Bemba ethnic group in Zambia has been linked to the relatively high status women enjoy in that society, where property is transferred and ancestral descent is traced along maternal lines (Kimuna and Djamba 2005). Although the traditional practice of mediating sexual behavior, marital fidelity in particular, by local cultural norms and gender power dynamics has declined in urban areas due to modernization, industrialization, and commercialism, it remains a possible model for emulation. Kimuna and Djamba (2005) recommend that researchers take a close look at this and other examples where cultural norms effectively mediate sexual behaviors to evaluate their suitability for HIV/AIDS prevention programs.

The studies cited above as well as others show that the Caldwellians' view of homogenizing African culture is oversimplified and unrealistic. As the diverse sub-cultures within Zambia and all other African countries illustrate, the Caldwellian argument of a grandiose African sexuality is uncritical at best and racially biased at worst. Mufune (2003) echoed these sentiments in a study in northern Namibia about changing patterns of sexuality and their significance in the spread of HIV/AIDS. Mufune pointed out the need to critically examine the categorical bashing and marginalization of traditional values and practices with the hope of distinguishing between those that are harmful and those that have potential for inclusion in HIV prevention programs.

Conclusion

This chapter, by examining different perspectives linking HIV/AIDS with tradition, culture, and religion, adds to the literature contextualizing HIV/AIDS in Sub-Saharan Africa. Although researches do not agree about the significance of religion in mediating HIV risk behavior, most studies hold that religiosity, particularly active adoption of a religious lifestyle, tends to restrain premarital sexual initiation. Prevailing counterviews indicate that religiosity does not necessarily indicate abstinence from premarital sex and that the nature and magnitude of the impacts depend largely on the stance of a particular religion toward the use of condoms, which tends to be either resisted or denounced in the major religious systems in Sub-Saharan Africa – Christian, Islamic, and traditional belief systems. Removing condom use from the list of possibilities renders negotiations about prevention strategies difficult for many sexually active young people.

Open dialogue on sexual orientation, especially homosexuality, is socially sanctioned under the influence of religious and moral teaching. Contentions regarding the origin of homosexuality in Africa are similarly value-laden, although little information exists about this topic, largely due to resistance to recognizing the prevalence of homosexuality in many African countries. Most of the discourse is dictated by religion, and leaders want to maintain the status quo. This stand has undermined any interest in understanding the nature and impact of sexual behavior in the spread of HIV, and development of strategies and services for men who have sex with men is bound to fail as long as the issue of homosexuality remains unaddressed.

This chapter examined a number of studies on the role of cultural norms pertaining to gender and sexuality that have bearing on the spread of the virus in Sub-Saharan Africa. Whereas notions of masculinity often involve engagement in premarital or extramarital sex, excessive consumption of alcohol, and the desire for many children, femininity is perceived as sexual passivity and subjugation to male partners that leaves females without sexual bargaining power. These cultural norms and values, together with the low social status of women, make females particularly vulnerable to HIV infection. Some cultural practices, such as early marriage, female genital cutting, abduction, ritual sex, and the belief that sex with a virgin girl cures HIV/AIDS, are integral parts of a male-dominated sex culture that exacerbate vulnerability for girls and women.

Criticism of studies that depict African culture as contributing to the spread of the virus has increased in recent years, largely because such studies fail to appreciate certain cultural norms and values that promote abstinence from premarital sex and fidelity between married couples. This neglect is not simply an oversight, but is due to a combination of continuing attacks by Western churches and scholars on African culture, modernization, and urbanization. Scholars in and outside of the region express strong concern over unqualified and categorical attacks that underestimate the agency of African societies to assess and adapt to changing situations.

Traditional medicine, another common cultural element in Sub-Saharan Africa, constitutes a major segment of medical pluralism that prevails throughout the region and affects HIV risk and health-seeking behavior. There is much evidence suggesting that healers can contribute to HIV prevention efforts and facilitate the referral of AIDS patients to treatment centers if they can be motivated to work within the framework of well-defined and accepted health policies and guidelines (UNAIDS 2000). In countries and communities where traditional medical organizations exist, these efforts may be systematized for possible greater integration of traditional healers into HIV/AIDS prevention programs, an area requiring further study.

References

Addai, I. 2000. Religious affiliation and sexual initiation among Ghanaian women. *Review of Religious Research* 41:328–343.

Ahlberg, B.M. 1994. Is there a distinct African sexuality? A critical response to Caldwell. *Africa* 64:220–242.

Ahmed, M.I., Tukur, M.H., Hundatu, M. et al. 2011. Lack of partner notification among seropositive patients: A serious threat to the success of HIV/AIDS prevention and control in Nigeria. *Abstracts of the International Conference on AIDS and STIs in Africa*, Addis Ababa. Abstract MOPE135.

Ampofo, A., Beoku-Betts, J., Njambi, W. et al. 2004. Women's and gender studies in English-speaking sub-Saharan Africa: A review of research in the social sciences. *Gender and Society* 18:685–714.

Bankole, A., Singh, S. and Woog, V. 2004. *Risk and Protection: Youth and HIV/AIDS in Sub-Saharan Africa*. New York: Alan Guttmacher Institute.

Barton, T.G. 1991. *Sexuality and Health in Sub-Saharan Africa: An Annotated Bibliography*. Nairobi: African Medical and Research Foundation.

Brown, J., Sorrell, J. and Raffaeli, M. 2005. An exploratory study of constructions of masculinity, sexuality and HIV/AIDS in Namibia, Southern Africa. *Culture, Health & Sexuality* 7:585–598.

Caldwell, J., Caldwell, P. and Quiggin, P. 1989. The social context of AIDS in sub-Saharan Africa. *Population and Development Review* 15:185–234.

Daly, J.L. 2001. AIDS in Swaziland: The battle from within. *African Studies Review* 44:21–35.

EECMY. 1999. *HIV/AIDS/STDs Prevention and Control Program-training Manual on HIV/AIDS/STDs Prevention and Control*. Addis Ababa: EECMY.

Ekanem, E. and Gbadegesin, A. 2004. Voluntary counseling and testing (VCT) for human immunodeficiency virus: A study on acceptability by Nigerian women attending antenatal clinics. *African Journal of Reproductive Health/La Revue Africaine de la Santé Reproductive* 8:91–100.

Ezumah, N.N. 2003. Gender issues in the prevention and control of STIs and HIV/AIDS: Lessons from Awka and Agulu, Anambra State, Nigeria. *African Journal of Reproductive Health/La Revue Africaine de la Santé Reproductive* 7:89–99.

Faigle, M. and Koijane, J. 2000. Economic, legal, political and cultural structural changes to support behavior change. *Abstracts of the 13th International Conference on AIDS*. Durban, South Africa. Abstract MoPeE2990. http://gateway.nlm.nih.gov/result_am?query=Faigle&id=102238778&itemnum=1&amhighlight=Yes&amsort=Relevance

Francis-Chizororo, M. and Natshalaga, N.R. 2003. The female condom: Acceptability and perception among rural women in Zimbabwe. *African Journal of Reproductive Health/La Revue Africaine de la Santé Reproductive* 7:101–116.

Garner, R.C. 2000. Safe sects? Dynamic religion and AIDS in South Africa. *Journal of Modern African Studies* 38:41–69.

Gbodossou, E.V.A., Floyd, V. and Fominyen Ngu, E. 2011. Right message, right messengers: Training African traditional healers as information, education and communication (IEC) agents. *Abstracts of the 16th International Conference on AIDS and STIs in Africa*, Addis Ababa. Abstract WEPE144.

Helman, C.G. 2007. *Culture, Health and Illness*, 5th ed. London: Hodder Arnold.

Kaler, A. 2004. The moral lens of population control: Condoms and controversies in southern Malawi. *Studies in Family Planning* 35:105–115.

Kimuna, S.R. and Djamba, Y.K. 2005. Wealth and extramarital sex among men in Zambia. *International Family Planning Perspectives* 31:83–89.

Leclerc-Madlala, S. 2001. Virginity testing: Managing sexuality in a maturing HIV/AIDS epidemic. *Medical Anthropology Quarterly* (New Series) 15:533–552.

Leclerc-Madlala, S. 2002. The mythology of virgin rape. *African Journal on HIV/AIDS* 1:87–95.

Makinwa-Adebusoye, P. and Tiemoko, R. 2007. Introduction: Healthy sexuality: Discourses in east, west, north and southern Africa. In Maticka-Tyndale, E., Tiemoko, R. and Makinwa-Adebusoye, P. (eds.), *Human Sexuality in Africa: Beyond Reproduction*, pp. 1–18. Johannesburg: Action Health Incorporated.

Maticka-Tyndale, E. 2007. Conclusion: Moving sexuality research forward. In Maticka-Tyndale, E., Tiemoko, R. and Makinwa-Adebusoye, P. (eds.), *Human Sexuality in Africa: Beyond Reproduction*, pp. 219–229. Johannesburg: Action Health Incorporated.

Mbulaiteye, S.M., Ruberandwari, A., Nakiyingi, J.S. et al. 2000. Alcohol and HIV: A study among sexually active adults in rural southwest Uganda. *International Journal of Epidemiology* 29:911–915.

Mekbib, T.A., Ferede, A., Tamiru, A. et al. 2011. Development bible: Theology and public health working hand in hand in the Ethiopian Orthodox Church. *Abstracts of the 16th International Conference on AIDS and STIs in Africa*, Addis Ababa. Abstract WEPE104.

Mufune, P. 2003. Changing patterns of sexuality in northern Namibia: Implications for the transmission of HIV/AIDS. *Culture, Health & Sexuality* 5:425–438.

Mwangi, R. 2006. Dialoguing with parents: Critical reflections on the cultural benefits of breaking the silence on issues of sexuality among the Maasai and the Meru people of Kenya. Unpublished.

Niang, C.I., Tapsoba, P., Weiss, E. et al. 2003. 'It's raining stones': Stigma, violence and HIV vulnerability among men who have sex with men in Dakar, Senegal. *Culture, Health & Sexuality* 5:499–512.

Noden, B.H., Gomes, A. and Ferreira, A. 2010. Influence of religious affiliation and education on HIV knowledge and HIV-related sexual behaviors among unmarried youth in central Mozambique. *AIDS Care* 22:1285–1294.

Nyanzi, S., Nassimbwa, J., Kayizzi, V. and Kabanda, S. 2008. 'African sex is dangerous!': Renegotiating 'ritual sex' in contemporary Masaka District. *Africa* 78:518–539.

Odimegwu, C. 2005. Influence of religion on adolescent sexual attitudes and behaviour among Nigerian university students: Affiliation or commitment? *Journal of Reproductive Health/La Revue Africaine de la Santé Reproductive* 9:125–140.

Olley, B.O., Seedat, S. and Stein, D.J. 2004. Self-disclosure of HIV serostatus in recently diagnosed patients with HIV in South Africa. *African Journal of Reproductive Health/La Revue Africaine de la Santé Reproductive* 8:71–76.

Oppong, J.R. and Kalipeni, E. 2004. Perceptions of AIDS in Africa. In Kalipeni, E., Craddock, S., Oppong, J.R. and Ghosh, J. (eds.), *HIV&AIDS in Africa: Beyond Epidemiology*, pp. 47–57. Oxford: Blackwell.

Otive-Igbuzor, E. 2007. Sexuality, violence and HIV/AIDS in Nigeria. In Maticka-Tyndale, E., Tiemoko, R. and Makinwa-Adebusoye, P. (eds.), *Human Sexuality in Africa: Beyond Reproduction*, pp. 199–218. Johannesburg: Action Health Incorporated.

Pelzer, K., Penpid, S. and Masheo, T.-A.B. 2006. *Youth Sexuality in the Context of HIV/AIDS in South Africa*. New York: Nova Science Publishers.

Pew Forum on Religion & Public Life. 2010. *Tolerance and Tension: Islam and Christianity in sub-Saharan Africa*. Washington, DC: Pew Research Center.

Romberg, C. 2001. Sacred sex, secret sex: Discourse and the experience of sexuality among adolescents in Rukungiri District, Southwest Uganda. MA thesis, University of Amsterdam.

Schatz, E. 2005. 'Take your mat and go!': Rural Malawian women's strategies in the HIV/AIDS era. *Culture, Health, and Sexuality* 7:479–492.

Schmid, B. 2007. Sexuality and religion in the time of AIDS. In Maticka-Tyndale, E., Tiemoko, R. and Makinwa-Adebusoye, P. (eds.), *Human Sexuality in Africa: Beyond Reproduction*, pp. 187–198. Johannesburg: Action Health Incorporated.

Schoepf, G.S. 1997. AIDS, gender, and sexuality during Africa's economic crisis. In Mikell, G. (ed.), *African Feminism: The Politics of Survival in Sub-Saharan Africa*, pp. 310–332. Philadelphia: University of Pennsylvania Press.

Smith, D.J. 2004a. Premarital sex, procreation, and HIV risk in Nigeria. *Studies in Family Planning* 35:223–235.

Smith, D.J. 2004b. Youth, sin and sex in Nigeria: Christianity and HIV/AIDS-related beliefs and behaviour among rural-urban migrants. *Culture, Health & Sexuality* 6:425–437.

Surur, F. and Kaba, M. 2000. The role of religious leaders in HIV/AIDS prevention, control, and patient care and support: A pilot project in Jimma Zone. *Northeast African Studies* 7:59–80.

Tadele, G. 2006. *Bleak Prospects: Young Men, Sexuality and HIV/AIDS in an Ethiopian Town.* Research Report 80/2006. Leiden: African Studies Center.

Tadele, G. 2008. Under the cloak of secrecy: Sexuality and HIV/AIDS among men who have sex with men (MSM) in Addis Ababa. Unpublished.

Tamale, S. 2011. Researching and theorizing sexualities in Africa. In Tamale, S. (ed.), *African Sexualities: A Reader,* pp. 11–36. Capetown, Nairobi, Oxford: Pambazuka Press.

Trinitapoli, J. and Regnerus, M.D. 2006. Religion and HIV risk behaviors among married men: Initial results from a study in rural sub-Saharan Africa. *Journal of the Scientific Study of Religion* 45:505–528.

Truter, I. 2007. African traditional healers: Cultural and religious beliefs intertwined in a holistic way. *SA Pharmaceutical Journal* 74(8):56–60.

UNAIDS. 2000. *Collaboration with Traditional Healers in HIV/AIDS Prevention and Care in Sub-Saharan Africa: A Literature Review.* Geneva: UNAIDS. http://data.unaids.org/ Publications/IRC-pub01/JC299-TradHeal_en.pdf.

UNAIDS. 2006. *Collaboration with Traditional Healers for HIV Prevention and Care in sub-Saharan Africa: Suggestions for Program Managers and Field Workers.* Geneva: UNAIDS.

UNAIDS. 2010. *Report on the Global AIDS Epidemic.* Geneva: UNAIDS.

Villanucci, A. 2010. Traditional healers in the context of health care. In Schirripa, P. (ed.), *Health System, Sickness and Social Suffering in Mekelle (Tigray-Ethiopia),* pp. 35–65. London: Transaction Publishers.

Wekwete, N.N. and Madzingira, N. 2008. Adolescent girls' susceptibility and vulnerability to HIV and AIDS: The case of Murehwa District, Zimbabwe. In OSSREA (ed.), *The HIV/AIDS Challenge in Africa, an Impact and Response Assessment: The Case of Zimbabwe,* pp. 111–172, Addis Ababa: OSSREA.

Wickström, A. 2010. Virginity testing as a local public health initiative: A 'preventive ritual' more than a diagnostic measure.' *Journal of the Royal Anthropological Institute* 16:532–550.

Wreford, J. 2009. The pragmatics of knowledge transfer: An HIV/AIDS intervention with traditional health practitioners in South Africa. *Anthropology Southern Africa* 32:37–47.

WHO. 2006. *The World Health Report 2006 – Working Together for Health.* Geneva: WHO.

Useful resources for further reading

Aniekwu, N. 2002. Gender and human rights dimensions of HIV/AIDS in Nigeria. *African Journal of Reproductive Health/La Revue Africaine de la Santé Reproductive* 6:30–37.

Becker, F. 2009. *AIDS and Religious Practice in Africa.* Leiden: Brill.

Feldman, D.A. 2008. *AIDS, Culture, and Africa.* Gainesville: University of Florida Press.

Gaydos, L.M., Smith, A., Hogue, C.J. and Blevins, J. 2010. An emerging field in religion and reproductive health. *Journal of Religion and Health* 49:473–484.

Nguyen, V.-K., Klot, J. and Pirkle, C. 2006. *Culture, HIV & AIDS: An Annotated Bibliography.* New York: Social Science Research Council.

Susser, I. 2009. *AIDS, Sex and Culture.* Chichester: Blackwell.

3
Gender Inequalities, Power Relations, and HIV/AIDS: Exploring the Interface

Ayalew Gebre, Tekalign Ayalew, and Helmut Kloos

Introduction

Although the HIV epidemic affects, directly or indirectly, all segments of the population regardless of age, sex, religion, and socioeconomic status, women are the most affected group in Sub-Saharan Africa and most other parts of the developing world. While slightly more than 50% of all HIV cases world-wide in 2010 were women, up to three times as many women as men aged 15–24 years were infected in Sub-Saharan African countries (UNAIDS 2010). The difference is the result of inequitable gender norms that influence male interactions with females on many issues, including HIV prevention, sexual intercourse, and physical violence (WHO 2007), as described in Chapters 1 and 2. Interventions to promote women's health and control HIV/AIDS and most laws and policies either neglect women's rights or, if they do mention them, are not implemented. This complacency is illustrated by the Protocol to the African Charter on Human and People's Rights on the Right of Women in Africa (the African Women's Protocol), which was adopted by the African Union in 2003. However, only 29 out of 52 countries had signed and ratified the protocol by 2011, and while it provides a strong framework for women's reproductive rights in the African context, it fails to include specific protections for girls and young women as it does for older and disabled women. Even for those countries that adopted the protocol, major hurdles remain in implementing its provisions (Gerntholz et al. 2011).

A global systematic review of 268 qualitative studies published between 1990 and 2004 demonstrated that gender stereotypes and differences in expectations about what is appropriate in sexual behavior of boys were evident in the sexual relations of youth (Marston and King 2006). The fact that progress in meeting Millennium Development Goals 3 (promote gender equality), 5 (reduce maternal mortality), and 6 (combat HIV/AIDS, malaria, and other diseases) lag behind progress in meeting other goals further bears out the failure to protect and promote women's reproductive rights (Gerntholz et al. 2011). According to Watkins (2010), misunderstandings about women and AIDS have impeded HIV prevention programs in Sub-Saharan Africa, an issue further examined in Chapter 8.

The inequitable nature of gender power relations that jeopardizes the rights and welfare of women is the major factor in the relatively greater vulnerability of Sub-Saharan women to HIV (Bah 2005; Foreman 2000; Jato 2002; Mekonnen et al. 2008) in an environment of predominantly heterosexual HIV transmission. Gender inequalities emanating from women's traditional socioeconomic dependence on men are manifested in their limited access to and control over political power and economic resources. The dependence and limitation in rights also affect women's sexual relations with men (ECA 2004; Kidane et al. 2004). The unequal power balance in gender relations that favors men is reflected in the unequal power relations in heterosexual interactions (Jato 2002; Mekonnen et al. 2008). Men usually decide when, how, and where to have sex. As a result, in many Sub-Saharan African countries, women have little power to negotiate safer sex, decide to seek reproductive health services, and insist on their male partners taking HIV-preventive measures (Bah 2005; Foreman 2000; Jato 2002). In addition, various gender norms, values, and assumptions regarding sex and sexuality, coupled with their physiological characteristics, make women more vulnerable than men to HIV infection (Foreman 2000; Njue and Kiragu 2006). From childhood, women and girls in Sub-Saharan Africa are made subservient to the risky sexual behaviors of men in the socialization process prescribed by gender norms, beliefs, and practices (Njue and Kiragu 2006), and these behaviors increase their HIV risk. Male sexual violence against women, another major vulnerability factor, is described in Chapter 2.

Although women are much more vulnerable to HIV than men for the aforementioned reasons, men are also at risk because of various socioeconomic and cultural factors. For example, less educated, younger, poor men living in high-risk neighborhoods are at relatively high risk of infection (Foreman 2000), as are miners and other workers living away from home for extended periods of time. This chapter examines gender-related HIV vulnerability factors in Sub-Saharan Africa with particular emphasis on unequal power relations between men and women. The chapter's objective is to explore the linkages between gender norms, values, and beliefs regarding sexuality and women's vulnerability to HIV infection. The authors assess the implication of women's limited decision-making power in sexual relationships, reproductive health matters, and HIV/AIDS issues. This chapter also examines men's risk of HIV infection and their potential role in more balanced sexual relations with women. Due to the ubiquity of gender issues in the discourse of HIV/AIDS in Africa, these and related themes pervade the discussions in the other chapters.

Conceptual framework

Gender inequalities, caused by women's socioeconomic dependence on men, are reinforced by gender norms, values, and assumptions pertaining to the notions of masculine and feminine behavior that subordinate women to an inferior position and assign men greater power to decide in all gender relations, including sexual matters (Baden and Wach 1998; Jato 2002; Mekonnen et al. 2008). Among the factors constraining women's sexual relations with men and increasing their vulnerability to HIV infection, women's physiology, the traditional role of sex in socialization, women's lower socioeconomic position, societal myths and misconceptions regarding HIV/AIDS, and harmful traditional practices deserve particular attention (Jato 2002; Seeley et al. 2004). These factors are compounded by the failure of various socializing agents to adequately communicate information to women on sexuality, greatly constraining their ability to negotiate and have a voice in when, how, and where to have sex. They heighten women's risk of contracting HIV, causing them to bear the burden of men's high-risk sexual behavior.

The linkages among these factors in women's vulnerability to HIV infection in Sub-Saharan Africa are depicted in Figure 3.1. The illustration is based on studies and hypotheses regarding gender inequalities and power relations offered by several investigators (Foreman 2000; Jato 2002; Mekonnen et al. 2008; Mookodi and Maundeni 2007; Njue and Kiragu 2006).

Although these relationships are primarily grounded in local socioeconomic and cultural contexts, gender-linked vulnerabilities to HIV may also be influenced by the international donor community. The ability of females to protect themselves may be compromised by some restrictive international AIDS funding regulations. For instance, the US President's Emergency Plan for AIDS Relief (PEPFAR), influenced by the American religious right, refused to fund the distribution of condoms and sex education for young people and commercial sex workers (Susser 2009). However, we do not show these influences in Figure 3.1 because PEPFAR has promoted other prevention programs that have, on balance, probably had no systematically negative effect on female HIV risk.

Gender, sex, and women's physiology in vulnerability to HIV infection

Gender is generally defined in terms of socially constructed roles and responsibilities that are assigned to men and women in a given society at a given time (Foreman 2000; Jato 2002). Thus, gender refers to widely shared expectations and norms within a cultural group or society about appropriate male and female behaviors, characteristics, and roles that ascribe to men and women differential access to power and decision-making capacity in

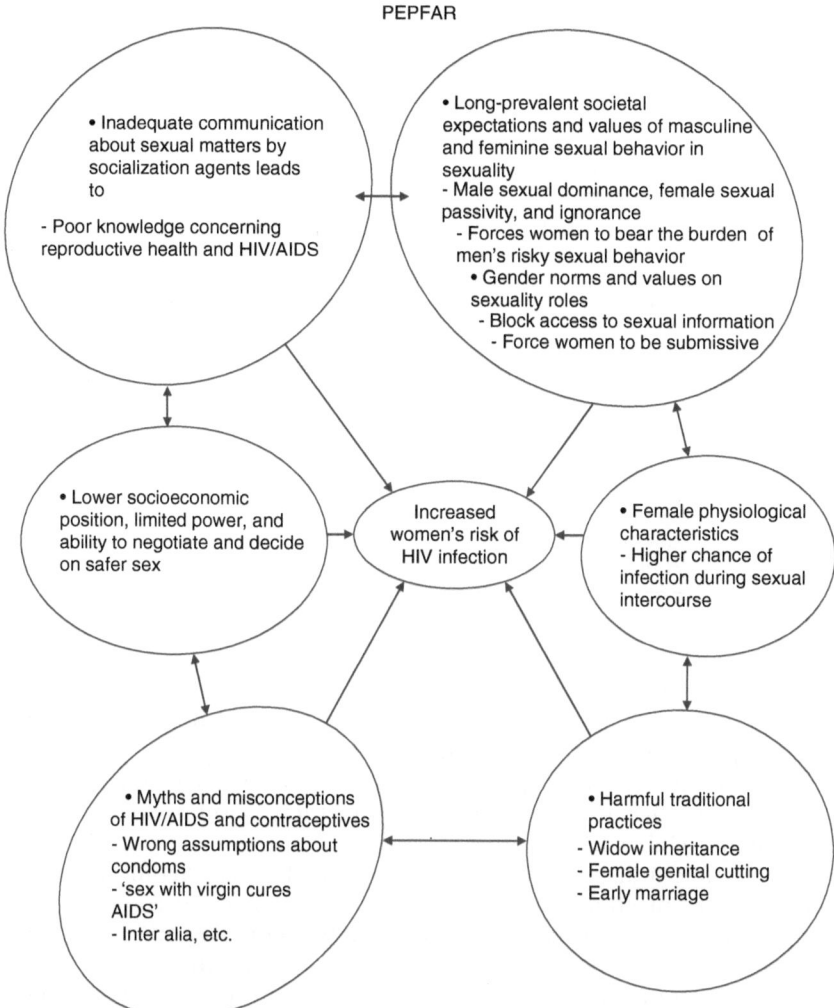

Figure 3.1   Conceptual framework of women's gender-based HIV vulnerability factors

all aspects of life, including production and access to resources (Mekonnen et al. 2008). Hence, the term 'gender' denotes the social creation and shaping of femininity and masculinity rather than the notion that relations between men and women are predestined by nature. Therefore, whereas gender defines the role relations between males and females, sex refers to the biological characteristics and abilities of men and women (Foreman 2000).

Due to women's biological characteristics and sociocultural factors, HIV/AIDS has different implications for the two sexes, particularly in

Table 3.1 HIV prevalence (%) of women and men aged 15–24 years in Sub-Saharan African countries with prevalence rates of 2.5% and above in 2009

Country	Women	Men
Botswana	11.8	5.2
Cameroon	3.9	1.6
Equatorial Guinea	5.0	1.9
Gabon	3.5	1.4
Kenya	4.1	1.8
Lesotho	14.2	5.6
Malawi	6.8	3.1
Mozambique	8.6	3.1
Namibia	5.8	2.3
Nigeria	2.9	1.2
South Africa	13.6	4.5
Swaziland	15.6	6.5
Tanzania	3.9	1.7
Uganda	4.8	2.3
Zambia	8.9	4.2
Zimbabwe	6.9	3.3

Source: UNAIDS (2010, p. 183).

Sub-Saharan African countries (Jato 2002; Mekonnen et al. 2008; UNAIDS 1999). In 2009, infection rates were between two and three times higher in young women than in men in the 15–24 age group in the 16 Sub-Saharan countries with HIV prevalence rates of 2.5% and above. The greatest gender differentials were reported in South Africa, Lesotho, Botswana, and Mozambique (Table 3.1).

The physiological characteristics of women make them significantly more vulnerable to infection than men (Baden and Wach 1998; Foreman 2000; Jato 2002). Several researchers have reported higher biological susceptibility of women to HIV infection than men. One study found that the risk of contracting HIV during intercourse with an infected partner is 11% for men but 20% for women (Baden and Wach 1998). Physiological susceptibility derives from the higher vulnerability of vagina than penis because of the vagina's wider, mucus membrane-lined surface (Foreman 2000). Semen stays in contact with the female genital tract for a longer period (Baden and Wach 1998). Semen typically contains higher concentrations of HIV virus than a woman's vaginal secretions, facilitating the entry of the virus into the female blood stream (Jato 2002). Tearing and bleeding during intercourse, often involving an immature cervix that emits only small amounts of vaginal secretion, further heightens female HIV infection risk. Thus 'rough', 'coercive', and 'dry' sex, as well as rape and female genital cutting, are particularly risky activities.

Gender-based violence is particularly widespread during wars, when mass rapes are perpetrated among refugees and displaced people (Foreman 2000). Apart from wars, rapes are routinely committed against women by familiar persons such as relatives and by strangers. And in a widespread practice in Sub-Saharan Africa, men lure and seduce women into sexual intercourse by offering them financial incentives and other advantages (Foreman 2002). In a study of young women in South Africa, 30% reported that their first sexual intercourse was forced, 71% reported having had sex against their will, but only 11% admitted to having been raped (UNAIDS 1999). The actual statistics are probably higher because of the stigma attached to being raped and the shame that keeps victims from disclosing this information. The need for stronger sexual violence legislation has often been voiced but inadequately acted upon by legislators and legal authorities (Kilonso et al. 2009).

Another factor that increases women's risk of HIV infection is poverty that compels girls to get involved in sexual relations with older men. Older men with financial means sometimes exploit the poverty of young girls in poor communities in Sub-Saharan Africa, paying the girls to engage in casual sex with them. They may do so in the belief that younger girls are not infected with HIV (Foreman 2000). Barker and Rich (1992) reported that older men in Nigeria and Kenya preferred sexual relations with adolescent girls because they were presumed to be virgins uninfected with HIV. This practice greatly raises the risk of infection to the girls, whose immature cervixes and thinner mucus membranes leave them especially vulnerable to the virus during rough sexual intercourse (Jato 2002).

Gender norms and values concerning sexuality and HIV/AIDS

Gender norms, values, assumptions, and practices regarding sexuality affect women's knowledge and ability to make informed decisions in sexual relations. In many societies in Sub-Saharan Africa, community and cultural norms relegate women to an inferior position in relation to men (Deutsch and Saxon 1998; Foreman 2000), increasing their risk of HIV infection (Kidane et al. 2004). Gender norms stipulate what men and women are supposed to know about sex and sexuality, and if the expectation is that women are to know little, the norms limit women's ability to determine their level of risk and acquire the information and means they need to protect themselves from HIV and other STIs (Jato 2002; Kidane et al. 2004). The subordinate position of women in most of Sub-Saharan Africa has its roots in the societal belief that women should have lower status and should not have the right to question or contradict males' risky sexual behaviors (MLHA 2001). In Ethiopia, it is considered a shame for married women to be found infected with HIV and to talk openly about contracting sexually transmitted diseases regardless of who the transmission agent was. Social stigma associated with HIV and resultant failure to disclose its presence are also common in Tanzania, Kenya, Uganda, Botswana, and South Africa (Mekonen 2004; Mekonnen et al. 2008).

Patriarchal societies tend to promote gender norms that subject women to the pressures of men's high-risk sexual behaviors. In many Sub-Saharan African countries, the common belief is that men's sexual desires are instinctive and uncontrollable (Seeley et al. 2004) and men have to express and satisfy their sexual impulses in a variety of ways. Women, on the other hand, are expected not to have or manifest strong sexual desires (Jato 2002). They are required to demonstrate marital fidelity and conform to the rules and norms of monogamy. For women, virtue in sexual matters is equated with passivity, silence, and compliance (Foreman 2000; Mekonnen et al. 2008). Women traditionally had no rights, opportunities, or access to appropriate formal and informal information channels for reproductive health and sexuality matters. This situation is gradually changing, especially in urban areas, where HIV/AIDS services are becoming increasingly available to women.

Gender norms that create unbalanced sexual relations are reinforced by masculine and feminine ideals. In Sub-Saharan Africa, men generally are expected to control women in sexual relations (Jafri 1997; Kidane et al. 2004). Masculine ideals equate virility with sexual prowess, adventure, aggression, control, and dominance in all aspects of sexual relations (Mekonnen et al. 2008). If men fail to live up to the expected sexual norms, their resentment and frustration are usually aggravated by alcohol and drug abuse, causing them to become even more sexually violent and aggressive toward women (Jato 2002). Hence men tend to perpetrate sexual violence and outrage against women (Foreman 2000; Mekonnen et al. 2008). As evidence of their sexual prowess, men are expected to have casual and multiple partners, and their infidelity is often tolerated. It is considered 'natural' for men to practice sex frequently and maintain many sexual partners as a sign of their virility; this expectation drives them to greater risk of HIV infection (Ahlberg 1994; Jato 2002).

These masculine ideals provide men with an excuse to engage in risky sexual activities. Men's superior socioeconomic position gives them the leverage to perpetrate gender-based violence, which takes the forms of sexual coercion and harassment, as well as sexual exploitation, transactional sex, taking multiple partners, and polygamy (Foreman 2000; Jato 2002). By contrast, women are expected to be ignorant, silent, and compliant concerning sex and sexual interactions. The sexual freedom of males and the relatively passive role of women are reflected in the finding that an estimated 60–80% of HIV-positive Sub-Saharan African women have had sexual intercourse solely with their husbands (UNDPI and UNAIDS 2001).

A study of gender inequalities and HIV/AIDS in Zambia (Bah 2005) provides further evidence for the above findings. Bah explored the links between gender inequalities emanating from sociocultural factors and women's vulnerability to HIV/AIDS based on data collected from informants in and around Lusaka. He found that Zambian women had lower positions in politics, economy, and the family sphere. The root causes of this inequality were cultural beliefs and perceptions of marriage and motherhood that confined women to the home, the traditional division of labor between men in production and women in reproduction, and the belief that women cannot be as productive as men. These assumptions and roles denied women access to education and reproductive health services in Zambia (Bah 2005).

Similarly, social norms do not allow married women in Sub-Saharan African countries to express curiosity about or explicitly discuss sexual issues (Jato 2002; Kidane et al. 2004). In the same vein, the ignorance of young girls about sex is viewed as a sign of moral purity, innocence, and chastity (Kidane et al. 2004). As part of the marriage contract, women are supposed to accommodate men's sexual impulses and not refuse sex, safe or otherwise. Worse still, where male sexual pleasure and power are dominant factors, the risks to the female partner are unlikely to be considered (Baden and Wach 1998). Women are expected to let men take sexual initiative and behave in ways that please men. To increase sexual pleasure for men, women in West, Central, and southern Africa administer vaginal stimulants, increasing their own risk of HIV infection. They insert external agents such as herbs, roots, and scouring powders to dry the vaginal passages so as to increase friction during intercourse, which is believed to be more sexually satisfying to males (Jafri 1997; Jato 2002). This practice causes inflammation, lacerations, and abrasions that can boost the opportunity for HIV transmission.

Another issue regarding sexuality that aggravates women's vulnerability to HIV infection in Sub-Saharan Africa is the high value attached to virginity and motherhood, polygamy, and harmful traditional practices related to marriage (Baden and Wach 1998; Foreman 2000; Mesfin 2007). The high value given to motherhood and fertility in particular seriously limits the ability of women to make decisions on matters related to HIV infection. These values are based on the feminine ideal that defines worth and social identity for women in traditional African societies (Mesfin 2007). The high value placed on fertility often conflicts with HIV prevention efforts. Couples who want to have children need to know their HIV status and then plan for mutually acceptable sexual relations and child bearing. This is all the more important as a number of common practices increase women's risk of HIV infection, including depriving widows of inheritances, female genital cutting, sexual cleansing, and early marriage (Baden and Wach 1998; Foreman 2000).

The practice of polygamy grants men authority over their wives, and currently has a broader dimension of allowing men to take as many partners as they wish as a matter of right (Foreman 2000; Kidane et al. 2004). This further reduces women's bargaining power and any measure of influence over the sexual behavior of their partners. In addition, the practice of paying large bride prices rests on the underlying belief that women are the property of men, bought through the marriage transaction. A consequence of this is that men in polygamous marriages feel their ownership of their wives gives them an excuse to inflict sexual violence on them, which adds to women's vulnerability of contracting HIV/AIDS (Jafri 1997; UNAIDS 1999).

The high value placed on virginity in many Sub-Saharan African countries, together with myths and misconceptions surrounding HIV/AIDS, directly and indirectly increases the vulnerability of women (Foreman 2000; Kalinda and Tembo 2010). The virginity of a girl is perceived by her partner, her family, and the community as proof of her innocence, purity, and passivity in sexual matters (Jato 2002). Seeking to preserve their virginity and meet social expectations, girls may engage in alternative forms of intercourse, such as anal sex (Jafri 1997; Thole and Caleb 2011), which carry a high risk of HIV infection (Kloos and Haile Mariam 2007). Anal sex is practiced between unmarried couples in parts of southern Africa as a way of deriving sexual gratification while preventing pregnancy and safeguarding virginity (Jafri 1997).

The temptation to participate in such risky behavior is aggravated by sexual pressure from uninformed peers and pornographic information in print and electronic media, including the Internet (Njue and Kiragu 2006). Due in part to exposure to pornographic material, young girls may consent to 'light sex.' This involves rubbing the penis against the vagina and can result in painful penetration. Young girls who practice light sex tend to believe they are protecting their virginity, but they are ignoring their risk of HIV infection. Semen ejaculated during light sex can expose the girl to HIV infection. Girls practicing light or anal sex are insufficiently informed and rarely seek information on the use of contraceptives. Moreover, the myth that sex with a virgin cures an infected man aggravates the vulnerability of young girls (Jafri 1997; Jato 2002). This discussion illustrates that gender norms, values, beliefs, and practices surrounding sexuality significantly limit women's power and opportunity to make independent decisions and informed choices about matters vital to their reproductive health and well-being.

Gender role socialization in relation to sexuality and HIV/AIDS

Gender-related and largely unbalanced socialization concerning male and female productive and reproductive roles has another set of factors that pose serious risks of HIV infections to women in Sub-Saharan Africa. From childhood, boys and girls grow up internalizing various stereotypes regarding gender roles in productive and reproductive activities (Njue and Kiragu 2006). Parents generally expect boys to become tough, independent, self-reliant, highly educated, ambitious, and hard-working individuals (Mekonnen et al. 2008). They also want boys to control the public sphere and aspire to great achievements in life (Jato 2002). Conversely, parents expect girls to be obedient, kind, attractive, decent, and successful in marriage as ideal wives and mothers (Njue and Kiragu 2006). The belief that girls are not as valuable as boys largely devolves from the socialization process that promotes men as the primary breadwinners and relegates women to a secondary role and dependency status (Foreman 2000).

Njue and Kiragu (2006) carried out research in Kenya and Uganda on gender role socialization pertaining to sexuality. Interviewing 2,332 students aged 9–19 in 31 primary and secondary schools, they found that young boys and girls learn gender roles in productive and reproductive relations mostly from families, teachers, and peer groups. Society expects girls to be obedient, submissive, and virgin before marriage. Boys, on the other hand, are expected to be tough, dominant, and educated. These findings underscored that boys and girls are inadequately informed about sex and sexuality, puberty and adolescence, and associated physiological changes. Due to the lack of information, boys and girls develop misconceptions regarding sex and HIV/AIDS. Among the misconceptions: 'Sex enlarges the breast.' 'HIV is not transmitted through anal sex.' 'Boys enjoy sex more than girls.' 'It is wrong to have a boyfriend or a girlfriend.'

It must be emphasized that gender role socialization in sex and sexuality puts both men and women at increased risks of HIV infection in Sub-Saharan Africa (Foreman 2000; Njue and Kiragu 2006). From childhood, men learn that they are expected to be brave and aggressive, and they are expected to conquer. Attempting to live up to these expectations may result in risky sexual behaviors. Boys are generally socialized with masculine ideals that value action and devalue the expression of emotions (Njue and Kiragu 2006). Matching up to this ideal tends to limit men's use of reproductive health and HIV/AIDS information (Foreman 2000; Jato 2002). The sexual information youngsters obtain from peers lacks appropriate kinds of reproductive health content and instead centers on encouraging and arousing their desires to engage in adventurous and risky sexual activities. As a result, boys often fail to exercise proper care and caution while engaging in sexual activities (Njue and Kiragu 2006). Sex education in schools often does not take into account male reproductive health needs and life skills training that would enable them to properly manage peer pressure (Mookodi and Maundeni 2007).

Women's socioeconomic dependence and HIV/AIDS

The socioeconomic dependence of women on men in the household and in society, although decreased somewhat in a number of sub-Saharan countries in recent years, remains strong, making women vulnerable to HIV and other sexually transmitted infections. Mekonnen et al. (2008) examined the implications of unequal power relations between men and women in Ethiopia. They explored how this factor curtailed women's access to awareness, knowledge, and communication about HIV/AIDS risks and their ability to negotiate for safer sex. The study was carried out among ethnic groups inhabiting densely populated zones in southern Ethiopia. The researchers selected Southern Nations and Nationalities Peoples Republic (SNNPR) due to its ethnic and religious diversity, women's low socioeconomic status, high HIV prevalence, and low level of HIV/AIDS knowledge and awareness. They found that women's lack of power in their socioeconomic and sexual relationships with men increased their vulnerability to HIV/AIDS. Women's powerlessness extremely limited their awareness of the different modes of HIV transmission and of prevention strategies. It also rendered them unable to openly discuss HIV/AIDS issues, negotiate safe sex, and undergo voluntary counseling and testing (VCT).

The researchers also investigated the socio-demographic factors (education, income, employment, religion, place of residence, and marriage) that influence women's power relations with men. They found that women who lived in rural areas were less educated, had no paid work, were usually married, were mostly Moslem, and were highly vulnerable to HIV/AIDS (Mekonnen et al. 2008). These findings suggest that major attitudinal and underlying socioeconomic changes rather than biomedical health interventions will be required to empower women and create a more equitable environment in the domestic and public spheres that may reduce their HIV risk.

Male risks of HIV infection and the role of men in balanced sexual relations

As indicated above, it is vital that men become actively involved in addressing gender issues undermining the socioeconomic status and health of women. But it is also important to note that male needs and constraints in sexual relations influence, to a large extent, their attitudes toward reproductive health. Men may feel threatened and alienated by the current discourse on women empowerment and ongoing efforts centered on the promotion of gender equality. Although women are highly vulnerable to HIV infection because of socioeconomic, cultural, and physiological factors related to sex and sexuality, men are also at risk for similar reasons, and they face additional risks from male-linked activities, such as men having sex with men and illicit drug use (UNAIDS 2010). A number of scholars have identified the involvement of men in promoting gender equality in sexual relations as an essential practical step in curbing the spread of HIV/AIDS. HIV/AIDS programs are increasingly recognizing the need for males to become part of the solution, as they are a major part of the problem (Mookodi and Maundeni 2007; UNAIDS 2011).

Different socioeconomic and cultural factors have made men vulnerable to HIV infection. Mookodi and Maundeni (2007) studied gender and HIV/AIDS in Botswana with particular emphasis on male risk factors. They

collected qualitative data from individual males and in male-based organizations in the Gaborone, Kasane, and Mauntlala areas. The researchers
identified the following as major social factors in male HIV infection risk
in Botswana: the way males learn to become men while growing up, the
way they learn about sex, the relative absence of traditional socialization
agents that prepare young people for adulthood, misconceptions about safer
sex, vulnerability to infection, and inadequate knowledge about HIV/AIDS.
In addition, they pointed out the following as lesser but important social
factors that expose men to HIV infection: peer pressure, boys' relationships
with older women, and reluctance of adults to discuss sexuality issues with
young males (Mookodi and Maundeni 2007).

In most cases, men are not aware of their own sexual behaviors that put
them at risk of HIV infection. An outstanding example of this is the presence of doubts about the reliability of condoms as a preventive measure and
the suspicion that condoms themselves contain or transmit the virus. Other
factors that put men at risk of HIV infection include the possibility of young
boys having sex with older women for the sake of financial and material
advantages, rural-to-urban migration, having multiple partners, drug and
alcohol abuse (Foreman 2000; Jato 2002), and men having sex with men
(UNAIDS 2010).

Mookodi and Maundeni (2007) lamented the fact that research on gender and HIV/AIDS and AIDS prevention programs and strategies have not
adequately incorporated male risk factors. They argued that not all men are
powerful and informed. The extent of men's knowledge and sexual experience varies, largely depending on where they reside, their level of education,
and their age. Certain male groups are not targeted by AIDS programs in
Botswana and other Sub-Saharan African countries: migrants, older men,
young adolescents, prison inmates, men having sex with men, injection
drug users, male children in primary schools, low-income individuals, and
residents of rural areas (Mookodi and Maundeni 2007; UNAIDS 2010).

In the discussion of male risk factors, the role of external agents and
processes should not be underestimated. For example, the global influence
exerted by pornography and the Internet on the sexuality of youngsters,
especially in urban areas, deserves to be mentioned. The potential impact
of socialization agents such as parents, community figures, religious leaders, and schools is great but still largely unexplored in the shaping and
determining of the sexuality of young and adult men.

Some have suggested that men can be involved in at least two ways in
addressing gender inequality and the fight against HIV/AIDS. They can be
targeted for interventions and they can partner with women to make a difference (Foreman 2000; Mookodi and Maundeni 2007). Partnering is about
securing men's acceptance of and support for the needs, choices, and rights
of their female counterparts in sexual relations and reproductive health
issues. Such partnerships also help to promote better understanding of men's

own identity, behaviors, and sexual health needs, as well as the challenges they face (Jato 2002; Mookodi and Maundeni 2007). A comparative review of 40 gender-integrated interventions in reproductive health in Africa and other developing regions reported positive outcomes of all programs. The study identified increased community awareness and dialogue around gender and reproductive health and improved communication between couples as the main outcomes (UNAIDS 2011). Another recently developed perspective on reducing gender power inequity holds that changing gender identities from what Jewkes and Morrell (2010) labelled 'hegemonically masculine men' and submissive, acquiescent women may be key to optimizing the goals of HIV prevention and care.

Conclusion

Researchers are generally in agreement that women in Sub-Saharan Africa are highly vulnerable to HIV because of their limited power to negotiate safe sex with their male partners. The socioeconomic and cultural factors that aggravate women's risk of HIV infection are closely interrelated: women's socioeconomic dependence on men, coupled with male-biased perceptions of masculinity and femininity in sex and sexuality, heightens women's chances of contracting HIV. Women might manage to negotiate safe sex with men in the interest of their reproductive health and well-being if they were socially and economically empowered with greater freedom to make decisions that protect their health. Therefore, a major component of HIV/AIDS prevention and broader socioeconomic development strategies must be the empowerment of women toward gaining greater access to gainful employment opportunities and income sources such as property ownership. As part of this process, gender equality issues need to be mainstreamed in health, education, and other development policy and program agenda to maximize women's involvement in local and national socioeconomic endeavors and to give them a voice in decision making regarding policy.

Similarly disturbing is the fact that women's sexual rights and their right to access reproductive health services are not incorporated in the legal instruments of some Sub-Saharan countries (Gerntholz et al. 2011; Mekonen 2004). The failure of socialization agents such as the family, schools, and religious organizations to keep young people informed about sex and sexuality has left women and young girls in these countries especially uninformed about the risks of HIV infection (see also Chapter 4 in this volume). Inclusion in school curricula of sex education that emphasizes objective information on sex and sexuality and broad life skills training can overcome this information gap. Also worth considering are community sensitization and empowerment programs aimed at redefining gender role socialization in the interest of educating and informing young boys and girls about sex and sexuality issues.

Communities in Sub-Saharan African countries are equally in need of redefining masculine and feminine sexual ideals in a way that promotes mutual responsibility, love, and care between men and women. In this process, important actors such as religious leaders and public officials have an indispensable role to play in the creation of awareness and the transformation of attitudes about gender equality, sexual and reproductive health rights, and balanced male and female power relations.

It should be noted that the failure of research endeavors and policy and program initiatives to adequately incorporate male risk factors for HIV infection and male sexual health needs has contributed to women's vulnerability to HIV infection. In light of this, it is essential that research as well as policy and program practices geared toward women empowerment also take male risk factors into account.

Further research also needs to be carried out on the range of socioeconomic and cultural factors in gender inequality related to HIV/AIDS that exists in different age, religious, and ethnic groups and social classes in Sub-Saharan African countries. Some of the factors that warrant investigation are the cultural diversity and complex nature of the social characteristics, perceptions, and values of gender and sexual roles along ethnolinguistic and cultural lines. Although a good number of studies have been conducted on these issues, most of them represent epidemiological research. Given that the issues under discussion are of a sensitive nature, we recommend that participatory, qualitative research methods be used whenever possible to gain increased understanding and insights on gender inequality and power relations between men and women that may reduce HIV transmission levels and facilitate prevention and treatment programs. This chapter also indicates that a human rights approach ensuring female control over their own body, decision making about their own sexuality, and access to information, education, and health services is a prerequisite to turning the epidemic around in Sub-Saharan Africa. Although a number of international laws clearly specify these and other rights, the road to achieving these goals is long and arduous (Tallis 2002, pp. 9–11).

References

Ahlberg, B.M. 1994. Is there a distinct African sexuality? A critical response to Caldwell. *Africa* 64(2):220–242.

Baden, S. and Wach, H. 1998. Gender, HIV/AIDS transmission and impacts: A review of issues and evidence. Briefing prepared for Swedish International Development Agency (SIDA). Brighton, UK: Institute of Development Studies, University of Sussex.

Bah, I. 2005. Gender inequality and HIV/AIDS in Zambia: A study of the links between gender inequality and women's vulnerability to HIV/AIDS. MA thesis, Department of Political Science, University of Zambia, Lusaka.

Barker, G. and Rich. S. 1992. Influences on adolescent sexuality in Nigeria and Kenya: Findings from focus group discussions. *Studies in Family Planning* 23:199–210.

Deutsch, F.M. and Saxon, S.E. 1998. Traditional ideologies, non-traditional lives. *Sex Roles* 38:331–362.

ECA. 2004. *Gender and HIV/AIDS. Commission on HIV/AIDS and Governance in Africa (CHG). Discussion on Outcomes.* Addis Ababa: Economic Commission for Africa.

Foreman, M. 2000. Masculinity and HIV/AIDS pandemic including gender-based violence. In Africa Development Forum (ed.), *Gender and HIV/AIDS, Report of the UNFPA-sponsored Panel Discussion on Gender and HIV/AIDS,* pp. 3–8. Addis Ababa: African Development Forum.

Gerntholtz, L., Gibbs, A. and Willan, S. 2011. The African Women's protocol: Bringing attention to reproductive rights and the MDGs. *PLoS Medicine* 8(4):e1000429, doi:10.1371/journal.pubmed.1000429.

Jafri, T. 1997. HIV, *Sexuality and Violence against Women.* A report to UNFPA CAST Directors, United Nations Development Fund for Women (UNIFEM). New York: UNIFEM.

Jato, M. 2002. Addressing the gender dimension in HIV/AIDS prevention in sub-Saharan Africa. Paper presented at the Center for Research Training and Information on Women in Development (CERTWID), Addis Ababa University, Addis Ababa.

Jewkes, R. and Morrell, R 2010. Gender and sexuality: Emerging perspectives from the heterosexual epidemic in South Africa and implications for HIV risk and prevention. *Journal of the International AIDS Society* 13:6, doi:10.1186/1756-2652-13-6.

Kalinda, T. and Tembo, R. 2010. Sexual practices and levirate marriages in Mansa District of Zambia. *Electronic Journal of Human Sexuality* 13 March 23, www.ejhs.org.

Kidane, A., Banteyerga, H., Noble, N. and Harada, Y. 2004. Gender and HIV/AIDS in Ethiopia: Focusing on selected woredas in Oromia and SNNPR regions. Miz-Hasab Research Center (MHRC). Sponsored by UNDP. Addis Ababa. Unpublished.

Kilonso, N., Ndung'u, N., Nthamburi, N. et al. 2009. Sexual violence legislation in sub-Saharan Africa: The need for strengthened medico-legal linkages. *Reproductive Health Matters* 17:10–19.

Kloos, H. and Haile Mariam, D. 2007. Some neglected and emerging factors in HIV transmission in Ethiopia. *Ethiopian Medical Journal* 45:103–107.

Marston, C. and King, E. 2006. Factors that shape young people's sexual behaviour: A systematic review. *Lancet* 368:1581–1586.

Mekonen, K. 2004. Women's vulnerability to HIV/AIDS. The need for legislation. IBERCHI. *Annual Journal of Ethiopian Women Lawyers Association* (Addis Ababa) 5:30–45.

Mekonnen, Y., Gugsa Y., Messele, T. et al. 2008. Gender relations and vulnerability regarding HIV/AIDS in Ethiopia: The role of power in relationships on HIV risk awareness and the ability to communicate and negotiate safer sex. In OSSREA (ed.), *The HIV/AIDS Challenge in Africa: An Impact and Response Assessment: The Case of Ethiopia,* pp. 311–353. Addis Ababa: OSSREA.

Mesfin, R. 2007. *The HIV/AIDS Challenge in Africa: An Impact and Response Assessment. Executive Summaries of Findings of Research Projects Carried out in Botswana, Tanzania, Uganda and Zambia.* Addis Ababa: OSSREA.

MLHA. 2001. *Report of the First National Conference on Gender and HIV/AIDS.* Gaborone, Botswana: Ministry of Labor and Home Affairs.

Mookodi, G.B., Maundeni, T., Kapunda, S.M. et al. 2007. Gender and HIV/AIDS: Male risk and male sector interventions in Botswana. In OSSREA (ed.), *The HIV/AIDS*

Challenge in Africa, an Impact and Response Assessment: The Case of Botswana, pp. 1–92, Addis Ababa: OSSREA.

Njue, C. and Kiragu, S. 2006. Gender differences in communication regarding sexual matters: Burdened girls and neglected boys. In Pertet, A. (ed.), *Re-thinking Research and Intervention Approaches that Aim at Preventing HIV Infection among the Youth,* pp. 33–42. Nairobi: Regal Press.

Seely, J., Garilleir, R. and Barnett, T. 2004. Gender and HIV/AIDS impact mitigation in sub-Saharan Africa: Negotiating the constraints. *Journal of Social Aspects of HIV/AIDS* 1:87–98.

Susser, I. 2009. *AIDS, Sex and Culture.* Chichester: Blackwell.

Tallis, V. 2002. *Gender and HIV/AIDS: Overview Report.* Sussex: University of Sussex, Institute of Development Studies.

Thole, K. and Caleb, F. 2011. HIV prevalence in women and girls indulging in anal sex in Malawi. *Abstracts of the International Conference on AIDS and STIs in Africa, Addis Ababa.* Abstract MOAC0104.

UNAIDS. 1999. *Gender and HIV/AIDS: Taking Stock of Research and Programs.* Geneva: Joint United Nations Program on HIV/AIDS.

UNAIDS. 2010. *UNAIDS Report on the Global AIDS Epidemic.* Geneva: UNAIDS.

UNAIDS. 2011. *A Summary Report of New Evidence that Gender Perspectives Improve Reproductive Health Outcomes.* Geneva: UNAIDS.

UNDPI and UNAIDS. 2001. *Fact Sheets: Global Crises, Global Action.* New York: UNDPI and UNAIDS.

Watkins, S.C. 2010. Back to basics: Gender, social norms, and the AIDS epidemic in sub-Saharan Africa. In Sahn, D.E. (ed.), *The Socioeconomic Dimensions of HIV/AIDS in Africa,* pp.134–162. Ithaca, NY: Cornell University Press.

WHO. 2007. *Engaging Men and Boys in Changing Gender-based Inequity in Health: Evidence from Programme Interventions.* Geneva: WHO.

WHO/UNAIDS/UNICEF. 2008. *Fact Sheet on HIV and AIDS: Ethiopia 2008 Update.* Geneva: World Health Organization.

Books, papers, and other resources for further reading

Boesten, J. and Poku, N. 2009. *Gender and HIV/AIDS: Critical Perspectives from the Developing World.* London: Ashgate.

Chant, S. (ed.). 2010. *The International Handbook of Gender and Poverty: Concepts, Research, Policy.* Cheltenham, UK: Edward Elgar Publishing.

Gibbs, A. 2010. Understanding of gender and HIV in the South African media. *AIDS Care* 22(S2):1620–1628.

Hunter, M. 2010. *Love in the Time of AIDS: Inequality, Gender and Rights in South Africa.* Bloomington, IN: Indiana University Press.

Population Council. 2008. *Sexual and Gender Based Violence in Africa: Literature Review.* http://www.popcouncil.org/pdfs/AfricaSGBV-LitReview.pdf

Tallis, V. 2012. *Feminism, HIV and AIDS: Subverting Power, Reducing Vulnerability.* Basingstoke, UK: Palgrave Macmillan.

4
Youth Sexuality and HIV/AIDS: Issues and Contentions

Woldekidan Amde and Getnet Tadele

Introduction

The vulnerability of youth to HIV infection, defined by the United Nations and the World Bank as persons between the ages of 15 and 24 years (World Bank 2011), has been receiving greater attention recently after years of neglect (UNAIDS 2012, pp. 26–28). The fact that nearly half of all new HIV infections worldwide occur in this age group indicates that youth may be central to the dynamics of the epidemic (Edström and Khan 2009). The need for further studies of youth in Sub-Saharan Africa is clearly indicated by their high vulnerability to HIV infection; youth prevalence rates are estimated to average 4.8% in the region but between 10% and 22.1% in the eight most affected eastern and southern African countries. Rates are significantly higher in some national and many local populations due to the relatively wider margins of error for youth than adults in estimated prevalence rates (UNAIDS 2010, p. 183). Studies of the vulnerability of youth are particularly urgent because of the intergenerational reproduction of structural disadvantages and social determinants of HIV vulnerability linked to lack of education, inequality, and orphaning (Edström and Khan 2009). Moreover, a better understanding of the changing knowledge, attitudes, and sexual behavior of youth may significantly contribute to shaping future interventions and coping behaviors in the region.

In spite of recent progress, social science research on youth sexuality and HIV/AIDS has been stifled by the unresolved structure versus agency debate. The debate is waged by two polarized groups: those who focus on agency and those who stress structure in the discussion of causes and solutions. Proponents of agency emphasize the significance of individuals making changes in their lives, and proponents of structure argue that contextual factors dictate individual choices and fate (McAnulla 2002, in Grix 2004). This ontological ambivalence in regard to how social reality is conceived is difficult to address since there is no clear agreement on whether one should dwell on agency or structure. Nonetheless, it is unavoidable that the ontological position dictates subsequent epistemological and methodological positions. While the former tends to adopt positivist perspectives and employ quantitative research methods, the latter adopt an interpretive perspective and use qualitative research methods. Accordingly, the former are criticized for insensitivity to contextual issues, and the latter for dwelling on a few individual cases that lack generalizability (Grix 2004, p. 121).

The two different viewpoints invariably affect studies of youth sexuality and HIV/AIDS; researchers from the two contending parties try to shed light on the sexuality of young people by relying exclusively either on the notion of agency in the form of the 'African sexuality thesis' or the notion of structure that focuses on the broader context in which the youth are located (Tadele 2006). When conceptualizing sexuality, advocates of the agency notion equate sexuality with sexual behavior. The narrowness of this understanding of the concept has led to the belief that reducing risky sexual behavior is a panacea for addressing HIV/AIDS. The agency approach to understanding HIV/AIDS has predominantly prevailed in the biomedical and behavioral approaches to the issue, which have long dominated HIV/AIDS prevention interventions. The biomedical approach promotes the treatment of HIV/AIDS as a medical issue and the behavioral approach assumes that provision of information will effect behavioral change. Consequently, these two approaches led to the development of the ABC strategy. This approach to preventing the sexual transmission of HIV has been broadly defined as abstinence, be faithful and use condoms, although different governments and organizations adopted different versions of the ABC slogan, particularly in regard to condom use (AVERT 2011).

However, there is growing resistance to the biomedical and behavioral approaches that emphasize individual agency. Recent studies demonstrate that HIV/AIDS is not just a medical or a behavioral issue, as it is mediated by social and cultural forces (Toubia 2004, in Tadele 2006; Walakira et al. 2006). The notion of HIV/AIDS as a development challenge is gaining popularity, changing researchers' focus from individual or behavioral matters to structural issues that are believed to be instrumental in mediating exposure to HIV/AIDS (Klein et al. 2002, in Walakira et al. 2006). A burgeoning body of literature highlights aspects of this gap in understanding HIV/AIDS and recognizes the role socioeconomic and cultural contexts play in putting young men and women in Sub-Saharan Africa at risk of HIV infection (Bankole et al. 2004; MOH/HAPCO 2005; Tadele 2006, 2007). However, some of the researchers who emphasize the role of culture in the spread of the virus in Sub-Saharan Africa have been accused of trying to depict culture in the region as being uniform and lacking dynamism (Nyanzi et al. 2008; Tamale 2011). As an example of the influence of the social context, Bankole et al. (2004, p. 9) identified a common challenge in research: male youth tend to overplay their sexual experiences to impress their peers and females cover up their sexual experiences for fear of social sanction. The high societal expectation that girls ought to abstain from sexual activities prior to marriage may explain why girls avoid sharing their premarital sexual experiences with others (Wekwete and Madzingira 2008).

This chapter aims to deepen understanding of a range of issues that address the link between youth sexuality and HIV/AIDS in Sub-Saharan Africa. The issues addressed here cover the ontological and methodological contentions in the field and the significance of cultural notions of masculinity and femininity in the region in putting youth at risk. We examine the link between early marriage and HIV/AIDS vulnerability; the connection between notions of masculinity (multiple sexual partners, polygamy, the desire to father many children, consumption of alcohol) and exposure to HIV/AIDS; and issues of homosexuality among youth and sexual violence involving youth (including boys as victims) as they pertain to HIV/AIDS. Finally, the chapter reviews perceptions of the efficacy of HIV/AIDS interventions, including public education and condom use.

Sexuality and vulnerability of youth to HIV/AIDS

Nearly all persistent inquiries in the gender discourse at the international and national levels exclusively apply the term 'gender' to women and girls; little consideration is given to men and boys. Approaching gender issues, even gender inequity, as female issues rather than societal concerns has long been deemed politically correct. A plethora of initiatives on sexual and reproductive health or against gender-based violence have held on to this outdated conception and to stereotypical notions of gender roles and relationships.

Cognizant of this skewed perspective, some investigators have tried to explore and understand gender and masculinity in the context of Sub-Saharan Africa. They have suggested that gender is a social construct and men and women reinforce existing stereotypes about gender by endorsing them in their daily interactions. They also point to the fluidity and plurality of concepts of manhood, challenging the tendency to view all men as culprits. Many consider a more realistic understanding of manhood, one that dismisses prevailing stereotypes, to be important in formulating public policy (Barker 2005; Silberschmidt 2001).

The one-sided discourse that accepts stereotypes about men and sees women's issues as only the concern of women also pervades programming of HIV interventions. Accordingly, despite several initiatives to empower women and girls, few attempts have been made to involve boys and men in initiatives and campaigns to bring about gender equality or tackle problems such as gender-based violence (see Chapter 3 in this volume). More recently, though, researchers and policy makers are realizing the importance of involving boys and men in bringing about a respect for the rights of women and girls, ensuring the empowerment of women, and enhancing the effectiveness of interventions (Barker 2005; Keeton 2007; Morrell and Jewkes 2011).

Masculinity

Involving males in interventions and changing stereotypical thinking requires an understanding of masculinity in the African context. The concept of masculinity, critical to an understanding of heterosexual relations in Sub-Saharan Africa, has been defined variously by different scholars. According to Connell (2005), masculinity is an aspect of gender that embodies a gamut of behaviors through which men and women interact, which in turn impact on individual and collective sense of being and experience. Researchers are beginning to examine the contribution of men's masculinity and sexuality to the HIV/AIDS epidemic in Sub-Saharan Africa (Lyncha and Visser 2010; Mookodi and Maunden 2007; Oguzane and Morrell 2005; Simpson 2009; Skovdal et al. 2011a, 2011b; Sorrel and Raffaelli 2005; Tadele 2011; Wyrod 2011) and explore possibilities for the formation of new or transformed masculine identities that can eliminate men's harmful and restrictive attitudes and behavior toward women and promote gender equitable practices (Morrell and Jewkes 2011; Silberschmidt 2001; VanKlinken 2011). Interest in these topics has been sparked by extensive literature depicting the repercussions of existing gender inequalities in Sub-Saharan Africa that perpetuate risky sexual practices and thereby contribute to the spread of HIV (Leclerc-Madlala 2001; see also Chapter 3 in this volume).

The culturally constructed perceptions of masculinity affect the behavior of men to a great extent (Brown et al. 2005). According to Waetjen (2004, in Brown et al. 2005), these notions are bound to differ depending on context such as rural or urban setting. However, a number of researchers, working in both rural and urban areas, have concluded that there is a close relationship between masculinity and sexuality. Price and Hawkins (2002, in Brown et al. 2005), for example, had typical findings. In their study, young men in Zambia indicated that being in a sexual relationship made them feel good about themselves and elevated their social status. Wood and Jewkes (2001, in Brown et al. 2005) found that having many sexual partners was an assertion of a boy's transition to manhood in a Xhosa neighborhood in South Africa. Waetjen (2004, in Brown et al. 2005) discovered that the notion of masculinity in Ovambo society in Namibia embraced issues of promiscuity, fathering many children, and drinking alcohol. All of these behaviors can increase vulnerability to HIV/AIDS infection.

Campbell (1997, in Brown et al. 2005) demonstrated that notions of masculinity not only increased risk but also undermined interventions aimed at bringing about behavioral change. Campbell found that the concept of masculinity among mine workers in South Africa was associated with having multiple sexual partners, fathering many children, and engaging in unprotected sex. Such notions of masculinity that embrace promiscuity and fertility fuel the spread of the virus.

Cultural notions of masculinity also embrace consumption of alcohol and other substances that impair decision making in some contexts in Sub-Saharan Africa. Use of these substances increases HIV risk by undermining the use of condoms and other preventive measures, and it contributes to sexual violence and coercion. Substance use is becoming a serious problem in the region because of their increasing availability and use of illicit drugs. Studies from various Sub-Saharan African countries have reported higher HIV risk or prevalence among consumers of alcoholic drinks (Brown and Wechsberg 2010), khat (*Catha edulis*) (Abebe et al. 2005; Beckerleg 2010), cannabis, and methamphetamine (Wechsberg et al. 2008), with early initiation of smoking often serving as a precursor or enhancer of harder drug use (Peltzer 2011). Little is known about HIV risk in youth associated with the recent spread of injection drug use in Sub-Saharan Africa (Beyrer et al. 2010), although the practice has been reported from Kenyan and Tanzanian towns and there is evidence that it is making inroads in Ethiopia as well (Kloos and Haile Mariam 2008). While most users of illicit drugs are young males, a considerable number of females are using substances in some countries, including South Africa (Ramobide 2011; Wechsberg et al. 2008). The dearth of research about the social and contextual factors associated with the use of most substances, including alcohol and cannabis, is impeding the development of interventions. Moreover, structural interventions directed at curbing the production and use of alcohol are difficult to implement because of the preponderance of homemade alcoholic beverages and resistance by the beverage industry (Hahn et al. 2011).

The social pressures of this cultural milieu are particularly strong for adolescents, who are in the developmental stage in which they naturally wrestle with questions of sexuality and identity. In the Sub-Saharan African context, girls are expected by their peers to have boyfriends, and boys are expected to have as many girlfriends as they can to live up to the expectation of being a man. Succumbing to the cultural pressure enables boys to raise their self-esteem and their reputation in society and girls to obtain various material benefits (Varga 1997, in Rutenberg et al. 2003). This scenario partly accounts for the ubiquity of sexual experience. Rutenberg et al. (2003) found among adolescents in a South African community in KwaZulu-Natal, where 38% of unmarried girls between the ages of 15 and 19 and 70% between the ages of 20 and 24 reportedly had at least one sexual partner.

Among sexually active youth, one intervention that would reduce the risk of infection is the use of condoms. However, the use of condoms does not fit well with the notion of masculinity in South Africa (Abdool-Karim et al. 1992, in Brown et al. 2005; Campbell 2003, p. 31). A review of studies of changes in condom use in different Sub-Saharan countries concluded that interventions aimed at increasing condom use among youth achieved limited increases in most cases (Foss et al. 2007). Despite having knowledge about HIV/AIDS and awareness of the value of condoms in preventing it, youth continued their risky sexual activities in their attempt to live up to the culturally prescribed role of masculinity.

Thus concepts of masculinity and expectations of sexual activity deeply rooted in culture impact both vulnerability of youth to HIV/AIDS and prevention and treatment behavior. Brown et al. (2005), reporting on several studies, suggested that researchers investigate how notions of sexuality and gender in Sub-Saharan Africa mediate the preventive behavior of individuals. Waetjen (2004, in Brown et al. 2005) underlined the need to offer alternative notions of masculinity to steer men away from risky practices and provide them with alternative media for expressing their manhood. At the very least, researchers must acknowledge the significance of these concepts for policy and programming.

Vulnerability of married adolescents

Although retaining virginity until marriage has traditionally been the norm in Sub-Saharan Africa, studies of differences in vulnerability to HIV of married and unmarried adolescents have received inadequate attention (Molla et al. 2008). Data obtained from antenatal clinics often indicate higher levels of HIV infection among unmarried female adolescents than their married peers (Kilian et al. 1999, in Clark 2004). However, the use of these data has been criticized because they are not representative of the total female population; the data exclude unmarried adolescents without any sexual experience and focus on sexually active and pregnant adolescents who use little protection (Zaba et al. 2000, in Clark 2004). However, epidemiological studies of HIV prevalence among different categories of adolescents based on marital status also report higher HIV prevalence among girls who have never been married than their married counterparts (Nunn et al. 1994, in Clark 2004). Some unmarried girls may exhibit low prevalence rates because virginity norms tend to delay age of sexual debut and therefore reduce vulnerability to HIV infection among younger rural youth (Molla et al. 2008).

Risk factors

Clark et al. (2006) explored factors contributing to the vulnerability of married women aged 15–19 to HIV/AIDS by analyzing Demographic and Health Survey (DHS) data from 29 countries in Africa and Latin America. Considering that the vast majority of sexually active adolescents in resource-poor countries are married, this study examined the popular perception that young women are safer in wedlock. Results showed certain individual and social factors render married female adolescents prone to HIV infection. Among the significant factors were the widely prevalent unsafe sexual practices of married adolescents; eight out of ten individuals who had unprotected sex during the previous week were married adolescents (Clark et al. 2006).

Another factor in the vulnerability of young married women is early marriage. In Malawi, as in many other Sub-Saharan African countries, parents want their daughters to marry early, partly in the hope that early wedlock will confer protection from HIV/AIDS (Bracher et al. 2003, in Clark 2004). Girls in their early teens are customarily given in marriage to much older men. The age difference increases vulnerability to HIV infection for the girls. A population-based study in Uganda focusing on adolescent women with sexual experience found higher HIV infection rates among 15- to 19-year-olds in wedlock than in their single counterparts, implying that exposure of the women to their infected older spouses was the cause of the infection in the women (Kelly et al. 2003, in Clark 2004). Some of the adolescent girls with sexual experience in a study in Zimbabwe claimed they were put at risk because their partners were not faithful (Wekwete and Madzingira 2008).

The higher risk to females in such asymmetrical unions is particularly acute in cultures that permit polygamy or men having multiple sexual partners. The inability of girls to negotiate safe sex with older husbands increases their risk of infection (Bankole et al. 2004; Clark 2004; MOH/HAPCO 2005). Unfortunately, in societies where verbal communication about sexuality is not allowed, the typical way a woman is able to communicate her desire for faithfulness and monogamy is to forego the use of condoms (Wekwete and Madzingira 2008).

In Kisumu district in Kenya and Ndola district in Zambia, married girls with sexual experience had 50% and 59% higher infection rates, respectively, than their unmarried counterparts (Glynn et al. 2001, in Clark 2004). Clark (2004), using DHS data for these two countries, described some of the behavioral differences between married and unmarried adolescent girls that might explain the difference in vulnerability. Married girls were more likely to be or plan to be pregnant than unmarried girls, particularly right after marriage, due to high societal expectation. Unmarried girls were more likely to engage in sexual activities in exchange for material gifts. On average, two of ten girls in Kenya and four in ten in Zambia traded sex for gifts or money. Clark's study underscores the high risk faced by married female adolescents and the dearth of interventions that address their situation.

Intervention

Clark (2004) decried the fact that existing interventions are not cognizant of the situation of married women, who often are not in a position to use the most popular prevention approaches, including limiting the number of partners, using condoms, or refraining from having sex. Existing HIV prevention strategies, which predominantly focus on the ABC acronym (abstinence, being faithful, and condom use), fail to capture the vulnerability of young women in general and of married women in particular; they do not take full account of the socioeconomic and cultural milieu (Farmer 2003, in Schatz 2005). Schatz (2005), studying strategies adopted by rural Malawian women against HIV infection, asserted that the ABC strategies are not effective in addressing the vulnerability of married women, particularly in a rural context, because women's involvement in intervention is confined, at best, to negotiating, and their negotiations are effective only if their male partners are willing to apply the interventions stringently.

This discussion suggests that HIV prevention programs should target the social structures and collective practices that shape sexual experiences as well as cultural norms, beliefs, and practices. Researchers need to understand the different forms of power that are based on gender, age, class, and religion and examine their impact on HIV/AIDS prevention programs aimed at young people (Holden 2003; Walakira et al. 2006). Clark (2004) stressed the need to revise existing HIV/AIDS policies and strategies and called for a country-specific multipronged approach to reduce vulnerability of married female adolescents, an approach that promotes later marriage and safe sex in marriage. We recommend that future studies about vulnerabilities of unmarried versus married be broadened to include additional categories of couples in sexual relationships such as nonmarried cohabiters, polygamous co-wives (Hattori and Dadoo 2007), and, as indicated above, unmarried girls with and without sexual experience. More detailed categorization will permit better focusing of HIV prevention programs on specific female risk groups.

Education, school attendance, and sexuality

One prevention strategy in the fight against the spread of HIV/AIDS is the promotion of educational opportunities for youth in general and for girls in particular. Participation in education provides adolescents with knowledge about preventive behaviors, delays the age of sexual initiation, and reduces the frequency of sexual experiences. Despite the association between school attendance and reduced vulnerability to HIV/AIDS, in Sub-Saharan Africa only one-fifth of girls and three out of ten boys between the ages of 15 and 19 have attained education above the primary level (Biddlecom et al. 2008).

The 20–30% of students who remain in school learn about the dangers of HIV/AIDS and how to prevent it. According to a national behavioral surveillance survey by the Ethiopian Ministry of Health (MOH/HAPCO 2005) involving 16,253 in-school youth and 1,275 out-of-school youth, awareness about HIV/AIDS and the different modes of prevention was higher among in-school youth than their out-of-school peers (MOH/HAPCO 2005). Tadele (2006) also reported a glaring lack of knowledge regarding HIV/AIDS and its transmission and prevention among Ethiopian male street youth, who relied solely on their peers for information. Similar differences prevailed across gender and males were more knowledgeable of HIV prevention than females (MOH/HAPCO 2005).

Greater knowledge is empowering, which is especially good news for women. Biddlecom et al. (2008) observed that the expansion of modern schooling in Sub-Saharan Africa means that an increasing number of adolescents spend a significant period of their adolescence in school. The school presents a whole new setting for bargaining the timing of first sex, which is a departure from previous generations. The MOH/HAPCO (2005) survey found that the average age of sexual initiation among young people in Ethiopia was 16 years. About 10% of the in-school youth had experienced sex, with the proportion higher among males (14.6%) than females (5.3%).

In a study of HIV/AIDS vulnerability of 538 adolescent girls in Zimbabwe, aged 15–19 years, far more out-of-school girls allegedly had sexual experience than their in-school counterparts (Wekwete and Madzingira 2008). The lower rate of sexual experience among these in-school girls may be due to the tendency of school girls in Sub-Saharan Africa to delay sexual debut (Gupta and Mahy 2003). Furthermore, Wekwete and Madzingira (2008) found lower condom use among out-of-school and older girls. Risk perception was also higher among out-of-school girls than in-school girls, a finding the researchers attributed to the fact that out-of-school girls comprise the bulk of the girls who had sexual experience. Out-of-school girls were more likely to feel that they had some chance of HIV infection than in-school girls. This can be explained by the inverse relationship that exists between school attendance and sexual activity: The majority of the sexually experienced girls were found among girls not attending school (Wekwete and Madzingira 2008). Similarly, Biddlecom et al. (2008) observed an inverse relationship between premarital sex and school attendance. Their summary of empirical data from national surveys of adolescents in 2004 in Burkina Faso, Ghana, Malawi, and Uganda revealed that girls are more likely to quit school if they engage in sex prior to marriage.

Competing concerns: pregnancy or HIV/AIDS?

The body of literature on youth sexuality depicts youth with a subculture of their own that defies conventional norms and values. Different sociocultural factors such as gender mediate the way sexuality is treated. Treatment of sexuality is often characterized by mutual reluctance to discuss the issue or concern that the reputation of the family would be jeopardized (Ramakrishna 2003, in Bukuluki et al. 2006). Reluctance to address the issue among youth has resulted in ineffective interventions. Policy makers have designed prevention strategies without regard for what motivates youth. They have assumed youth are concerned with avoiding HIV/AIDS, and this presumption has dictated program design and allocation of resources. The fact is, however, that young people are more concerned with pregnancy than with disease (Bukuluki et al. 2006). And conventional approaches to HIV/AIDS prevention concentrate on the disease.

Bukuluki et al. (2006) found that youth in Jinja Town (Uganda) practiced sex uninhibited by stringent social or moral constraints. For many girls, pregnancy, not HIV/AIDS, was the main concern. To deal with the contradiction between social expectations and their behavior, the youth in Jinja as well as throughout much of the region tend to keep their sexuality secret. Girls have greater reason than boys for secrecy as becoming pregnant or even revealing that they are sexually active could bring disrepute to their family; therefore, they engage in clandestine sexual activities. The cloak of secrecy surrounding their sexuality prevents girls from benefiting from widely available sexual and reproductive health services, increasing their HIV risk. Their failure to access these services further complicates their situation as they are ambivalent about the subsequent decisions they have to make in the face of social rejection and the disrepute they could bring to their families. The fear of rejection by their community and disgracing their families is the underlying reason girls in high-HIV-prevalence areas are far more concerned about pregnancy than HIV/AIDS (Bukuluki et al. 2006).

The possibility of pregnancy is generally very scary to girls, prompting them to take dangerous routes, such as undergoing unsafe abortions. WHO (2007, cited in Plummer et al. 2008) estimated the prevalence rate of unsafe abortions among women aged 15–44 years in East Africa to be 3%. As a study in Tanzania showed, East African women who have unsafe abortions often take dangerous substances to induce the abortion and consequently experience health complications. The use of traditional medicine to prevent unwanted pregnancy is rife among most of these women (Plummer et al. 2008). Despite the serious consequences, women choose these procedures rather than suffer stigma and rejection from others, including their partners.

On the other hand, some women in some areas want to be pregnant because of cultural pressures to give birth early. At the same time, they know that pregnancy and subsequent motherhood would undermine their academic or occupational aspirations and they also want to avoid becoming infected by HIV. This obviously results in ambivalence. In a study of 1,426 adolescent girls in 110 communities in KwaZulu-Natal, South Africa, a district where HIV is hyper-endemic, Rutenberg et al. (2003) found that growing numbers of female adolescents, increasingly aware of the HIV risk in their community, were considering the risks involved in becoming pregnant and questioning the cultural value of early birth. Despite the ambivalence, women in Sub-Saharan Africa find it difficult to avoid pregnancy, even during the HIV epidemic.

Homosexuality

As discussed in Chapter 2, a sizeable body of literature documents that homosexuality prevails even in the most 'traditional societies' of Sub-Saharan Africa despite denial of its presence (Niang et al. 2003) and despite being criminalized in the majority of the countries in the region (Johnson

2007). Nonetheless, in many countries, the issue is ignored in HIV/AIDS interventions, perpetuating the myth that it does not exist. Any discussion of the issue has a homophobic tone. Tadele (2008, 2010, 2011) explored sexuality and HIV/AIDS among males having sex with males (MSM) in Addis Ababa and found that a growing number of young men engaged in sex with other men. He also observed an increasing number of young MSM sex workers and clients with a high demand for younger boys. The MSM in Tadele's study harbored erroneous conceptions about prevention and transmission of HIV. The most disconcerting finding of the study was that many MSM believe that HIV cannot be transmitted through anal intercourse and therefore do not take any protective measures. Similar perceptions have been reported from other African countries, and many researchers associate these erroneous beliefs with higher HIV prevalence among MSM than in the general population (see Adebajo et al. 2008; Allman et al. 2007; Carter 2008; Johnson 2007).

The implications of denying the existence of homosexuality are staggering. In order to avoid any backlash from society or the state, MSM are secretive about their sexual orientation and often become involved in heterosexual relationships as a strategy for avoiding any suspicion. This behavior has been confirmed by studies showing that 88% of the MSM in Senegal and 69% in Kenya reported having experienced heterosexual relationships (Horizons Program, cited in Johnson 2007). This fact that MSM feel a need for secrecy and deception makes it all the more urgent to recognize and deal with the HIV risk facing not just MSM, but also the heterosexual population; appropriate prevention programs are needed.

In response to the neglect of homosexuality in HIV/AIDS interventions throughout Sub-Saharan Africa, Tadele (2008) urged adoption of a holistic approach that recognizes all risky sexual behavior, including intercourse between individuals of the same sex, and the role of socioeconomic and cultural factors in mediating individuals' sexual behavior. Failure to acknowledge these could undermine progress made thus far in the fight against the pandemic.

Sexual violence

Sexual violence is one of the drivers of HIV/AIDS in Africa, and sexual violence against adolescents is a serious problem (Abrahams et al. 2006; ECSA-HC 2011; Jewkes and Morrell 2010). Wekwete and Madzingira (2008) confirmed the connection between sexual violence and infection in adolescent girls. They examined the vulnerability to HIV/AIDS of 538 girls between the ages of 15 and 19 years in the Murehwa district of Zimbabwe. The research was precipitated by the results of an earlier study showing that even though they constituted the majority of HIV-infected people in the area, adolescents did not consider themselves to be at risk of HIV infection and AIDS. Although only a small proportion (15%) admitted to having had sexual experience, many said they had experienced sex against their will. Thirty percent of the girls with sexual experience claimed they were raped, coerced, or tricked into having sex (Wekwete and Madzingira 2008). In the Behavioral Surveillance Survey in Ethiopia, 15.3% of young females reported that they had been coerced into having their very first sex (MOH/HAPCO 2005), a figure that is probably an underestimate. Tadele (2006) found that gang rape, manipulation, coercion, assault, and verbal threats were common features of young people's sexual relationships and the main concern of street and school girls in a regional town in Ethiopia.

Sexual abuse against male adolescents has not received the attention it merits in Sub-Saharan Africa, where myths and stereotypes surrounding male-to-male sex and masculinity are abundant. The attention sexual abuse of boys has received is underwhelming to the extent that the problem is hardly talked about, it is seldom brought to the attention of law enforcement agencies, and there are few studies focusing on it, all of which reinforce the prevailing misconception that no such problem exists.

Reasons abound for the cloak of secrecy surrounding the sexual abuse of boys in the region: cultural factors such as stereotypes about masculinity and the belief that males cannot be sexually victimized, especially by women. The impact of sexual abuse on boys is underestimated; and if an incidence of abuse is reported, it is not appreciated, or at least not deemed worthy of condemnation. The shadowy nature of the issue is further aggravated by the relative dearth of research on sexual abuse of boys, which allows misperceptions and myths to go unchallenged and leaves many sexually abused boys unattended and unprotected from pedophiles (Watkins and Bentovim 1992).

Contrary to popular perception, the few studies that do exist expose a higher incidence and a darker side of the state of sexual abuse against boys. For instance, a small-scale study in Addis Ababa found that male street children are increasingly targeted for sexual abuse (29% prevalence) (Tadele 2009). The street boys were vulnerable to the sexual abuse, inter alia, due to the culture of secrecy surrounding sexuality in general and homosexuality and pedophilia in particular, the lack of awareness regarding the prevalence and magnitude of the problem, drug abuse, pornography, the precarious nature of street life, the cultural stereotype of denying that men can be victimized, and the absence of legal measures. Sexual abuse of boys is hardly reported, and thus it evades public attention and recognition. Accordingly, victims receive no support and experience a number of negative consequences (Tadele 2009).

The case against conventional HIV/AIDS prevention strategies

Public education regarding HIV/AIDS

Many researchers have drawn attention to the knowledge gap among youth regarding HIV/AIDS and methods of prevention, particularly among young people living in rural areas, and emphasized the need for intervention (MOH/HAPCO 2005). There is a huge lack in the provision of HIV/AIDS related services to youth, including access to condoms. Bankole et al. (2004) observed that most youth in Sub-Saharan Africa lack access to information that could help them practice safe sex or protect themselves from HIV/AIDS. Where the information is available, many young people do not know where or how to access it or they cannot afford to pay any attendant expenses. Although new approaches to HIV prevention have resulted in increasing access to condoms in recent years especially among adults, persisting imbalance between the needs of young people and investment in youth-targeted HIV prevention continues to limit their availability to this age group (UNAIDS 2010, pp. 65, 70).

In a survey examining knowledge about HIV/AIDS and sexual practices among secondary school students in Benin City, Nigeria, Wagbatsoma and Okojie (2006) found a disturbing lack of awareness coupled with risky sexual practices. Although the level of general awareness was high, only 16.2% knew the cause of the disease and the students lacked information about HIV transmission. Students listed kissing HIV-infected persons, living with persons with HIV, and communal use of apparatuses as routes of transmission, demonstrating their lack of proper information about HIV transmission. Only two out of five students mentioned sex as the main mode of transmission. In addition, the adolescents in the survey were reportedly exposed to HIV by using sharp instruments and having their heads shaved regularly at barber shops (Wagbatsoma and Okojie 2006).

On the other hand, some researchers questioned the effectiveness of awareness raising interventions. Knowledge does not always produce the desired action. In situations where the age-old gender inequality issue is not addressed, mere awareness and knowledge of HIV/AIDS usually does not promote behavioral change (Tallis 2000, in Leclerc-Madlala 2001). One reason awareness has not produced behavioral change is the manner in which the information has been presented. Shoveller et al. (2004) identified two issues in intervention approaches that are relevant to youth in their journey to understand their sexuality: the relationship between sex and disease and the degree of openness permitted in discussions about sex. The researchers suggested that the way in which these two issues are treated in educational interventions either antagonizes youth or makes them feel at ease. They argued that treating sex in close relationship with HIV/AIDS irritates youth, as does denying them the opportunity for open discussion about sex. These educational approaches fail to recognize the significance of the social milieu in mediating behavior; instead, they produce anxiety rather than empower young people to better manage their feelings, including sexual feelings.

Alienated partly by these conventional prevention approaches, youth employ different coping strategies. One strategy is avoidance, whereby they shun or remain oblivious to any education dealing with sexuality or HIV/AIDS, and they keep engaging in risky sexual practices with little reservation. This is in sharp contrast to the expectation of educators that provision of information to youth will result in a decrease in their risky sexual behavior. As a case in point, a concentrated public education effort to promote awareness was made in Rakai district, a high prevalence area in Uganda. Contrary to the aims of the education campaign, the adolescents did not appear to be bothered by the issue of HIV/AIDS (Nangendo et al. 2006). Researchers termed their nonchalant attitude toward this serious threat a sense of 'normalization' and linked it with the resignation that nothing can be done about it (Nangendo et al. 2006).

In response to all the fear-inducing messages they receive about HIV/AIDS, young people have developed a variety of coping strategies to lessen their fear and anxiety regarding the virus. Nangendo et al. (2006) grouped the coping strategies the youth employ into different categories: anticipatory coping, demystification, avoidance and denial, behavioral disengagement, and preventive coping. Anticipatory coping involves some of the risky sexual behavior of youth. For instance, they may engage in sex as a means of eking out a living or to infect others as a form of retaliation.

Demystification is a strategy that reduces fear of the pandemic by removing any seriousness from discussions of the issue of HIV/AIDS. One way of doing this is to devise terms that strip the disease of its fearsomeness. Another is to make it a subject of mockery, assigning humorous names to it. Other means of demystification are to equate HIV/AIDS with other curable diseases, or to overplay or fabricate how protective certain practices, such as being circumcised, are in avoiding HIV/AIDS.

Demystification is closely linked with another coping strategy: avoidance and denial. An example of community avoidance occurs when girls are hired in bars under the pretext of waiting on tables but are actually made to attract customers and sleep with them. Once they become infected with HIV or other sexually transmitted agents – as is inevitable – the girls are dismissed so they will not alarm clients. Avoidance and denial are also evident at the individual level. Youth do not avail themselves of opportunities to learn more about HIV/AIDS, or they do not get tested under the guise that the cost of testing is prohibitive or the claim that their lives would change for the worse if they learn their sero-status. The logical companion to avoidance is behavioral disengagement, whereby young people are characterized by inertia despite finding themselves in risky scenarios, and they seem to resort to accepting whatever may come their way.

Youth employ preventive coping to protect themselves against HIV/AIDS; the primary preventive strategy is getting married. Parents frequently arrange for early marriage for their daughters. However, despite being depicted as a safe haven by HIV/AIDS education, marriage gives a false sense of security from HIV. As discussed above, married girls increasingly find it difficult to protect themselves from the virus, as they find it problematic to negotiate the use of condoms and it is common for married people to engage in extramarital relationships. Although these coping strategies in no way reduce the risk of HIV/AIDS, they produce a perception among youth that they are at low risk (Nangendo et al. 2006).

Walakira et al. (2006) reported that young people adopt normalization of HIV/AIDS as a strategy to deal with the anxiety they develop from anti-HIV/AIDS messages and communication that advocate behavioral change and condom use and often arouse fear of the disease. The researchers suggested that educators change their approach and focus on dialogue as a proper and more effective response to the nuances of the context in which the youth find themselves. Nangendo et al. (2006), also concerned about the sense of normalcy among the youth, went further, claiming that public education has failed to instill awareness about sexuality and HIV/AIDS; they recommended moving away from sexual education in public schools toward public health interventions that strategically address evolving notions of vulnerability among this group.

Manuel (2005) was also critical of HIV/AIDS education interventions that adopt a uniform approach in addressing different groups in society. She made a case for recognizing differences among youth in terms of what, in the social milieu, engages and fascinates them, which may depend on whether they go to school or not, whether they live in an urban or a rural area, or what their income level is. Her observations, as well as those of others, illustrate that despite the fact that youth comprise one of the most highly HIV-affected groups, there is a need to appreciate the different categories of youth in regard to their exposure to the virus (see also Tadele 2006). Instead of delivering generic messages, educators and health care workers need to develop more focused programs that address the needs of young people in different age and gender groups, of different socioeconomic statuses, in different geographic locations and of different HIV statuses (Mekonnen et al. 2011).

Contextual factors that impede condom use among youth

The level of condom use remains low among youth in Sub-Saharan Africa. Condom use in the region differs across countries, with higher use reported in Central and West Africa and lower use in eastern and southern Africa (Bankole et al. 2004). As many studies show, a number of factors, including age, sex, gender, and income, are associated with rates of condom use among young people. One reality that undermines condom use is the male–female power imbalance and resulting inability of young women to negotiate safer sex with their older partners. Young people believe it is important that both partners agree on using condoms, but consensus is difficult when there are differences in age, socioeconomic status, power, perception about protection, or trust (Walakira et al. 2006).

Data for 24 Sub-Saharan African countries show the proportion of young people using condoms during last intercourse to be far smaller than the proportion of those who claim to have the experience of using condoms. Condom use is more popular among unmarried teenagers who are engaged in sexual activity than married couples. There is a stark difference in the reported rates of condom use among young men and women, with far higher proportions of young men reporting to have used condoms (Bankole et al. 2004). Researchers examining HIV/AIDS vulnerability of girls between the ages of 15 and 19 in Zimbabwe's Murehwa district found that two out of five (39.0%) of the sexually active adolescent girls admitted that they had not used condoms as protection from HIV or STIs. This finding illustrates that the girls were either unable to demand safer sex or were giving in to the common perception that abdicating the use of condoms is an expression of trust toward a partner (Wekwete and Madzingira 2008).

While the majority of adolescent girls in the Zimbabwe study had a positive attitude toward the use of condoms, distinct differences in the way condom use was perceived were found among different groups. A higher proportion of sexually inexperienced girls than sexually experienced girls embraced the use of condoms, which the authors partly attributed to the inability of the latter to effectively negotiate their use. The study also found that older girls were less positive about the use of condoms than their younger peers. The implications of sexually active adolescent girls not eager to use condom is unsettling (Wekwete and Madzingira 2008).

Subjective perceptions and interpretations about proposing condom use during sex tend to stifle actual use. In a relationship, using condoms can be considered a sign of distrust or infidelity, as noted among youth in Uganda. Walakira et al. (2006) found the inclination of the Ugandan youth to quit using condoms when they felt they were in real or trusting relationships to be the main factor that impeded their use. The authors traced the perception that using condoms is irrelevant when one is in a trusting relationship to previous HIV/AIDS awareness raising campaigns in Mozambique that gave the impression that the use of condoms should be confined to passing sexual relationships. Other factors that inhibit the use of condoms are gender disparity and lack of capacity of girls to negotiate condom use (Manuel 2005).

Varga (1997) investigated the symbolism associated with the use of condoms and factors that mediate their use among 100 female commercial sex workers in South Africa. The researcher identified several factors influencing the use of condoms. For example, financial concerns and other impediments could hamper negotiation for condom use with clients. On the other hand, the use of condoms with partners is undermined, regardless of awareness about HIV/AIDS, by all the derogatory connotations connected with their use, namely promiscuity, sickness, suspicion, and lewdness (Varga 1997).

Walakira et al. (2006) observed that normalization is a barrier to condom use whereby out-of-school youth, without undergoing HIV testing, are often resigned to the belief either that they are infected or that there is nothing they can do to prevent infection. Hence, many young people may be devoid of motivation to use condoms. The researchers identified other barriers: among men, the strong desire for condom-less sex; among women the pressure to give birth. Misinformation and misperceptions regarding reliability of condoms and their impact on sexual gratification also impede consistent condom use. Incidents such as the ban in Uganda against distribution of a particular brand of condom that did not meet quality standards reinforce beliefs about the unreliability of condoms and nurture a sense that risk and risky behavior are normal (Wendo and Nakaayi 2004, in Walakira et al. 2006). Some youth are reluctant to use condoms because they dislike their smell or their size (Walakira et al. 2006). Some adolescent girls are ashamed to use condoms or find them difficult to use (Wekwete and Madzingira 2008). Most southern African countries have launched innovative approaches to address negative perceptions toward condoms and are increasing their accessibility through the use of media and community spots such as barbers.

Relatively little information is available on the use of female condoms by youth, although they have been marketed in pilot projects in Sub-Saharan Africa since 1996 to provide women with more independent protection from HIV and STIs and as a contraceptive. Although sex workers accepted female condoms, the larger population of married couples and men in general did not (Deniaud 1997). The distribution of female condoms began increasing in the 1990s, and in 2009, 36.2 million female condoms were dispersed throughout Sub-Saharan Africa (UNAIDS 2009), but no information is available on their use by youth or other population groups. A study of 74 male students in South Africa showed that males considered it their responsibility to have male condoms; very few had ever used female condoms (Mantell et al. 2011).

In light of their complacency toward HIV/AIDS prevention, youth are often considered rebellious or stubborn. However, Walakira et al. (2006) suggested the issue is not stubbornness, but the inadequacy of intervention initiatives to make a difference in the behavior of young people. And sometimes the initiatives have the opposite effect from what is intended: the youth normalize the pandemic and pay little heed to the information they receive. Walakira et al. called for replacing approaches that focus exclusively on individual behavior with comprehensive measures that take account of aspects of the young people's social environment including perceptions regarding sexual relations and socioeconomic status, which determine whether the youth use condoms.

Conclusion

In this chapter we attempted to broaden understanding of issues concerning the relationship between youth sexuality and HIV/AIDS in Sub-Saharan Africa. Literature on the topic is fragmented, owing much to ontological and methodological differences in the way researchers approach the issue. This complicates efforts to compare results. For a long time, research in the region was in the behavioral and epidemiological traditions. Increasingly studies are addressing the structural barriers that hamper individuals from applying their knowledge to prevent HIV/AIDS. This trend has prompted studies on the significance of notions of masculinity and femininity in the vulnerability to HIV infection.

The practice of early marriage exposes female adolescents to HIV risk, as they often marry older men with a history of multiple sexual partners. Girls often lack the skills and are culturally inhibited from negotiating safe sex, and there are negative meanings attached to the use of condoms, such as notions of infidelity and mistrust.

Homosexuality is criminalized in many Sub-Saharan countries and the topic is off limits for discussion in the region, despite research confirming its wide prevalence and the risky sexual behavior among MSM, who often erroneously think that sex with other men is safe. MSM often engage in heterosexual relationships to disguise their sexual orientation. This disconcerting scenario was highlighted in some of the literature reviewed here, and researchers have called for recognition of the role of homosexuality in the spread of HIV and urged the provision of HIV/AIDS-related services to MSM, services that are acutely lacking in the region. The homophobic social milieu has also undermined visibility of the problem of sexually abused boys and men. Considering that discussion of homosexuality and sexual abuse against boys and men is taboo in Sub-Saharan Africa, their presence and extent poorly documented, and epidemiological impact not well understood, it is imperative to support research in this direction.

References

Abebe, D., Debella, A., Dejene, A. et al. 2005. Khat chewing habit as a possible risk behaviour for HIV infection: A case-control study. *Ethiopian Journal of Health Development* 19:174–181.

Abrahams, N., Jewkes, R., Laubscher, R. and Hoffman, M. 2006. Intimate partner violence: Prevalence and risk factors for men in Cape Town, South Africa. *Violence and Victims* 21(2):247–264.

Adebajo, S. et al. 2008. Men, Sexuality and HIV/AIDS in the context of HIV/AIDS in Nigeria. Paper presented at the Africa Regional Sexuality Resource Centre Seminar Series (ARSRC), Lagos, Nigeria.

Allman, D., Adebajo, S., Myers, T. et al. 2007. Challenges for the sexual health and social acceptance of men who have sex with men in Nigeria. *Culture, Health and Sexuality* 9:153–168.

AVERT. 2011. *The ABC of HIV Prevention*. htpp://www.avert.org/abc-hiv.htm

Bankole, A., Woog, V., Singh, S. and Wulf, D. 2004. *Risk and Protection: Youth and HIV/AIDS in Sub-Saharan Africa*. New York: Alan Guttmacher Institute.

Barker, G. 2005. Engaging boys and young men in promoting gender equality: Reflections on masculinities in Sub-Saharan Africa and program responses. Background paper for the first Pan African Seminar on Working with Boys and Young Men to Address Gender-based Violence and HIV/AIDS, May 15–16, Addis Ababa.

Beckerleg, S. 2010. East African discourses on khat and sex. *Journal of Ethnopharmacology* 132:600–606.

Beyrer, C., Wirtz, A.L., Baral, S. et al. 2010. Epidemiological links between drug use and HIV epidemic: An international perspective. *Journal of Acquired Immune Deficiency Syndromes* 55(Suppl. 1):S10–S16.

Biddlecom, A., Gregory, R., Lloyd, C.B. and Mensch, B.S. 2008. Associations between premarital sex and leaving school in four sub-Saharan African countries. *Studies in Family Planning* 39:337–350.

Brown, F.A. and Wechsberg, W.M. 2010. The intersecting risk of substance abuse and HIV risk among substance-using South African men and women. *Current Opinion in Psychiatry* 23:205–209.

Brown, J., Sorrell, J. and Raffaelli, M. 2005. An exploratory study of constructions of masculinity, sexuality and HIV/AIDS in Namibia, Southern Africa. *Culture, Health & Sexuality* 7:585–598.

Bukuluki, P., Walakira, E. and Muasya, I. 2006. Implications of the research findings for policy development. In Pertet, A.M. (ed.), *Re-thinking Research and Intervention Approaches that Aim at Preventing HIV Infection among the Youth*, pp. 91–102. Nairobi: Regal Press Kenya.

Campbell, C. 2003. *'Letting them Die': Why HIV/AIDS Prevention Programmes Fail*. Oxford: International African Institute in association with James Currey.

Carter, M. 2008. Activists arrested during attempt to highlight Uganda's neglect of HIV prevention for men who have sex with men. Aidsmap news. http://www.aidsmap.com/en/news/15781220-1B04-45C5-A68F-04AF86CD94BE.asp

Clark, S. 2004. Early marriage and HIV risks in Sub-Saharan Africa. *Studies in Family Planning* 35:149–160.

Clark, S., Bruce, J. and Dude, A. 2006. Protecting young women from HIV/AIDS: The case against child and adolescent marriage source. *International Family Planning Perspectives* 32:79–88.

Connell, R.W. 2005. *Masculinities* (2nd edition). London: Polity Press.

Deniaud, F. 1997. Current status of the female condom in Africa (in French). *Santé* 7:405–415.

ECSA-HC (East, Central and Southern African Health Community). 2011. *Child Sexual Abuse in Sub-Saharan Africa: A Review of the Literature*. Arusha, Tanzania: ECSA-HC.

Edström, J. and Khan, N. 2009. Perspectives on intergenerational vulnerability for adolescents affected by HIV: An argument for voice and visibility. *IDS Bulletin* 40:41–50.

Foss, A.M., Hossain, M., Vickerman, P.T. and Watts, C.H. 2007. A systematic review of published evidence on intervention impact on condom use in sub-Saharan Africa. *Sexually Transmitted Infections* 83:510–516.

Grix, J. 2004. *Foundations of Research*. Basingstock, UK: Palgrave Macmillan.

Gupta, N. and Mahy, M. 2003. Sexual initiation among adolescent girls and boys: Trends and differentials in sub-Saharan Africa. *Archives of Sexual Behavior* 32: 41–53.

Hahn, J.A., Woolf-King, S.E. and Muyindike, W. 2011. Adding fuel to the fire: Alcohol's effect on the HIV epidemic in sub-Saharan Africa. *Current HIV/AIDS Report* 8:172–180.

Hattori, M.K. and Dadoo, F.N. 2007. Cohabitation, marriage, and 'sexual monogamy' in Nairobi's slums. *Social Science and Medicine* 64:1067–1078.

Holden, S. 2003. *AIDS on the Agenda: Adapting Development and Humanitarian Programmes to Meet the Challenge of HIV.* Oxford: Oxfam.

Jewkes, R. and Morrell, R. 2010. Gender and sexuality: Emerging perspectives from the heterosexual epidemic in South Africa and implications for HIV risk and prevention. *Journal of the International AIDS Society* 13:6.

Johnson, C.A. 2007. *Off the Map: How HIV/AIDS Programming Is Failing Same-sex Practicing People in Africa.* New York: International Gay and Lesbian Human Rights Commission.

Keeton, C. 2007. Changing men's behavior can improve women's health. *Bulletin of the World Health Organization* 85:505–506.

Kloos, H. and Haile Mariam, D. 2008. Some neglected and emerging factors in HIV transmission in Ethiopia. *Ethiopian Medical Journal* 45:103–107.

Leclerc-Madlala, S. 2001. Virginity testing: Managing sexuality in a maturing HIV/AIDS epidemic. *Medical Anthropology Quarterly*, New Series 15:533–552.

Lyncha, I., Brouard, P.W. and Visser, M.J. 2010. Constructions of masculinity among a group of South African men living with HIV/AIDS: reflections on resistance and change. *Culture, Health & Sexuality* 12:15–27.

Mantell, J.E., Smit, J.A., Beksinska, M. et al. 2011. Everywhere you go, everyone is saying condom, condom. But are they being used consistently? Reflections of South African male students about male and female condoms. *Health Education Research* 26:859–871.

Manuel, S. 2005. Obstacles to condom use among secondary school students in Maputo City, Mozambique. *Culture, Health & Sexuality* 3:293–302.

Mekonnen, T., Getachew, T. and Abera, M. 2011. Youth reproductive health services (VCT, STI and FP) utilization and service preference in Fantale Woreda, East Shoa Zone 2009. International Conference on AIDS and STIs in Africa, Addis Ababa, December 4–6. Abstract MOAD0104.

MOH/HAPCO. 2005. *HIV/AIDS Behavioral Surveillance Survey (BSS) Ethiopia 2005. Round Two.* http://www.etharc.org/resources/download/finish/33/50

Molla, M., Berhane, Y. and Lindtjorn, B. 2008. Traditional values of virginity and sexual behaviour in rural Ethiopian youth: Results from a cross-sectional study. *BMC Public Health* 8:9.

Mookodi, G.B. and Maunden, T. 2007. Gender and HIV/AIDS: Male risk and male sector interventions in Botswana. In OSSREA (ed.), *The HIV/AIDS Challenge in Africa, an Impact and Response Assessment: The Case of Botswana*, 1–92, Addis Ababa: OSSREA.

Morrell, R. and Jewkes, R. 2011. Carework and caring: A path to gender equitable practices among men in South Africa. *International Journal of Equity in Health* 9:17.

Nangendo, F. et al. 2006. Coping by normalizing: Implications for HIV and AIDS prevention in young people from the Rakai District, Uganda. In Pertet, A.M. (ed.), *Re-Thinking Research and Research and Intervention Approaches that Aim at Preventing HIV Infection among Youth*, pp. 81–90. Nairobi: SOMA-Net.

Niang, C.I., Tapsoba, P., Weiss, E. et al. 2003. 'It's raining stones': Stigma, violence and HIV vulnerability among men who have sex with men in Dakar, Senegal. *Culture, Health & Sexuality* 5:499–512.

Nyanzi, S., Nassimbwa, J., Kayizzi, V. and Kabanda, S. 2008. 'African sex is dangerous!' Renegotiating 'ritual sex' in contemporary Masaka District. *Africa* 78:518–538.

Oguzane, L. and Morell, R. (eds.). 2005. *African Masculinities: Men in Africa from the Late Nineteenth Century to the Present.* Durban: UKZN Press.

Peltzer, K. 2011. Early smoking and associated factors among in-school male and female adolescents in seven African countries. *African Health Science* 11:320–328.

Plummer, M.L., Wamoyi, J., Nyalali, K. et al. 2008. Aborting and suspending pregnancy in rural Tanzania: An ethnography of young people's beliefs and practices. *Studies in Family Planning* 39:281–292.

Ramobide, D. 2011. *Substance Abuse in South Africa. Central Drug Authority Briefing, 6 September 2011.* Parliamentary Monitoring Group. http://www.pmg.org.za.

Rutenberg, N., Kaufman, C.E., Macintyre, K. et al. 2003. Pregnant or positive: Adolescent childbearing and HIV risk in KwaZulu Natal, South Africa. *Reproductive Health Matters* 11(22):122–133.

Schatz, E. 2005. Take your mat and go! Rural Malawian women's strategies in the HIV/AIDS era. *Culture, Health, and Sexuality* 7:479–492.

Shoveller, J.A., Johnson, J.L., Langille, B.D. et al. 2004. Socio-cultural influences on young people's sexual development. *Social Science and Medicine* 59:473–487.

Silberschmidt, M. 2001. Changing gender roles and male disempowerment in rural and urban East Africa: A neglected dimension in the study of sexual and reproductive behaviour in East Africa. *Aidsnet Newsletter* (Danish NGO Network on AIDS and Development) No. 10.

Simpson, A.J. 2009. *Boys to Men in the Shadow of AIDS: Masculinities and HIV/AIDS Risk in Zambia.* New York: Macmillan.

Skovdal, M., Campbell, C., Madanhire, C. et al. 2011a. Masculinity as a barrier to men's use of HIV services in Zimbabwe. *Globalization and Health* 7:13.

Skovdal, M., Campbell C., Nyamukapa, C. and Gregson S. 2011b. When masculinity interferes with women's treatment of HIV infection: A qualitative study about adherence to antiretroviral therapy in Zimbabwe. *Journal of the International AIDS Society* 14:29.

Sorrel, J.B.J. and Raffaelli, M. 2005. An exploratory study of constructions of masculinity, sexuality and HIV/AIDS in Namibia, Southern Africa. *Culture, Health & Sexuality* 7:585–598.

Tadele, G. 2006. *Bleak Prospects: Young Men, Sexuality and HIV/AIDS in an Ethiopian Town.* Research Report 80/2006. Leiden: African Studies Centre.

Tadele, G. 2007. Male street youths and the HIV/AIDS pandemic in Dessie, Ethiopia: What are their rights? Who cares for them? And where is their citizenship? Unpublished.

Tadele G. 2008. Under the cloak of secrecy: Sexuality and HIV/AIDS among men who have sex with men (MSM) in Addis Ababa. Unpublished.

Tadele, G. 2009. Unrecognized victims: Sexual abuse against male street children in Merkato area, Addis Ababa. *Ethiopian Journal of Health Development* 23:174–182.

Tadele, G. 2010. Boundaries of sexual safety: Men who have sex with men (MSM) and HIV/AIDS in Addis Ababa. *Journal of HIV/AIDS and Social Services* 9:261–280.

Tadele, G. 2011. Hetronormativity and 'troubled' masculinities among men who have sex with men (MSM) in Addis Ababa. *Culture, Health & Sexuality* 13:457–469.

Tamale, S. 2011. Researching and theorizing sexualities in Africa. In Tamale, S. 2011 (ed.), *African Sexualities: A Reader*, pp. 11–36. Capetown, Nairobi, Oxford: Pambazuka Press.

UNAIDS. 2009. Annual Report 2009. http://data.unaids.org/pub/Report/2010/2009_annual_report_en.pdf

UNAIDS. 2010. *Report on the Global AIDS Epidemic.* Geneva: UNAIDS.

UNAIDS, 2012. *Together We Will End AIDS.* Geneva: UNAIDS.

VanKlinken, A. 2011. The need for circumcised men: The quest for transformed masculinities in African Christianity in the context of the HIV epidemic. PhD thesis, Utrecht University.

Varga, C.A. 1997. The condom conundrum: Barriers to condom use among commercial sex workers in Durban, South Africa. *African Journal of Reproductive Health/La Revue Africaine de la Santé Reproductive* 1:74–88.

Wagbatsoma, V.A. and Okojie, O.H. 2006. Knowledge of HIV/AIDS and sexual practices among adolescents in Benin City, Nigeria. *African Journal of Reproductive Health* 10:76–83.

Walakira, E., Bukuluki, P., Sengendo, J. and Mugumya, F. 2006. The untapped knowledge in condom promotion: A case of young people in Uganda. In Pertet, A.M. (ed.), *Re-Thinking Research and Research and Intervention Approaches that Aim at Preventing HIV Infection among the Youth*, pp. 73–80. Nairobi: SOMA-Net.

Watkins, B. and Bentovim, A. 1992. The sexual abuse of male children and adolescents: A review of current research. *Journal of Clinical Psychology & Psychiatry* 33:197–248.

Wechsberg, W.M., Luseno, W., Rieman, K. et al. 2008. Substance abuse and sexual risk within the context of gender inequality in South Africa. *Substance Use and Misuse* 43:1186–1201.

Wekwete, N. and Madzingira, N. 2008. Adolescent girls' susceptibility and vulnerability to HIV and AIDS: The case of Murehwa District, Zimbabwe. In OSSREA (ed.), *The HIV/AIDS Challenge in Africa, an Impact and Response Assessment: The Case of Zimbabwe*, pp. 111–172, Addis Ababa: OSSREA.

World Bank. 2011. *Children and Youth: Who Are Youth?* http://go.worldbank.org/2ESS9SO270

Wyrod, R. 2011. Masculinity and the persistence of AIDS stigma. *Culture, Health and Sexuality* 13:443–456.

Books, papers, websites, and other resources for further reading

Appleton, P. and Parker, R. (eds.). 2010. *Routledge Handbook of Sexuality, Health and Rights.* London: Routledge.

Children Affected by AIDS Electronic Discussion Forum, hosted by USAID and the Synergy Project: http://www.syngergyaids.com

Handa S., Devereux S. and Webb, D. (eds.). 2008. *Social Protection for Africa's Children.* London: Routledge.

Lalor, K. 2004. Child sexual abuse in sub-Saharan Africa: A literature review. *Child Abuse and Neglect* 28:439–460.

Marston, C. and King E. 2006. Factors that shape young people's sexual behaviour: A systematic review. *Lancet* 368:1581–1586.

McGrath, N., Nyirenda, M., Hosegood, V. and Newell, M.-L. 2009. Age at first sex in rural South Africa. *Sexually Transmitted Infections* 85(Suppl. 1):i49–i55.

UNAIDS' resources about young people aged 15–24: http://www.unaids.org/young people/index.html

UNICEF's Voices of Youth. http://www.unicef.org.voy/explore/aids/explore_aids.php

5

Food Insecurity, Poverty, and HIV/AIDS

Ayalew Gebre, Sebsib Belay, and Helmut Kloos

Introduction

Most socioeconomic studies of HIV/AIDS in Sub-Saharan Africa have emphasized impacts and responses, particularly regarding issues surrounding household welfare, broad socioeconomic consequences, and social responses (Bukusi 2008; Kapunda 2005; Muiruri 2008; Nuwagaba 2005; Pankhurst et al. 2008). A number of studies have examined the interfaces between food insecurity, poverty, and HIV/AIDS (see for example Crush et al. 2011; d'Adesky 2007; Gillespie 2008; Ogunbayo 2004; Oxfam-International and Save the Children-UK 2002; Russell 2005; UNAIDS 2008; USAID and PEPFAR 2007; Weiser et al. 2007). Most of the studies have failed to consider different agricultural, socioeconomic, and cultural environments, thus failing to capture context-specific dynamics. Drimie and Casale (2009) warned that a combination of HIV/AIDS, food insecurity, a weakened capacity of governments to deliver basic social services, and compromised resilience or ability of households to cope threaten the current and future welfare of people, particularly children, in several southern African countries.

Concerns about food security have been widely reported during recent decades in Sub-Saharan Africa, where chronic food insecurity is more intense and widespread than in other parts of the world (Tadesse et al. 2008). This is the only region where food insecurity is projected to increase between 2010 and 2021 (USDA 2011, p. 10). The situation has assumed critical levels in many parts of Sub-Saharan Africa. Although international organizations have seen chronic and seasonal food insecurity largely as a rural issue, it has increasingly impacted urban livelihoods since the 1980s, mainly as a result of rapid urbanization and lagging employment (Crush et al. 2011; Maxwell 2000). The spread of food insecurity from the drought-prone areas of eastern and southern Africa to the many mushrooming cities throughout

Sub-Saharan Africa is a cause for concern. Food insecurity was at the top of the agendas of West African regional organizations in 2010 (OECD 2011); 77% of 6,500 households in 11 cities in southern Africa were classified as food insecure in 2008, including 83% of households surveyed in Cape Town and 42% of households in Johannesburg (Frayne et al. 2009, pp. 6, 13). Crush et al. (2011) considered the urban and rural spheres to be highly interdependent and interactive in the context of the political economy of migration in southern Africa, with far-reaching implications for HIV/AIDS impacts on food security in both urban and rural communities.

The situation is projected to deteriorate further in much of Sub-Saharan Africa, largely as a result of continued rapid population growth and poverty levels that are the highest worldwide (Thomas and Zuberi 2012). Food production, availability, and consumption, hampered by inefficient technologies, weak distribution systems, and low demand for food by poor populations, are expected to remain low or decline further, particularly in the eastern, central, and western subregions. A number of factors in food insecurity, including climate change, shortage of arable land, water shortages, high food prices, high fertility rates among the poor, and extremely high urbanization rates, may differentially affect the four subregions. However, while Central Africa is projected to experience the highest level of malnutrition during the next four decades and southern Africa the lowest (IFPRI 2010; Thomas and Zuberi 2012), predictive modeling of food insecurity under different scenarios has not been attempted at the national or district levels.

This chapter examines the nexus among food insecurity, poverty, and HIV/AIDS in Sub-Saharan Africa with a focus on the eastern and southern subregions. This nexus is most prominently visible at the individual and household levels. Food-insecure and impoverished individuals and households are often pressured into adopting high-risk coping strategies, compelling them to engage in survival activities that can expose them to potentially dangerous situations. This often involves migrating in search of food, additional sources of income, or transactional and high-risk sex (IBDR 2007; Weiser et al. 2007). In the wider Sub-Saharan population, food insecurity increases maternal and child HIV/AIDS vulnerability and secondary infections of children (Jones 2011).

The central argument that runs through this chapter is that there is an overlapping and reinforcing link among the three major epidemics of food insecurity, poverty, and HIV/AIDS in the countries under discussion. The interplay is manifested in a range of agricultural systems, socioeconomic conditions, and cultural contexts in both rural and urban settings. The chapter addresses the following principal questions: (1) What is the magnitude of food insecurity, poverty, and HIV/AIDS in eastern and southern Africa? (2) How do these calamities influence one another? and (3) What are their impacts?

Conceptualizing the relationships among food insecurity, poverty, and HIV/AIDS

Food insecurity

Food security exists in a population when all people at all times have physical and economic access to sufficient, safe, and nutritious food to meet their dietary needs and food preferences for an active and healthy life (FAO 1996). The core concept this definition embodies is secure access at all times to sufficient food. The FAO definition centers on four core elements: *sufficiency* (defined as the calories required for an active, healthy life); *access* to food (through production, purchase, exchange, or in the form of gifts); *security* (defined by the balance between vulnerability, risk, and insurance); and *time* (food insecurity can be chronic, transitory, or cyclical) (Maxwell and Smith 1992, in Zegeye and Debebe 1995).

Food security, therefore, has three components: a safe and nutritionally adequate food supply at both national and household levels; a reasonable degree of stability in the seasonal and annual supply of food; and physical, social, and economic access of each household to enough food to meet its needs. Hence, the definition integrates availability of nutritious food, stability in the supply of food, physical access to food, and the biological utilization of food (Lovendal and Knowles 2007). Given these parameters, a major indicator of food insecurity in a society is the number of people whose food consumption level is below the minimum intake deemed necessary for maintenance of good physical health. The U.S. Department of Agriculture defined food-insecure people as individuals consuming fewer than 2,100 calories per day (Shapouri et al. 2009).

The 2,100 calories-per-day measure does not consider differences in the nutritional needs of different age groups, of the two genders, or the health statuses of different population groups. For example, people living with HIV/AIDS (PLWHA) commonly experience malabsorption and altered metabolism that may necessitate nutritional supplements (de Pee and Semba 2010). And co-infection with tuberculosis and intestinal pathogens further increases nutritional requirements for PLWHA (Semba et al. 2010). Moreover, recommended daily caloric intakes are up to one-third higher for persons engaging in heavy work than for those performing light activity. Similarly, calorie requirements are about 10% higher in asymptomatic PLWHA but 20–30% and 50–100% higher in symptomatic adults and children, respectively (WHO 2003, pp. 4, 9).

Two serious physiological effects of AIDS are reduced appetite (and thus lower food intake) and impaired nutrient absorption from food consumed. These effects contribute to malnutrition, which weakens the immune system of HIV-infected persons and in turn increases their susceptibility to malaria, tuberculosis, and other opportunistic infections. In addition, malnutrition leads to faster progression from symptomless infection to full-blown AIDS (IBDR 2007).

Extensive household expenditure surveys (HES) conducted by Smith et al. (2006) in 12 Sub-Saharan countries shed further light on the higher food requirements of vulnerable populations. The researchers found that substantially higher percentages of female- than male-headed households reported low diet diversity in 8 of 12 sub-Saharan countries. Quality and diverse diets, important to ensure food security, are often compromised by AIDS morbidity. Morbidity results in a reduction in the labor supply, which often causes a shift from cultivating labor-intensive but nutritious crops to less labor-demanding, less nutritious crops (de Waal 2003, in Akrofi et al. 2010). Smith et al. (2006) found strong associations between the two dietary parameters of quality and diversity and household expenditure in all countries, and diet diversity was significantly lower in rural than urban areas. Both energy deficiency and diet diversity rates varied significantly among regions and districts in individual countries due to variations in rainfall, socioeconomic development, and levels of security.

De Waal and Whiteside (2003) observed that AIDS caused widespread and rapid deterioration of food security that continued long after the 2001–2002 food crisis in southern Africa. They attributed this phenomenon to reduced community capacity because of reduced farm labor availability caused by declines in customary household and community support in farming activities and high AIDS mortality, especially among women. The absence of the labor and skills of these productive adults greatly diminished resilience, coping behavior, and household and community capacity to withstand food stress, the core of their 'new *variant* famine' hypothesis (de Waal and Whiteside 2003). Multinational studies by de Waal et al. (2010) of the relationship between HIV prevalence and state fragility, or state insecurity, in the more affluent southern African states indicate that these impacts tend to be underestimated at the household and community levels. At the state level, however, resilience tends to be increased by the beneficial effects of national and international responses to HIV/AIDS on national security and governance. Perhaps even more important in explaining the prolongation of food insecurity in southern Africa may be the realization that the HIV/AIDS pandemic is a long-term event that is projected to continue to suppress life and development for a number of years to come (de Waal 2010).

Many local people have associated poor diets with AIDS and are now also coping with the higher food intake requirements for antiretroviral therapy (ART) in food-scarce areas. Zimbabweans, for instance, are aware of the association between weather-related food shortages and full-blown AIDS (Rödlach 2011), and ethnographic research in a South African community found that many PLWHA modify their adherence to or refuse ART to get their CD4 counts to dangerously low levels in order to qualify for disability grants (Jones 2011).

The Kenya Institute for Public Policy Research and Analysis (KIPPRA 2009) observed that food security status in eastern and southern African countries has continued to deteriorate since the 1990s. USAID (2009), citing an FAO report, stated that more than 17 million people faced food insecurity in eastern Africa in 2007. The proportion of underweight children increased by 36% between 1990 and 2005 in East Africa and 35% of children in South Africa, 65% in Mozambique, and 75% in Zimbabwe were estimated to be food insecure in 2007 (IFAD 2006). These data largely reflect the low agricultural productivity in these countries and recent droughts (USDA 2009).

Researchers estimate that consumption levels, even among high-income groups, generally fell below two-thirds of the nutritional requirement in 2008. In southern Africa, rising domestic food prices reportedly affected an estimated 8.7 million people in 2008–2009, including 5.1 million people in Zimbabwe, 353,000 people in Lesotho, and 239,000 people in Swaziland (Shapouri et al. 2009). According to an USAID (2009) report, the number of food-insecure people in southern Africa increased by nearly one-third between the 2007/2008 and 2008/2009 market years.

Efforts to improve food security and livelihoods of HIV/AIDS- affected households through the integration of HIV and nutrition programs have been hampered by lack of information on how to effectively implement these programs in resource-poor areas (Ivers et al. 2009). Several researchers noted the difficulty in enlisting poor and HIV-affected people in programs and in reducing stigma and discrimination. Swaans et al. (2009) recommended that service providers and researchers engage themselves as active participants in collaboration with service recipients to explore livelihood systems in the search for appropriate solutions. This approach may yield a better understanding of the linkages between food insecurity and HIV transmission, treatment, and care and improve the effectiveness of food assistance and livelihood strategies (Anema et al. 2009), but adequate responses must also be tailored to specific socioeconomic settings (Frega et al. 2010).

Poverty

According to UNDP (2011), the number of poor people will continue to increase, particularly in the least developed countries, if social inequalities and environmental deterioration continue to intensify, economic growth continues to slow, and income inequalities deepen further. Most countries in Sub-Saharan Africa are characterized by severe and widespread poverty; more than three-quarters of the poor live in rural areas and depend primarily on subsistence agriculture (Pinstrup-Andersen and Pandya-Lorch 2001, in Hitzhusen 2007). The poverty of the region is evident when applying the UNDP Multidimensional Poverty Index, which measures poverty using multiple indicators of deprivation at the individual level in education, standard of living, and health. On this index, values were higher than 0.3 in 27 countries and higher than 0.5 in the poorest countries (Guinea, Mozambique, Central African Republic, Burundi, Burkina Faso, Mali, Ethiopia, and Niger, in that order) between 2000 and 2010. Only two countries outside Sub-Saharan Africa (Nepal and Timor-Leste) had values above 0.3 (UNDP 2011, pp. 23–25). These national statistics provide only a crude picture of the distribution of poverty in the region because poverty disproportionately affects the most disadvantaged population groups, namely women, children, the elderly, and people with disabilities (Corbett 2008).

Definitions of poverty vary depending on disciplinary approaches and ideologies, and there is no single definition that captures all the facets of human deprivation emanating from poverty (Handley et al. 2009). UNDP-Lesotho (2007) defined poverty as a state of deprivation in which individuals or groups of people are denied the opportunities and choices most basic to human development. Poverty may refer not only to the lack of the necessities for material well-being but also to the denial of opportunities for living a tolerable life. Therefore, poverty can be conceived of as being absolute or relative. Absolute poverty is a consumption-based state of deprivation and refers to the inability to secure the minimum basic needs for human survival (World Bank 1991, in Corbett 2008). On the other hand, relative poverty is a type of deprivation that implies degrees of income inequality among household groups or communities. It describes the condition of the lower 30–40% of income groups in any society and generally includes the majority of people who lack access to adequate social services. Absolute and relative poverty can be defined by using quantitative parameters such as per capita income, per capita provision of social amenities, per capita food consumption, or a variety of other measures (Corbett 2008; UNDP-Lesotho 2007).

The dominant Western definition conceptualizes poverty in terms of income or consumption (Handley et al. 2009) and is therefore widely thought of as 'income poverty.' One of the most rudimentary dimensions of poverty, or deprivation, is equated with chronic food insecurity. Hence, the term 'poorest of the poor' (the 'ultra-poor' or the 'indigent') is widely applied to those who cannot afford the bare minimum caloric intake of 2,100 kcal/day (UNDP 1997, in Corbett 2008).

In general, poverty can be viewed from three perspectives: income, basic needs, and capability. From the income perspective, a person is poor if his/her income level is below the widely accepted poverty threshold of around US $1 per day. The basic needs perspective considers poverty a deprivation of material resources necessary to meet basic human needs, including food. The capability perspective looks at poverty as the absence of some basic capacity to function – a person with a low level of functionality is considered poor (Corbett 2008).

The causes of poverty are multidimensional and center around inadequate access to and uneven distribution of resources. Political economy drivers and maintainers of poverty include weak nations; weak civil societies; corruption; and denial of human rights such as the rights to education, health, and livelihoods (Handley et al. 2009). Ethnic and gender inequalities, limited access to education and employment opportunities, environmental degradation, health services, war, social upheavals, and absence of welfare assistance further contribute to poverty. Common consequences of poverty – malnutrition, infectious diseases, high infant and maternal mortality, and lower life expectancy – are particularly rife in Sub-Saharan Africa. In extreme cases, poverty situations may deteriorate even further into a state of chronic malnutrition, poor physical health, and chronic depression (Corbett 2008; Handley et al. 2009).

HIV/AIDS

HIV infection and mortality rates from AIDS are the highest in the countries of eastern and southern Africa, as described in Chapter 1, and they have a significant reciprocal and synergistic relationship with poverty parameters and food insecurity. Health care workers are increasingly recognizing that PLWHA require a high level of food security before and after starting ART to reduce mortality risk and optimize treatment results. HIV infection tends to reduce all three components of food security: availability, accessibility, and security. Declines in food production and decreases in income at individual and family levels affect food availability and accessibility as well as the ability of PLWHA to follow dietary recommendations, further discussed below. Many HIV-infected individuals, affected households, and those weakened by AIDS find it hard to access food and tend to become food insecure when they are unable to earn income or grow crops. HIV/AIDS is also likely to cause or worsen food insecurity by impacting the productive members of society, reducing household productivity, increasing the number of dependents, and disrupting the transfer of local knowledge and skills. In addition, the epidemic results in the loss of farming skills, decline in agricultural activities, reduced capacity to work, shifts in cropping patterns, reduced household earnings, and drastic increases in health care and medical costs (Steinberg et al. 2002).

Just as HIV/AIDS is intertwined with food insecurity, it is closely related to poverty, both as a cause and as a result. Ill health in general and the HIV epidemic in particular strike the poorest segments of society hardest. In rural settings, poor households affected by ill health risk losing their land, farm implements, and livestock, pushing them deeper into poverty. HIV/AIDS tends to disrupt the division of labor in traditional households, creating the possibility whereby the wife or AIDS orphans may assume the role of household head/breadwinner. Furthermore, ill health can impoverish households through income losses and medical expenses that trigger a spiral of asset depletion, indebtedness, and cuts to essential consumption processes (Kabir et al. 2000). Thus, HIV/AIDS tends to exacerbate poverty and worsen food insecurity, thereby increasing the vulnerability especially of rural households and undermining their capacity to withstand shocks (ECA and CHGA 2004, p. 14).

In sum, HIV/AIDS poses an enormous challenge to poverty reduction efforts, exerting a profound impact on the achievement of the Millennium Development Goals, particularly in eastern and southern Africa. Countries in these regions have to deal with the highest HIV infection rates, recurrent famines, and chronic food insecurity as well as widespread poverty, all synergistically interacting with one another (WHO and UNAIDS 2009).

The nexus between food insecurity, poverty, and HIV/AIDS

In order to illustrate the complexity of the nexus between food insecurity, poverty, and HIV/AIDS, we center the discussion on HIV/AIDS as a force cutting across the two focal issues. Thus, the interactions between HIV/AIDS and food insecurity and HIV/AIDS and poverty are discussed separately.

Food insecurity and HIV/AIDS

The relationship between HIV/AIDS and different aspects of food insecurity is revealed in a number of ways in Sub-Saharan Africa. Manifestations of this relationship are found in the reduction in the amount of time farmers spend on farm plots, the shrinking of the agricultural workforce, the diminishing area of cultivated land, the smaller number of crop varieties planted, decreasing crop yields and livestock production, and the loss of agricultural skills (Muller 2004). The National Agricultural Advisory Services of Uganda (NAADS 2003, p. 1), examining the agricultural impacts of AIDS, estimated that AIDS-affected households in Ethiopia spend 50–60% less time on agriculture than nonaffected households. Moreover, FAO (2001, in NAADS 2003) projected that AIDS would reduce the agricultural workforce by 17% in Kenya, 14% in Uganda, and 13% in Tanzania during the period from 1985 to 2020 and even more sharply in southern African countries. However, these projections are no longer tenable due to the massive roll-out of antiretroviral drugs throughout the region since about 2005 that sharply reduced AIDS-related mortality (see Chapter 8). Nevertheless, food insecurity linked to HIV/AIDS continues to affect the lives of farmers throughout Sub-Saharan Africa. In addition to undermining the capacity of HIV-affected households to work, food-related problems compel households to divert their financial, material, and human resources to the mitigation of HIV/AIDS impacts, worsening and perpetuating food insecurity and thus their vulnerability to the epidemic.

Ngowi (2006) noted that the HIV epidemic threatened all spheres of life in Tanzania. In addition to reducing agricultural productivity and consequently increasing food insecurity, AIDS negatively affected the quality of services provided by agricultural extension workers in Moshi district of Tanzania who were burdened by HIV/AIDS in their families. Many farmers could not be trained and advised by extension agents, causing declines in agricultural productivity and food security (Ngowi 2006).

Citing a 2001 FAO report, Ngowi (2006) noted that in Kenya substantial amounts of financial resources at national, regional, district, household, and individual levels had been diverted from the agricultural sector to deal with various aspects of HIV/AIDS. For example, time was diverted from agricultural pursuits to activities and processes related to the treatment of HIV/AIDS. Consequently, farmland that could be used for food production lay idle and uncultivated. Financial resources that could have been utilized for agricultural work were diverted to covering the costs of AIDS impact mitigation in the form of nutritional, medical, and educational support to the infected and affected. A later study by FAO (2003) of impacts of and responses to HIV/AIDS in Uganda found that whereas two-thirds or more of households in agricultural and fishing communities used household income and assistance from relatives to pay for medical and burial expenses, about four-fifths of pastoralist households sold assets and cattle for these purposes and thus incurred significantly greater productivity losses.

Related to this, food insufficiency often increases HIV transmission, risk behavior, and susceptibility to HIV infection among women using sex work as a means of survival. Several studies have reported that women who do not get sufficient food are far more likely than others to sell sex for money or resources and engage in unprotected and intergenerational sex (Gillespie 2008; Gillespie and Kadiyala 2005; Piot et al. 2007). Women's low socioeconomic status and food insufficiency in southern African countries and throughout Sub-Saharan Africa play important roles in causing many to become sex workers.

Another link between food insecurity and female HIV vulnerability was reported from Ethiopia, where food insecurity during famines caused destitute women to flee their homes in search of assistance, and they were reportedly taken advantage of in return for support (IRIN 2003). On the other hand, several reports from Zimbabwe indicate that the economic crisis in the country reduced risky behavior and multiple sexual partnerships because men could not afford to pay for transactional sex (Mate 2005).

In Namibia and Zambia, FAO (2003) recorded significantly greater impacts on female- than male-headed households in several rural communities. In Namibia, male-headed households unaffected by HIV/AIDS had the largest number of cattle, followed by affected male-headed households, unaffected female-headed households, and affected female-households, in that order. Similarly, in Zambia, male-headed households without orphans had the largest average landholdings and cultivated areas, followed by male-headed households with orphans, female-headed households without orphans, and those with orphans.

In Uganda, a study of rural communities where livelihoods are based on farming and fishing identified another link to food insecurity. AIDS-affected households were found to be using poor or obsolete implements for their farming and fishing activities because they could not afford access to or utilization of information services recommended by agricultural extension agents. Competing cash needs and limited income constrained the ability of many affected Ugandan households to adopt modern farming methods. The use of inferior tools and methods reduced production, contributing to food insecurity and malnutrition (Guerny 2002, in NAADS 2003). In some cases, recommended agronomic practices such as compost preparation and proper crop spacing proved to be too difficult and time-consuming for HIV-infected people to manage, and farmers lacked the strength to till the land properly in preparation for cropping. Limited labor availability and physical weakness tended to delay planting and harvesting activities, resulting in preharvest losses. Moreover, the heavy demands of care of the sick prevented infected and affected farmers from attending seminars on improved farming practices provided by agricultural extension workers (NAADS 2003).

Appleton (2001, in NAADS 2003) noted that AIDS-affected households fostering orphans or headed by widows, widowers, or orphans have limited ability to add value to farm produce because they lack resources and access to farm inputs. In addition, increased medical and funeral costs reduce household investment on livestock and farm inputs and implements, resulting in low-quality farm production.

Further contributing to food insecurity is the fact that limited extension services are available to orphan household heads, usually not included in community-level sensitization sessions because they are considered too young to benefit from the service. Fishing activities are similarly affected. NAADS (2003) reported a significant increase in the percentage of AIDS-affected households (43%) whose fish catch dropped sharply from 1997 to 2002 as compared to nonaffected households (20%). Low quality and volume of fish catches for affected households were attributed to reduced amount of time spent fishing, loss of labor to illness, physical weakness, and inadequate investment in modern fishing equipment (NAADS 2003).

Gender-based division of many agricultural activities in Sub-Saharan Africa aggravates the impact of HIV/AIDS on agricultural productivity because it lowers labor input and reduces the area of land cultivated and food availability. For example, NAADS (2003) pointed out that weeding and pruning in coffee fields and mulching banana trees are considered male activities in Iganga district in Uganda. Production of these crops therefore declines when male household members experience HIV-induced ill health or when they die. Moreover, infected and affected men spend less time grazing and watering animals, an activity traditionally regarded as in the male domain. NAADS (2003) reported that men's involvement in livestock production fell by 38% in agro-pastoral communities and by 25% in pastoral communities in Uganda between 1997 and 2002.

HIV/AIDS further impacts the food security of affected and infected families by forcing distressed households to sell assets such as land and crops at low prices. In Ugandan and other patrilineal societies, AIDS-affected food insecurity is exacerbated by the custom of families of the deceased appropriating the household assets of widows and orphans. Patrilineal tradition also requires that surviving brothers of the deceased inherit the deceased's wife and children as well as his household resources. Wives who refuse to be inherited are customarily sent away and dispossessed of the household property, leaving them and their children helpless and food insecure (NAADS 2003).

Food production and security may be indirectly affected by HIV/AIDS in land-scarce areas. For instance, the increasing scarcity of land due to the diversion of agricultural land to burial sites is a little-researched linkage between food insecurity and HIV/AIDS. This effect is particularly acute in rural areas in Tanzania, where the impact of HIV/AIDS on agricultural production and productivity is particularly severe due to extremely high population densities. This situation is exacerbated by cultural values requiring that the dead be buried on the most fertile land, usually on the household compound, to give them the highest respect (Ngowi 2006). Land scarcity aggravated by AIDS-related increases in the amount of agricultural land diverted to burial grounds has also been reported from Durban, Johannesburg, and other urban areas, contributing to the eviction of peri-urban farmers, who typically have no tenure rights, and competition with housing and industrial development (Kironde Lusugga 2008; Roelf n.d.). The scarcity of new land and expected increases in urban populations and AIDS-related mortality have sparked municipal information campaigns that address cultural conservatism by suggesting cremation, recycling of graves, and other alternative burial methods (Kironde Lusugga 2008; Roelf n.d.).

Recent increases in food prices in eastern Africa have further impacted the livelihoods of food-insecure rural households, which must augment their food supply by buying grains from local markets. Households are forced to spend a large part of their income on food commodities whose prices continue to soar. Thus the impact of the HIV epidemic, compounded by the rise in food prices, low level of agricultural productivity, and low level of household income, exacerbate the poverty of already food-insecure and needy HIV-affected households in the countries of the region (Brahmbhatt and Christiansen 2008).

Poverty and HIV/AIDS

Gillespie (2008) described what he called the 'upstream and downstream' sides of the relationship between poverty and HIV/AIDS in eastern and southern Africa. This is a useful way of picturing the reciprocal relationship between the two phenomena. The upstream side refers to the pathways by which poverty acts as an HIV risk factor for vulnerable people. The downstream side of the relationship encompasses those elements of the postinfection situation by which HIV/AIDS precipitates or exacerbates poverty for the infected and affected. The fact that poverty fuels the spread of HIV/AIDS and HIV/AIDS aggravates poverty (Oxfam-International and Save the Children-UK 2002) requires that discussions of poverty and HIV/AIDS consider this two-way relationship.

Socioeconomic determinants of HIV infection are difficult to study holistically and remain inadequately understood at the individual, household, and community levels (Muthengi 2007). In an extensive review of economic and cultural factors of the epidemic, Nattrass (2009) concluded that the role of poverty in HIV/AIDS is usually less important than social and behavioral factors. This opinion contrasts with the extreme position in the poverty/AIDS debate that malnutrition, and thus poverty, drives HIV infection (Stillwaggon 2006). Although several studies have found an inverse relationship between nutrition levels and HIV prevalence, per capita income has not been demonstrated to be significantly associated with HIV infection. Instead, cultural variables, particularly religion, and country-level variations appear more important, and a number of studies reported that better-off people were as vulnerable to HIV as poorer people or even more so (Gillespie et al. 2007; Nattrass 2009).

The most extensive socioeconomic data examined, from the Demographic and Health Survey (DHS) datasets, show an overall direct relationship between HIV prevalence and education, a strong indicator of socioeconomic status in Sub-Saharan Africa. In Kenya and Tanzania, education was the variable most strongly correlated with HIV, regardless of sex, age, or place of residence. Infection rates in adults with six years of schooling were up to 50% higher than in people without education, a statistic Fortson (2008) attributed to higher likelihood of premarital sex in the former group and a larger number of lifetime sexual partners due to greater autonomy and mobility of wealthier people. The wealth gradient in HIV, by contrast, showed no consistent pattern in these and other Sub-Saharan countries, due in part to deficiencies in the DHS database, including different definitions, samples, and study methods; the use of risk behavior rather than HIV prevalence data; and the changing nature of the epidemic in different countries (Beegle and de Walque 2009; Fortson 2008).

Another review, of nine national demographic, health, and serobehavioral surveys in eastern and southern Africa, revealed that many wealthy people are at high risk of infection and that the relationship between wealth and HIV infection tends to change over time in different social groups (Parkhurst 2010). Muthengi (2007), examining the DHS data for Kenya, found a significant association between wealth and HIV infection among women nationwide but between wealth, ethnic group, and

HIV only among Kalenjin women, suggesting that wealth and education have different effects on HIV risk in that population, with the wealth effect predominating. However, in recent years education has become protective against HIV infection, apparently due to the relatively greater behavioral changes among educated people (Muthengi 2007). Temporal changes in socio-epidemiological variations remain understudied. Further studies may elucidate structural factors of poverty and wealth that can inform policy makers and program health managers regarding how to identify, support, and monitor high-risk groups.

Poverty has increased in many Sub-Saharan countries during the last few decades and persists at high levels in many communities. In 2011, all but 11 of the 46 countries in the low human development category were in Sub-Saharan Africa; only seven Sub-Saharan countries – five of them in southern Africa – were in the medium human development group. The Democratic Republic of the Congo had the lowest human development index (HDI), followed by Niger, Burundi, and Mozambique. The value of the HDI for Ethiopia was 0.406 (0.363), for Kenya 0.521 (0.509), for Tanzania 0.467(0.466), and for Uganda 0.505 (0.446); the average per capita gross domestic products for these four countries were $1,055, $1,240, $744, and $1,454, respectively (UNDP 2011). Incomes increased worldwide except in sub-Saharan Africa between 1990 and 2005, where some 300 million people lived on less than $1 per day during that period and where the proportion of people in the bottom income category more than doubled between 1980 and 2005 (UNDP 2006, p. 269). In a study of adolescent sexuality in Dessie Town in Ethiopia, Tadele (2006) described how broader structural factors such as poverty greatly increase the spread of HIV/AIDS among young adolescents.

Poverty affects young people's sexuality and the spread of HIV/AIDS in various complex ways. It results in a dearth of romantic love. It forces young people to migrate in search of jobs elsewhere, thereby resulting in a disruption of family and community norms related to sexuality. It affects the societal response to HIV/AIDS. It delays marriage. It forces young women to exchange sex for money and gifts, often without using condoms. It produces a paucity of information and hence a plethora of misunderstandings. It makes young people fatalistic, thereby encouraging unsafe sex. And it determines who falls ill most quickly once infected and who will have access to treatment, including ARTs (Tadele 2006, p. 15).

Tadege (2005), in her study conducted in Addis Ababa, concluded that there are bi-causal relationships between poverty and HIV/AIDS. Firstly, the relationship between poverty and HIV/AIDS can be seen in light of the spatial and socioeconomic distribution of HIV infection and poverty-related factors that affect coping capacities of households and communities. The poor have weak endowments of human and financial resources, few marketable skills, and generally poor health, all contributing to low productivity. Secondly, the relationship between HIV/AIDS and poverty can be understood by considering processes through which household and community experiences of HIV/AIDS intensify poverty. The disease, through a complex socioeconomic process, tends to aggravate poverty by reducing household coping capabilities, thus increasing vulnerability to the health consequences. FAO (2003) reported these impacts among farming, pastoral, and fishing communities in Namibia, Uganda, and Zambia. Thus poverty fosters the spread of the virus, while getting infected with HIV, in turn, increases the poverty of already affected people, households, and communities. Tolera (2006) examined the relationship between risk environment (poverty, gender inequality, low income, poor access to health and education services, and low employment opportunities) and vulnerability to HIV infection in Addis Ababa. He found that disadvantaged community groups, particularly poor people, women, and the least educated, tend to be at an elevated risk of HIV infection.

Poverty is strongly gendered in eastern and southern Africa as a result of prevailing social norms and practices, above all the economic dependence of women on men and sexual inequities in the predominantly patriarchal societies. Otive-Igbuzor (2010) considered patriarchy and poverty to be in an unholy alliance that increases the burden of the disease on African women. The sexual exploitation of female workers in many types of employment by male supervisors and managers is an example of gendered sexual inequity and poverty (Bukusi 2008). This and other aspects of the problem of female subordination and exploitation are described in Chapters 2, 3, 4, and 6.

The sale of household and other family assets and illegal 'property grabbing' are other disturbing components of the relationship between poverty and HIV/AIDS. In rural areas, distress sales of livestock, grain, and other household assets to pay for the costs of illness and burial and to maintain households often diminishes food production and weakens the ability of AIDS-affected households to cope with shocks. Ugandan females who lose their husbands, whether to AIDS or other causes, have livestock and other household assets taken by relatives. In the worst-case scenarios, women's property rights are violated when infected female heads of households are evicted from their houses, forcing them into poverty (FAO 2003; Kamusiime and Rugadya 2007). The resultant depletion of resources further impoverishes affected households, plunging them further into the downward spiral of the poverty–HIV/AIDS relationship.

Naidu and Booysen (2008) estimated that 18–24% of the South African population live in a state of chronic poverty. Available data show that HIV/AIDS-affected households in Soweto are likely to move into and out of poverty for a certain period of time because of insecure and fluctuating income. Several studies indicate a strong correlation between extreme poverty and high HIV prevalence in South Africa. Naidu and Booysen (2008) underscored that the epidemic cannot be examined in isolation from the state of poverty in the country.

Studies in southern African countries suggest that HIV incidence is highest among the poorer groups in any given country (Lopman et al. 2007). Researchers attribute the high HIV prevalence rates in southern Africa, which is wealthier than the eastern African countries, to a strong association between social inequality in income and employment and HIV prevalence in that region. Countries with greater inequalities have higher HIV prevalence, with the most extreme disparity evident in South Africa (Fassin and Schneider 2003; Gillespie et al. 2007).

While the poor are undoubtedly hit hardest by the downstream impacts of AIDS, their chances of being exposed to HIV in the first place are not necessarily greater than the chances of some wealthier individuals or households, as noted above. This pattern indicates that while socioeconomic and gender inequalities exacerbate the spread of HIV, AIDS-related disease and death increase these inequalities – a potentially vicious cycle (Gillespie 2008).

Conclusion

The magnitude of the impacts of HIV/AIDS in Sub-Saharan Africa is closely linked with food insecurity and poverty, leaving countries in these regions more vulnerable than those in other regions. As a result, food insecurity, poverty, and HIV/AIDS – often intertwined and exacerbated by rapid population growth, inefficient food production systems, and environmental degradation – pose a tremendous development challenge in these regions. Thus, any development policy or program intervention aimed at addressing these challenges needs to consider an integrated, multidisciplinary, and multisectoral approach that takes into account the intricate and overlapping characteristics of these and related problems as well as the connections among them.

Now, nearly four decades after the first AIDS cases were reported from Africa, the long wave of intergenerational impacts of the epidemic is becoming starkly evident. Lessons have been learned about the intertwining of HIV/AIDS with poverty, malnutrition, and agriculture. It is becoming clear that if the Millennium Development Goals for poverty, hunger, and HIV/AIDS are to be met in Sub-Saharan Africa, governments must address the mutually reinforcing and converging dynamics of the epidemic proactively through more effective AIDS-responsive and context-sensitive food policy and poverty reduction programs (von Braun et al. 2005). By viewing food aid through an 'HIV/AIDS lens' and in the context of people's livelihoods, organizations can reduce both susceptibility to HIV infection and vulnerability to AIDS impacts (Kadiyala and Gillespie 2004).

We hope the information that can guide the integration and effective implementation of HIV, nutrition, food production, and food security programs, still scarce (Ivers et al. 2009), will be generated in the near future. We conclude that any development intervention that aims at revealing the intricate linkages between food insecurity, poverty, and HIV/AIDS must harmonize or unify the cumulative impacts of the epidemics with sustainable food production and poverty alleviation in both rural and urban communities in Sub-Saharan Africa. To ensure the achievement of this goal, there is a need for studies that pay due attention to the local and regional agroecological, socioeconomic, and cultural contexts that facilitate the implementation of appropriate and properly targeted economic development and HIV/AIDS policies and programs.

References

Akrofi, S., Brouwer, I.D., Price, L.L. and Struik, P.C. 2010. Home gardens contribute significantly to dietary diversity in HIV/AIDS afflicted households in rural Ghana. *Journal of Human Ecology* 31:125–134.

Anema, A., Vogenthaler, N., Frongillo, E.A. et al. 2009. Food insecurity and HIV/AIDS: Current knowledge, gaps, and research priorities. *Current HIV/AIDS Reports* 6:224–231.

Beegle, K. and de Walque, D. 2009. *Demographic and Socioeconomic Patterns of HIV/AIDS Prevalence in Africa*. World Bank Policy Research Working Paper Series, No. 5076. Washington, DC: World Bank.

Brahmbhatt, M. and Christiansen, L. 2008. *Rising Food Prices in East Asia: Challenges and Policy Options. Safety Net Measures*. Rome: Food and Agriculture Organization.

Bukusi, E. 2008. Assessing the magnitude and perceived impact of HIV/AIDS on the sugar sub-sector: A case study of western Kenya. In OSSREA (ed.), *The HIV/AIDS Challenge in Africa, an Impact and Response Assessment: The Case of Kenya*, pp. 1–73. Addis Ababa: OSSREA.

Corbett, T.J. 2008. *Poverty. Encarta Encyclopedia (DVD)*. Redmond, WA: Microsoft Corporation.

Crush, J., Frayne, B., Drimie, S. and Caesar, M. 2011. *The HIV and Urban Food Security Nexus*. Urban Food Security Series, No. 5. Capetown: African Food Security Urban Network.

d'Adesky, A. 2007. *Overlapping Epidemics: HIV/AIDS, Hunger and Poverty*. Boston: WE-ACTX.

de Pee, S. and Semba, R.D. 2010. Role of nutrition in HIV infection: Review of evidence for more effective programming in resource-limited areas. *Food and Nutrition Bulletin* 31:S313–S344.

de Waal, A. 2010. Governing a world with HIV/AIDS: An unfinished success story. In Sahn, E. (ed.), *The Socioeconomic Dimensions of HIV/AIDS in Africa: Challenges, Opportunities and Misconceptions*, pp. 42–56. Ithaca, NY: Cornell University Press.

de Waal, A. and Whiteside, A. 2003. New variant famine: AIDS and food crisis in southern Africa. *Lancet* 362:1234–1237.

de Waal, A., Klot, J.F. and Mhajan, M. 2010. *HIV/AIDS, Security and Conflict: New Realities, New Response*. New York: Social Science Research Council and Clingendael Institute.

Drimie, S. and Casale, M. 2009. Multiple stressors in Southern Africa: The link between HIV/AIDS, food insecurity, poverty and children's vulnerability now and in the future. *AIDS Care* 21:28–33.

ECA and CHGA. 2004. *Impact of HIV/AIDS on Rural Livelihoods and Food Security: Interactive Ethiopia Discussion Outcomes*. Addis Ababa: Economic Commission for Africa and Commission on HIV/AIDS and Governance for Africa.

FAO. 1996. *Rome Declaration on World Food Security and World Food Summit Plan of Action. World Summit 96/3b*. Rome: U.N. Food and Agriculture Organization.

FAO. 2003. *HIV/AIDS and Agriculture: Impacts and Responses: Case Studies from Namibia, Uganda and Zambia*. Rome: U.N. Food and Agriculture Organization.

Fassin, D. and Schneider, H. 2003. The politics of AIDS in South Africa: Beyond the controversies. *British Medical Journal* 326:495–497.

Fortson, J.G. 2008. The gradient in sub-Saharan Africa: Socioeconomic status and HIV/AIDS. *Demography* 45:303–322.

Frayne, B., Battersby-Lennard, J., Finchman, R. and Haysom, G. 2009. *Urban Food Security in South Africa: Case Studies of Cape Town, Msunduzi and Johannesburg*. Working Paper No. 15. Halfway House, South Africa: Development Bank of Southern Africa.

Frega, R., Duffy, F., Rawat, R. and Grede, N. 2010. Food insecurity in the context of HIV/AIDS: A framework for a new era of programming. *Food and Nutrition Bulletin* 31(Suppl.):S292–S312.

Gillespie, S.R. 2008. *Poverty*, food insecurity, HIV vulnerability, and the impacts of AIDS in sub-Saharan Africa. *IDS Bulletin* 39:5.

Gillespie, S.R. and Kadiyala, S. 2005. *HIV/AIDS and Food and Nutrition Security: From Evidence to Action*. Washington, DC: International Food Policy Research Institute.

Gillespie, S.R., Kadiyala, S. and Greener, R. 2007. Is poverty or wealth driving HIV transmission? *AIDS* 21(Suppl. 7):S5–S16.

Handley, G., Higgins, K., Sharma, B. et al. 2009. *Poverty and Poverty Reduction in Sub-Saharan Africa: An Overview of Key Issues*. London: Overseas Development Institute.

Hitzhusen, J. 2007. Context, concepts and policy on poverty and inequality. In Lal, R., Hansen, D.O., Uphoff, N. and. Slack, S.A. (eds.), *Food Security and Environmental Quality in Developing World*, pp. 162–182. London: CRC Press.

IBDR. 2007. *HIV/AIDS, Nutrition, and Food Security: What We Can Do. A Synthesis of International Guidance*. Washington, DC: International Bank for Reconstruction and Development/World Bank.

IFAD. 2006. *Rural Poverty Portal*. New York: International Fund for Agricultural Development.

IFPRI. 2010. IFPRI food security CASE maps. Generated by IFPRI in collaboration with Statplanet. http://www.ifpri.org/climate-change/casemaps.html

IRIN. 2003. Ethiopia: Drought exposing women to abuse, says UNICEF. *IRIN Newsletter* (Office of the Coordination of Humanitarian Affairs), United Nations.

Ivers, L.C., Cullen, K.A., Freenberg, K.A. et al. 2009. HIV/AIDS, undernutrition and food security. *Clinical Infectious Diseases* 49:1096–1102.

Jones, C. 2011. 'If I take my pills I'll go hungry': The choice between economic security and HIV/AIDS treatment in Grahamstown, South Africa. *Annals of Anthropological Practice* 35:67–80.

Kabir, A., Rahman A., Saliway, S. and Pryer, J. 2000. Sickness among the urban poor: A barrier to livelihood security. *Journal of International Development* 12: 707–722.

Kadiyala, S. and Gillespie, S. 2004. Rethinking aid to fight AIDS. *Food and Nutrition Bulletin* 25: 271–281.

Kamusiime, H. and Rugadya, M.A. 2007. HIV/AIDS in Uganda's national land policy. Paper presented at the Poverty Social Impact Assessment (PSIA) Training, Jinja, 7 July.

Kapunda, S.M. 2005. Socio-economic impact of HIV/AIDS on rural small-scale industrial sub-sector: The case of selected villages in Botswana. A research report submitted to OSSREA for the 2004 HIV/AIDS Challenge for Africa Competition. Unpublished.

KIPPRA. 2009. *Low Agricultural Productivity and Food Insecurity in the Nile Basin Countries*. Nairobi: Kenya Institute for Public Policy Research and Analysis, Project Management Unit, Socio-Economic Development and Benefit Sharing, Nile Basin Initiative (NBI).

Kironde Lusugga, J.M. 2008. Governance of communal land and resources in Africa. Paper presented at the 18th International Anti-Corruption Conference, Athens, Greece, 30 October–2 November.

Lopman, B., Lewis, J., Nyamukapa, C. et al. 2007. HIV incidence and poverty in Manicaland, Zimbabwe: Is HIV becoming a disease of the poor? *AIDS 2007* 21(Suppl. 7):S57–S66.

Lovendal, C.R. and Knowles, M. 2007. Tomorrow's hunger: A framework for analysis of vulnerability to food security. In Guha-Khasnobis, B., Acharya, S.S. and Davis, B. (eds.), *Food Security. Indicators, Measurement and the Impact of Trade Openness*, pp. 62–94. Oxford: Oxford University Press.

Mate, R. 2005. *Making Ends Meet the Margins? Grappling with Economic Crisis and Belonging in Beitbridge Town, Zimbabwe*. CODESRIA Monograph Series. Dakar: CODESRIA.

Maxwell, D. 2000. *Urban Food Insecurity in Sub-Saharan Africa*. Ottawa: International Development Research Center.

Muiruri, P. 2008. A situational analysis on responses to HIV/AIDS challenges in the food, beverages and tobacco manufacturing sectors in Nairobi city, Kenya. In OSSREA (ed.), *The HIV/AIDS Challenge in Africa, an Impact and Response Assessment: The Case of Kenya*, pp.191–245. Addis Ababa: OSSREA.

Muller, T.R. 2004. *HIV/AIDS and Agriculture in Sub-Saharan Africa*. AWLEA Series No. 1. Wageningen, The Netherlands: Wageningen Academic Publishers.

Muthengi, E. 2007. Socioeconomic status and HIV infection among women in Kenya. Paper presented at the Fifth African Population Conference, Arusha, Tanzania, 10–14 December.

NAADS. 2003. *The Impact of HIV/AIDS in the Agricultural Sector and Rural Livelihoods in Uganda: Baseline Report*. Rome: Integrated Support to Sustainable Development and Food and Agriculture Organization.

Naidu, V. and Booysen, F. 2008. Poverty dynamics in HIV/AIDS affected households in Soweto, South Africa: A pilot study of income-earning households. In OSSREA (ed.), *The HIV/AIDS Challenge in Africa, an Impact and Response Assessment: The Case of South Africa*, pp. 117–212. Addis Ababa: OSSREA.

Nattrass, N. 2009. Poverty, sex and AIDS. *AIDS and Behavior* 13:833–840.

Ngowi, H.P. 2006. The way HIV/AIDS affects the agricultural sector in Tanzania. A research report submitted to OSSREA for the 2004 HIV/AIDS challenge for Africa competition. Economics Department, Mzumbe University, Morogoro, Tanzania. Unpublished.

Nuwagaba, A. 2005. HIV/AIDS in armed conflict situation in northern Uganda. Research report, Department of Social Work and Social Administration, Makerere University, Kampala. Unpublished.

OECD (Organization for Economic Co-operation and Development). 2011. West African futures: Settlement, market and food security, conceptual note. Report SWAC (2011)(1). http://www.oecd.org/dataoecd/12/30/47427140.pdf

Ogunbayo, O. 2004. Food security, poverty reduction and HIV/AIDS. Presented at the 15th International Conference on AIDS, Bangkok, Thailand. Unpublished.

Otive-Igbuzor, E.J. 2010. Patriarchy and poverty: Rethinking African women's vulnerability to HIV/AIDS. http://werhcafrica.org/index.php/resources/48-papers/50–patriarchy-and-poverty-rethinking-african-womens-vulnerabilities-to-hivaids

Oxfam-International and Save the Children-UK. 2002. HIV/AIDS and food insecurity in southern Africa. http://www.oxfam.org.uk/resources/policy/hivaids/downloads/hiv_food_insecurity.pdf

Pankhurst, A., Tesfaye, A., Gebre, A. et al. 2008. Social responses to HIV/AIDS in Addis Ababa, Ethiopia with reference to commercial sex workers, people living with HIV/AIDS and community-based funeral associations in Addis Ababa. In OSSREA (ed.), *The HIV/AIDS Challenge in Africa, an Impact and Response Assessment: The Case of Ethiopia*, pp. 141–309. Addis Ababa: OSSREA.

Parkhurst, J.O. 2010. Understanding the correlations between wealth, poverty and human immunodeficiency virus in African countries. *Bulletin of the World Health Organization* 88:519–526.

Piot, P., Greener, R. and Russell, S. 2007. Squaring the circle: AIDS, poverty and human development. *PLoS Medicine* 4:e314.

Rödlach, A. 2011. 'AIDS is in the food: Zimbabweans' association between nutrition and HIV/AIDS and their potential for addressing food insecurity and HIV/AIDS. *Annals of Anthropological Practice* 35:219–237.

Roelf, W. n.d. Durban runs out of space for the dead. *Mail and Guardian (South Africa)*, May 14. http://www.amren.com/news04/05/18/durbancementery.html

Russell, S. 2005. *Illuminating Cases: Understanding the Economic Burden of Illness through Case Study Household Research.* London: Oxford University Press in association with the London School of Hygiene and Tropical Medicine.

Semba, R.D., Darnton-Hill, I. and de Pee, S. 2010. Addressing tuberculosis in the context of malnutrition and HIV coinfection. *Food and Nutrition Bulletin* 31: S345–S364.

Shapouri, S., Rosen, R.S., Meade, B. and Gale, F. 2009. *Food Security Assessment, 2008–09.* Washington, DC: US Department of Agriculture, Economic Research Service.

Smith, L.C., Alderman, H. and Aduayom, D. 2006. *Food Security in Sub-Saharan Africa: New Estimates from Household Expenditure Survey.* Washington, DC: International Food Policy Research Institute.

Steinberg, M., Johnson, M.S., Schierhout, G. and Ndewa, D. 2002. *Hitting Home: How Households Cope with the Impact of HIV/AIDS in South Africa.* Menlo Park, California: Henry J. Kaiser Family Foundation.

Stillwaggon, E. 2006. *AIDS and the Ecology of Poverty.* Oxford: Oxford University Press.

Swaans, K., Broerse, J., Meinke, M. et al. 2009. Promoting food security and well-being among poor and HIV/AIDS affected households: Lessons from an interactive and integrated approach. *Evaluation and Program Planning* 32:31–41.

Tadege, A. 2005. The impact of HIV/AIDS on poverty at household level: The case of two kebeles in Addis Ababa. M.A. thesis, Institute for Regional and Local Development Studies, Addis Ababa University, Addis Ababa.

Tadele, G. 2006. Bleak prospects: Young men, sexuality and HIV/AIDS in an Ethiopian town. Research Report 80/2006. Leiden: African Studies Center.

Tadesse, T., Haile, M., Snay, G. et al. 2008. The need for integration of drought monitoring tools for proactive food security management in sub-Saharan Africa. *Natural Resources Forum* 32:265–279.

Thomas, K.J.A. and Zuburi, T. 2012. *Demographic Change, the IMPACT Model, and Food Security in Sub-Saharan Africa*. New York: UNDP.

Tolera, A. 2006. Poverty and vulnerability to HIV infection in Addis Ababa: Exploring the relationship. Department of Sociology and Social Anthropology, Addis Ababa University, Addis Ababa, and Christian Michelson Institute. Bergen, Norway. Unpublished.

UNAIDS. 2008. *Report on the Global AIDS Epidemic*. Geneva: UNAIDS/WHO.

UNDP. 2006. *Human Development Report 2006*. New York: UNDP.

UNDP. 2011. *Human Development Report 2011*. New York: UNDP.

UNDP-Lesotho. 2007. *Lesotho National Human Development Report – 2006*. Maseru: UNDP-Lesotho.

USAID. 2009. *Global Food Insecurity and Price Increase*. Situation Report No.1, Fiscal Year 2009 – May 22, 2009. Washington, DC: USAID.

USAID and PEPFAR. 2007. *HIV and Food Security Conceptual Framework*. Washington, DC: Office of U. S. Global AIDS Coordinator and the Bureau of Public Affairs, U.S. State Department.

USDA. 2009. *Food Security Assessment, 2008–09*. Washington, DC: US Department of Agriculture, Economic Research Service.

USDA. 2011. *International Food Security Assessment, 2011–21*. Washington, DC: US Department of Agriculture, Economic Research Service.

von Braun, J., Swaminithan, M.S. and Rosegrant, M.W. 2005. *Agriculture, Food Security, Nutrition and the Millennium Development Goals*. IFPRI Essay. http://www.ifpri.org/sites/default/files/publications/ar03e.pdf

Weiser, S.D., Leiter, K., Bangsberg, D.R. et al. 2007. Food insufficiency is associated with high-risk sexual behavior among women in Botswana and Swaziland. *PLoS Medicine* 4(10):e260.

WHO. 2003. *Nutrient Requirements of People Living with HIV/AIDS*. Geneva: WHO.

WHO and UNAIDS. 2009. *Partnership with Faith-based Organizations: Strategic Framework. Report UNAIDS/10.02E*. Geneva: WHO and UNAIDS.

Zegeye, T. and Debebe, H. 1995. Food security: A brief review of concepts and indicators. In Demeke, M., Amha, W., Ehui, A. and Zegeye, T. (eds.), *Food Security, Nutrition, and Poverty Alleviation in Ethiopia: Problems and Prospects. Proceedings of the Inaugural and First Annual Conference of the Agricultural Economics Society of Ethiopia*, pp. 19–36. Addis Ababa: United Printers.

Books, papers, and other resources for further reading

Abebaw, D., Yibeltal, F. and Belay, K. 2010. The impact of a food security program on household food consumption in Northwestern Ethiopia: A matching estimator approach. *Food Policy* 35:286–293.

Ansell, N., Robson, E., Hajdu, F. et al. 2009. The new variant famine hypothesis: Moving beyond the household in exploring links between AIDS and food insecurity in southern Africa. *Progress in Development Studies* 9:187–207.

Barnett, T. and Whiteside, A. 2006. *AIDS in the Twenty-First Century: Disease and Globalization*, Chapters 7 and 9. London: Palgrave Macmillan.

Barnett, T. and Whiteside, A. 2007. Poverty and HIV/AIDS: Impact, coping and mitigation policy. In Cornia, G.A. (ed.), *AIDS, Public Policy and Child Well-being*. Florence, Italy: UNICEF Innocenti Research Centre.

Byron, E., Gillespie, S.R. and Hamazakaza, P. 2006. Local perceptions of risk and HIV prevention in southern Zambia. Renewal Working Paper. http://www.ifpri.org/renewal

Lamptey, P.R., Johnson, J. L. and Khan, M. 2006. The global challenge of HIV and AIDS. *Population Bulletin* 61(1):1–28.

Little, P., McPeak, J, Barrett, C. and Kristjanson, P. 2006. The multiple dimensions of poverty in pastoral areas of East Africa. Overview paper for Pastoralism and Poverty Reduction in East Africa: A Policy Research Conference, Nairobi, Kenya, 27–28 June.

Mano, R. and Matshe, I. 2006. *Impact of HIV & AIDS on Agriculture and Food Security from Zimbabwe: Empirical Analysis of Two Districts in Zimbabwe.* FANRPAN Working Document: Series Ref. Number: NAT ZIM001. Harare: Department of Agricultural Economics & Extension, University of Zimbabwe.

Mazzeo, J., Rödlach, A. and Brenton, B. 2011. Introduction: Anthropologists contront HIV/AIDS and food security in Sub-Saharan Africa. *Annals of Anthropological Practice* 35:1–7.

Mishra, V., Bignami-Van, S., Green, R. et al. 2007. HIV infection does not disproportionately affect the poorer in sub-Saharan Africa. *AIDS 2007* 21(Suppl. 7): S17–S28.

Population Department of the Ministry of Finance and Economic Development. 2008. *An Annotated Bibliography of Population and Reproductive Health Researches in Ethiopia, 2002–2007.* Addis Ababa, Ethiopia: Ministry of Finance and Economic Development (MoFED).

Pribram, V. 2011. *Nutrition and HIV.* Chichester: Wiley-Blackwell.

Various articles in the journal *Food Security: The Science, Sociology and Economics of Food Production and Access to Food.*

Part II

Impacts and Responses to HIV/AIDS

6
Socioeconomic and Psychosocial Impacts of HIV/AIDS and Responses at Different Levels of Society

Ayalew Gebre, Damtew Yirgu, and Helmut Kloos

Introduction

The security, economic stability, and social fabric of Sub-Saharan African countries have been seriously threatened by HIV/AIDS (ILO 2001; UNAIDS 2009). Foremost among the severe impacts are high morbidity and mortality rates, consequent economic hardship at all levels of society, social stigma, and discrimination toward the infected and affected. Different community groups experience the impacts of HIV/AIDS differently. The impacts are most direct at the individual and household levels (Barnett and Whiteside 2006, p. 198), but many structural impacts are similarly severe at the community level (ECA n.d.). Although the incidence of HIV declined in 22 Sub-Saharan African countries by more than 25% between 2001 and 2009 as a result of antiretroviral (ARV) treatments and behavioral changes (UNAIDS 2010, p. 8), it is becoming increasingly clear that the cumulative impacts of AIDS on existing and potential human and social capital and on the livelihood of future generations will extend over the long term (ECA n.d.). Nevertheless, the full socioeconomic, cultural, demographic, and political implications for Sub-Saharan African countries, communities, and households are still poorly understood.

It took national governments and various actors a number of years to evaluate the full extent and far-reaching impacts of the HIV/AIDS epidemic beyond the infected individuals and immediate family members. In the course of time, perspectives and perceptions about HIV/AIDS have significantly changed in response to its multidimensional and extensive impacts; the pandemic is no longer being considered a personal and/or family health problem, but a national public health and multisectoral development concern. The complex nature of the epidemic's impacts has required infected and affected individuals and families to adopt comprehensive strategies for coping with the biomedical and psychological health problems as well as with socioeconomic and cultural challenges. At the national level, governments have increasingly responded to the need to prevent and treat the underlying infection while caring for the growing number of patients on treatment by devising and implementing multisectoral interventions comprising prevention, treatment, care and support, and overall impact mitigation strategies, with encouraging results (UNAIDS 2010). This chapter examines the socioeconomic and cultural impacts of HIV/AIDS at different levels of social organization and the responses of actors and stakeholders at the individual, community (including the workplace), and national levels.

Impacts at different levels

Impacts on individuals

Infected individuals bear the most direct and severe consequences of HIV infections and the painful challenges of having to cope with the resultant impact as they experience direct biomedical and psychosocial health challenges. People living with HIV/AIDS (PLWHA) typically suffer from multidimensional effects of HIV/AIDS, ranging from physical to emotional challenges involving debilitating and painful illness, fear of imminent death, social stigma and discrimination (Taylor 1999), and impairment of children's psychosocial development (Moime 2009). The impacts of the pandemic are compounded and aggravated by the long-term challenges associated with heavy medical, psychological, and socioeconomic burdens, all of which severely undermine the ability of infected and affected individuals to cope with the difficulties they face and maintain their livelihoods.

The devastating HIV/AIDS-related morbidity and mortality seriously erode the social capital and economic base of infected individuals and their families and can induce consequences reaching far beyond personal health problems. Individuals with long-term morbidity incur social, emotional, and economic costs in the course of the illness trajectory in the form of increasing medical costs and reduced income and food production, especially in the labor-intensive subsistence economies of Sub-Saharan Africa and in households where the infected person is the primary income earner. A study in rural and urban communities in South Africa revealed that 80% of households would lose over half of their monthly income if the primary income earner were to die (Collins and Leibbrandt 2007).

As a social disease, AIDS impacts individuals and households through prevailing cultural values and social norms that tend to generate stigma. HIV/AIDS-related social stigma is inextricably linked with its predominantly sexual transmission in Sub-Saharan Africa. PLWHA most commonly experience external (or attributed) and internal (self) stigma, known in the 'hidden distress model' as enacted and felt stigma, respectively (Alonzo and Reynolds 1995; Scambler 1984). Internal/self-stigma, characterized by the shame of being sero-positve, results in self-blaming, and external/attributed stigma is marked by oppressive fear and often results in discrimination and socioeconomic marginalization.

Recent studies are shedding light on the relationship between social capital and stigmatizing attitudes. One study in a South African community, for instance, found the social capital components of empowerment, trust, and group membership to be associated with self-stigma and safety and trust with attributed stigma (Chiu et al. 2008). In such a context, stigma can seriously affect HIV-positive persons both socioeconomically and psychologically, further aggravating their poor physical health.

The menace of AIDS as a highly stigmatizing disease is exacerbated by its power to draw a strong negative societal response against infected individuals (Clarke 2001). As a result, infected persons are likely to be socially stigmatized to the extent they may be rejected, discriminated against, or forced into isolation, often leading to depression and denial of essential services and support. PLWHA themselves have reported that the challenges of AIDS-related social stigma can be far more painful and damaging than the disease itself (McKee et al. 2004). A number of studies have found high exposure to stigma by PLWHA in a wide range of settings in Sub-Saharan Africa (Mhloyi 2008; Mugabe 2005; Muiruri 2008; Pankhurst et al. 2008). The stigma occurred in the family and household, the neighborhood, workplaces, public institutions including health facilities and schools, community organizations, and the wider society. Therefore, infected people are likely to encounter stigmatization and discrimination in both family and community settings. Indeed, AIDS-induced stigma and discrimination are so pervasive that PLWHA suffer these challenges even at the hands of those they expect or trust to be their providers of care and protection. In this regard, many of the study reports coming particularly from eastern and southern Africa have shown that, contrary to cultural expectations, many HIV-positive persons experience blame, rejection, and other negative attitudes meted out by close relatives, including both affines and consanguines. Accordingly, the best-known sociocultural capital available in traditional societies, including kinship ties, may fail to function as networks of trust and help for PLWHA because of the stigma attached to the disease.

Men have been widely blamed for bringing the virus into their households, as illustrated by findings from a study in Zimbabwean towns (Mhloyi 2008). Those in the study who disclosed their HIV-positive status to their wives complained of suffering consequences in the form of constant blame and accusation from relatives of their wives. The study also described some incidents in which children, reportedly under the influence of in-laws, bitterly accused their fathers of infecting and killing their mothers. The study indicated that in the context of sociocultural beliefs and attitudes that accuse wives of sorcery when their husbands die, mothers-in-law and other relatives of the diseased tend to accuse AIDS widows of having bewitched their husbands who died of AIDS.

A study from Addis Ababa, Ethiopia, suggests that despite some recent improvements made in connection with external stigma, HIV-positive people continue to be stigmatized, shunned, and discriminated against by family members and close relatives (Pankhurst et al. 2008). Such attitudes resulted in ostracism; forced confinement to the home; and refusal to eat together or share clothes, utensils, and space with the infected individuals.

Beyond the family environment, PLWHA experience similarly pervasive social stigma and discrimination at workplaces and public institutions. The discrimination may come even from health professionals who are supposed to provide service and assistance as a matter of professional ethics. Studies conducted in Western countries revealed that some physicians avoided treating HIV-infected persons if they had the choice, and they were not comfortable being around high-risk groups (Taylor 1999). Similarly, studies from Ethiopia and Uganda report that HIV-positive people experience stigmatization and discrimination at health institutions at the hands of health workers. According to a study by Nuwagaba (2008), 10.5% of people in a group of PLWHA interviewed in Uganda were not able to access medical services at health facilities because of the negative attitudes of physicians. Similar incidents of stigmatization and discrimination against PLWHA at health service facilities and by community organizations, particularly by funeral associations (*iddirs*) have been documented in Ethiopia (Pankhurst et al. 2008).

Stigma and discrimination can seriously curtail PLWHA's use of health services and participation in community organizations; they may withdraw their membership or decide against joining new organizations because of felt or actual neglect and rejection or outright exclusion. Pankhurst et al. (2008) showed that some *iddirs* in Addis Ababa went to the extent of forcing PLWHA to discontinue their membership or denying membership to others. In some cases, the worry that their sero-status might be exposed (self-stigmatization) kept PLWHA from joining these community organizations or caused them to withdraw from them. Thus enacted AIDS stigma at both family and community levels can have profound and complex consequences on infected and affected individuals that severely affect their ability to cope with the emotional and physiological challenges of the disease.

Besides its adverse effects on the emotional health and morale of infected people, AIDS-related stigma acts as an enormous barrier to making positive changes in social and individual behavior (McKee et al. 2004). In respect to sero-status disclosure, many studies (Mhloyi 2008; Muiruri 2008; Pankhurst et al. 2008) from Sub-Saharan African countries reported that because of fear of enacted stigma, PLWHA commonly delayed revealing their infection status or did so only to a limited number of trusted people. The same studies pointed out that many PLWHA were reluctant to disclose their status even to immediate family members and relatives such as spouses, siblings, children, and in-laws. They were discouraged from coming forward primarily for fear of blame, rejection, and other negative consequences. Some PLWHA who disclosed their HIV status even reported having experienced blame and rejection by the very people in whom they confided.

As a result, PLWHA commonly find it difficult to choose between two coping strategies: They are torn between keeping their situation secret to avoid becoming the target of enacted stigma, discrimination, and abandonment by the family and revealing the truth in the expectation that being open makes it easier for them to find psychosocial and economic support. Because of this dilemma, it is common for infected persons to experience emotional and psychosocial problems resulting from both enacted and felt stigma, also known as 'self-stigmatization', and associated discrimination. Thus AIDS-related stigma seriously undermines the capacity of PLWHA to effectively cope with the impacts of AIDS, with adverse consequences on their care, treatment, and support-seeking behavior. Fear of stigma prevents them from disclosing their sero-status, hindering them from approaching kin groups, friends, or service providers for treatment services and psychosocial and economic support (Clarke 2001; McKee et al. 2004).

Impacts on households

The socioeconomic interaction between HIV-affected and nonaffected households has been changing to the disadvantage of the former in recent years (Mhloyi 2008; Muiruri 2008). It is common for affected households to exhaust their resource and savings on HIV-induced health care expenditures. Many end up selling their assets and borrowing from formal and informal credit institutions, incurring huge debts. Consequently, the socioeconomic status of affected households changes, as does their relationships with the nonaffected. This situation often necessitates a reallocation of resources within and between households. In an effort to mitigate the effects of AIDS, many affected households divert resources from economically viable activities to covering AIDS-related health care expenses and funeral costs. In regard to interhousehold relationships, AIDS has induced the reallocation of resources from the affected to the nonaffected, aggravating the level of poverty of the former and negatively impacting on their welfare (Mhloyi 2008; Mugabe 2005).

Social inequities are major drivers of HIV/AIDS, with marginalized females especially vulnerable to infection, as pointed out in previous chapters. Once poor individuals or household are infected, they are more likely to remain poor or even regress to more chronic conditions of poverty. This two-way link between poverty and HIV/AIDS represents a peculiar development dilemma about which little has been written. Addressing one necessitates addressing the other also. Poverty contributes to the spread of AIDS and therefore needs to be addressed in any discussion of solutions to the HIV/AIDS crisis. On the other hand, because HIV infection often leads households to chronic and perpetual poverty, it must be given attention in devising poverty alleviation efforts (Nattrass 2004; see also Chapter 5 in this volume).

Although the traditional African nuclear and extended family system continues as the central social unit responsible for ensuring the emotional bond of caring and overall well-being of members, the AIDS epidemic has burdened families with enormous psychosocial and economic consequences. The AIDS crisis has necessitated adaptive changes in structure, size, and social roles, but these adaptations have adversely affected the resilience and coping capacity of families and households. Many studies in eastern and southern Africa have found that affected households come under heavy socio-demographic and economic pressures; they experience the loss of social support networks, household disintegration, conflict between and separation of spouses, disagreements with children and in-laws, widowhood, and orphanhood (Barnett and Whiteside 2006, p. 197; Collins and Leibbrandt 2007; Mhloyi 2008; Mugabe 2005; Pankhurst et al. 2008). AIDS-afflicted household members, children of PLWHA in particular but also caregivers, face social stigma and discrimination at school and in other community settings that extend from infected parents, further discussed in Chapter 9.

AIDS mortality has changed household characteristics, particularly size and composition, and given rise to new types of families, including child-, widow-, and grandparent-headed families. For instance, 3% of the sample households studied by Mhloyi (2008) in a rural district in Zimbabwe were sibling-headed and 7% were grandparent-headed. The predominance of single-parent- and dual-orphan-headed households render these units particularly vulnerable socioeconomically. Dual AIDS orphans – those bereft of both mother and father – headed some households. Mugabe (2005) found that in Uganda 5% of the grandparents heading households were aged 73–77; they had lost their sons and daughters to AIDS and were taking care of their grandchildren.

By inducing the emergence of new types of households, the HIV/AIDS epidemic has also caused reallocation of traditional social roles, rights, and obligations among family members. Many AIDS orphans are forced to take the burden of adult responsibilities prematurely. They are increasingly assuming adult roles as caregivers of infected household members before and after the death of parents. In a high-prevalence rural district in western Kenya, children helped care for their ill parents, grandparents, siblings, and other people in the community either because of sociocultural reasons, because there was nobody else to provide care, or because they felt a family or moral duty to do so (Skovdal 2011). A number of studies from Sub-Saharan Africa report that new households that emerge after the death of one or both household heads are highly vulnerable; their ability to survive as socioeconomic units is tenuous because their income-producing capacity tends to be weaker as they are managed by orphaned children or elderly grandparents, who are dependent members under normal circumstances. In its most severe form, AIDS can cause households to dissolve as parents die and children are sent to relatives for care and upbringing (AVERT 2011a; UNAIDS 2006).

However, the adverse effects of HIV/AIDS are neither equally distributed nor uniformly felt among the different types of households. Rather, the scope and intensity of the impacts are more likely to be wider and more severe on poor households headed by females, children, and elderly persons. Moreover, impacts of AIDS are not equally distributed even among members of the same household. Infected and affected household members are differentially impacted along gender, age, and socioeconomic lines. HIV-infected and affected women, for example, are burdened with the multiple responsibilities of caregivers of the sick, widowed household heads, and guardians of orphaned grandchildren. Affected girls experience more severe impacts than boys due to the different social roles they customarily have to play. If orphaned, they are more likely to drop out of school than boys, and as breadwinners of affected households they sometimes resort to engaging in high-risk sexual activities to produce an income. Similarly, many mothers, grandmothers, and other female family members themselves are vulnerable because they remain sexually active, partly through the cultural institution of widow inheritance, as reported in a study in Kampala (Nyanzi 2011). Mhloyi (2008) found in Zimbabwe that many affected women, especially grandmothers and young girls, engage in commercial sex to support their families. As the main caregivers of bedridden AIDS patients in the family, women are also directly exposed to infection. The Mhloyi study revealed that in most instances, husbands fall sick and die before their wives, burdening the women with the responsibility of providing care and support not only for their sick husbands but also for paternal orphans.

Orphanhood is one of the most outstanding demographic and socioeconomic impacts of AIDS. In many Sub-Saharan communities, grandparents and other female relatives provide by far the most support to AIDS orphans, yet they are highly vulnerable to deprivations, abuse, and food insecurity (UNAIDS 2006). Orphans placed under the guardianship of extended family members are likely to encounter a number of challenges. Poor guardians may give priority to their own children in schooling and providing other necessities, subjecting orphans to exploitation, neglect, and abuse, including sexual violence. Mhloyi (2008) found in Zimbabwean communities that even uncles, who are culturally expected to be custodians of deceased brothers' children and wives, may inherit the property of the dead fathers of AIDS orphans and then abandon them. Mhloyi also found that orphans, especially girls, neglected and abandoned by kin guardians are further exposed to labor exploitation and sexual abuse, mostly from families employing them to do domestic work, increasing their risk of HIV infection. Other challenges faced by orphans in foster homes and orphanages are described in Chapter 9.

AIDS orphans are differentially impacted based on their orphanhood status as single or dual, maternal or paternal orphans. Mugabe (2005) reported from Ugandan communities that dual orphans are more severely impacted than single-parent orphans, while maternal orphans are likely to fare far better than their paternal counterparts. Similarly, Mhloyi (2008) found that more dual orphans dropped out of school in Masvingo Province in Zimbabwe than paternal and maternal orphans. In terms of overall well-being, paternal orphans tend to be more adversely affected than maternal orphans, and dual orphans more than single-parent children.

Continuing AIDS-associated morbidity, treatment, care, and mortality create a wave of intergenerational impacts on the well-being of households and orphans. Mugabe (2005) reported that the welfare of affected rural households in Uganda deteriorated noticeably due to AIDS-induced permanent loss of employment, exhaustion of savings, increased borrowing, mounting debt, and depletion of productive assets. Eventually, many households were left with little means of survival and no resources to meet medical expenses for the treatment of AIDS-related health problems or to send their children to school.

As important household resources are depleted to meet health care and funeral costs, AIDS orphans face difficulties surviving by themselves into adulthood. They may become a burden to relatives, who may relocate from their neighborhood or community setting and siblings, resulting in the separation of family members (AVERT 2011b). Studies of HIV/AIDS impacts in nine of the ten regions of Ghana (Sory et al. 2011), in Zimbabwe (Mugabe 2005), and among rural households in Uganda (Mhloyi 2008) found that significantly fewer children from AIDS-affected than unaffected households attended school. Similarly, children from affected households who attended school missed more classes, were less attentive when present, and suffered from self-imposed isolation and stigmatization (Mhloy 2008; Mugabe 2005). These trends are likely to exacerbate socioeconomic inequalities and AIDS impacts into future generations.

Impacts on communities

The impacts of the AIDS pandemic at the individual, household, and community levels are closely interrelated. The sociocultural and demographic impacts of HIV/AIDS are multifaceted and pose serious challenges to the social fabric of communities, endangering the stability and continuity of cultural norms, social networks, institutions, and organizations. As a long-term event, the pandemic can severely disrupt the functioning of informal community institutions. Mortality and morbidity stretch and then break traditional support systems and threaten the economic, social, and cultural viability of households and communities, permitting a sense of fear, fatalism, and helplessness to reign.

The major impacts of HIV/AIDS at the community level include changes in population structure, increased orphanhood and dependency ratios, loss of labor and production time, stepped-up exploitation of natural resources, and the undermining of traditional institutions. A study of the socioeconomic impacts of HIV/AIDS in Zimbabwe identified rising orphanhood, increases in morbidity and mortality, deepening poverty, and family disintegration as the principal consequences of HIV/AIDS at the community level and noted that community time and labor were diverted from productive economic activities to voluntary home-based care, visiting the sick, and attending funerals (Mhloyi 2008).

Changes in the demographic structure of many HIV/AIDS-affected communities have increased the dependency ratio through the loss of economically productive members of the population, leaving a rising number of AIDS orphans and elderly without family support. Also seriously endangered by the pandemic is social capital such as customary institutions and community-based organizations. In particular, increased HIV/AIDS morbidity and mortality directly affect funeral associations and institutions caring for orphans. Pankhurst et al. (2008) drew attention to this situation, emphasizing that traditional funeral associations (*iddirs*), the most affected community-based organizations in Ethiopia, are threatened to the point of disintegration. The researchers underscored that *iddirs* suffered high death rates among their members, which in turn required increased payouts to families and expenditure of resources and labor for funerals. Shiferaw (2002) and Pankhurst and Haile Mariam (2004) also noted that *iddirs* were increasingly disintegrating under the pressures of high AIDS-induced death rates among their members and the resultant depletion of resources.

There is mounting evidence that the HIV/AIDS-related demographic and socioeconomic changes in Sub-Saharan Africa are contributing to nonsustainable use of natural resources (Oromasionwu et al. 2011). For instance, households and communities experiencing AIDS-related mortality of their main income earners become more dependent on natural resources, particularly fuel wood, wild foods, and water, as low-cost substitutes for more sustainable resources. According to the Africa Biodiversity Collaboration Group, this coping strategy, which was confined in the pre-AIDS era mostly to times of seasonal food shortages, famines, and war, is resulting in accelerated degradation and destruction of often-scarce natural resources and undermining environmental stewardship. The urgency of ensuring sustainability of common-property natural resources in Sub-Saharan Africa calls for further studies and mitigation of this understudied problem (Hunter et al. 2011).

Another human–environment relationship bearing on HIV is transactional sex of fishermen around Lake Victoria. Due to increasing lake water pollution around towns, commercial fish have migrated to cleaner areas of the lake, requiring more extensive fishing excursions that require fishermen to spend longer periods away from their wives. A thriving 'sex for fish' relationship, known as *'jaboya'* in Nyanza, has developed between fishermen and local women at distant fish-landing sites, where the fishermen must sell their catch quickly in the absence of refrigeration on boats. These sexual relationships with multiple partners, combined with widespread resistance to condom use, have greatly increased HIV risk in the area, a situation reported also from other parts of Africa (Mojola 2010). The two studies summarized here reveal complex relationships among HIV/AIDS, livelihoods, and the environment that must be expected to exist in many other forms in Sub-Saharan Africa and that demand the attention of researchers and planners who try to contextualize HIV/AIDS in African subsistence economies.

Impacts on the private sector workplace

The workforce and the production of many private firms have been significantly affected by HIV/AIDS. Small-scale enterprises and manufacturing firms in high-prevalence HIV communities have experienced a decline in productivity, profitability, and welfare of employees due to long-term illness and deaths among the labor force, management, and business owners. Moreover, debilitating illnesses and deaths present great challenges to infected workers in the form of health problems and resulting stigma and discrimination. In terms of economic impact, increased direct and indirect costs and declines in productivity, profitability, and competitiveness are common burdens for companies in affected communities (UNAIDS 2006). These relationships in southern African companies are examined in Chapter 7.

Infected workers are likely to encounter workplace discrimination meted out by employers and managers or coworkers. In Addis Ababa, Pankhurst et al. (2008) reported incidents in which microenterprise owners dismissed HIV-positive employees for fear customers would stigmatize their businesses. In Nairobi, Muiruri (2008) found that employers discriminately urged infected workers to retire early, denied them promotion and training opportunities, and imposed compulsory HIV testing when hiring. On the other hand, worker attrition due to prolonged sickness and resultant death, provision of health benefits, and costs of replacing employees are enormous challenges for the affected firms.

The economic impact of HIV/AIDS poses a serious threat to the labor market in heavily infected communities, depleting the labor pool of trained and experienced manpower and limiting employment opportunities. Loss of workers and workdays due to AIDS-related diseases and the need to care for the sick are bound to result in significant decline in productivity, loss of earning, and attrition in skill and experience (Rosen 2003, cited in Muiruri 2008). Studying food, beverage, and tobacco factories in Nairobi, Muiruri (2008) reported the common perception that firms were primarily concerned about the financial cost of HIV/AIDS. Firm owners considered reduced productivity, profit, and management performance to be among the most common consequences of the HIV pandemic and labor efficiency and productivity to be directly or indirectly affected by HIV/AIDS-induced morbidity and mortality.

Fear of the disease and associated stigma adversely affect interactions and social relationships among workers. The practice of discriminating against PLWHA causes sero-positive employees to enter into a constrained relationship with employers, managers, and other coworkers. A study of rural microenterprises in Botswana found that troubled relationships between infected workers and employers/managers affected management performance (Kapunda 2007). The study described the refusal of some HIV-positive employees to be transferred to sections considered suitable for them. Widespread absenteeism due to attendance at funerals and workers taking time off to care for infected family members or relatives as well as deterioration of workers' physical and mental capacities added to the problems managers and owners faced in dealing with HIV-infected workers. The worsening relationships often contributed to low labor productivity and poor management performance (Kapunda 2007). Labor productivity is often further reduced because AIDS-related demands on workers' time tend to reduce the supply and quality of labor and force firms to incur increasing production costs and loss of profit.

Although microenterprises and large manufacturing firms are both vulnerable to the impacts of AIDS, they tend to be differentially affected by the pandemic. Being primarily family- or household-managed, microenterprises are more seriously impacted than larger firms. Kapunda (2007) noted that the relatively greater impacts on microenterprises were particularly severe for businesses with five and fewer workers. Because women, children, and other household members are often the workforce of small businesses, these enterprises suffer greatly when workers are HIV-infected or affected; owners cannot afford to replace them with paid workers.

Responses to HIV/AIDS at different levels

Individual- and household-level responses

The active involvement of the directly affected social actors (individuals and families) is critical in sustaining collective efforts in the prevention of HIV through voluntary counseling and testing (VCT), the reduction of vulnerability and high-risk behavior, and impact mitigation (Wegelin-Schuringa 2006). The discussion in this section revolves around documented local experiences of the adaptive responses of infected individuals and affected social actors at the family level.

As PLWHA deal with the various challenges they encounter, they develop and use different adaptive and coping strategies, as described by Pankhurst et al. (2008), including emotion-focused and problem-focused responses. At the individual level, a common initial response to being diagnosed

HIV-positive is shock, usually with short-term psychological distress and sometimes with severe depression involving thoughts of suicide. However, the negative psychosocial response to testing positive tends to change over time, and sero-positive people try to manage mainly through active or positive coping mechanisms (Taylor 1999). Individual coping strategies are also likely to change due to changing psychological, sociocultural, and economic factors. Alonzo and Reynolds (1995) argued that the nature of stigma HIV-positive persons experience and the coping strategies they develop vary based on the stigma trajectory, which in turn depends on the development of their biophysical health status, that is, the trajectory of their illness.

Several studies (Mhloyi 2008; Mugabe 2005; Pankhurst et al. 2008) reveal that PLWHA develop and employ a number of mechanisms to cope with the sociocultural, psychological, and economic impacts of HIV/AIDS. Pankhurst et al. (2008) found that the major coping strategies of PLWHA in Addis Ababa included disclosing sero-status to family members, friends, employers, or the community; joining PLWHA associations; seeking help from care and psychosocial support organizations; and seeking religious healing.

As an important negative accessory of HIV/AIDS, stigma poses incapacitating challenges for PLWHA. Felt stigma especially has important behavioral implications in terms of influencing people's response to testing HIV-positive and their coping behavior (Scambler 1984). Depending on the type of coping strategy they chose in relation to status disclosure, PLWHA are faced with the problem of 'information management' if they decide to keep their sero-status secret or 'impression management' if their status is known (Clarke 2001).

Concerning the disclosure of sero-status, the coping strategy adopted by PLWHA may take one of three forms: absolute secretiveness, selective disclosure, and full disclosure. Pankhurst et al. (2008) found that the majority of a PLWHA sample population in Addis Ababa employed the selective disclosure mechanism, disclosing their status to spouses, close relatives, and friends. Many others kept their status an absolute secret. Only a few made public their HIV-positive status and became involved in mass educational campaigns to sensitize and inform the population about HIV risk. Mugabe (2005) described similar proactive behavior of some PLWHA who, with the help of some nongovernmental organizations (NGOs), set up drama groups to sensitize community residents to HIV/AIDS issues and generate income for their survival. In the quest for spiritual and psychological remedy, some joined 'born-again' churches.

Most affected households adopt a range of coping mechanisms in response to social and economic challenges. These responses may involve demographic changes in the size, structure, and function of households as well as economic changes, including alterations in labor organization, consumption, and spending patterns. Evidence from Zimbabwe and Uganda indicates that affected households are more likely to use different strategies to deal with the multifaceted effects of the epidemic. Mugabe (2005) found in a rural Ugandan community that responses to deteriorating food security included resorting to cheaper and lower quality consumption items, reducing the number of meals, borrowing cash or in-kind items, and selling assets. To cope with the loss of household labor due to long-term illness and/or death, some households forced children to quit school and become involved in the care of the sick and help generate income. Mangoma et al. (2008) and Mhloyi (2008) reported that in towns in Zimbabwe some female orphans felt compelled to engage in commercial sex work to meet family needs. Another strategy for coping with AIDS-related food insecurity was to reduce family size by putting some of the children under the care of relatives and migrating to take new jobs.

Although extended family networks have been weakened in many high HIV-prevalence African societies due to AIDS-induced socioeconomic and demographic changes, they continue to be the most important sociocultural resource available to AIDS orphans and affected families. Typically, siblings, grandparents, uncles, and aunts are responsible for caring for AIDS orphans and orphan-headed households. In the case of the death of either spouse or both, affected households make readjustments to cope with the resulting difficulties. Usually, the responsibility for the care of orphaned children rests with close relatives, underscoring the role that the extended family plays in coping with the impacts of HIV/AIDS on households (Mhloyi 2008).

In the subsistence farming economies of Sub-Saharan Africa, HIV/AIDS impacts societies at the livelihood and household levels. The immensity of the burden of the epidemic in this region is largely due to prevailing socioeconomic conditions: (1) the great majority of the population in these countries is poor and inadequately informed about the causation and treatment of HIV and lives in rural areas, (2) most countries depend on agriculture or mining, and (3) the heaviest burden of the epidemic falls on rural areas when migrants return home once they develop full-blown AIDS. These and other population movements, together with variable vulnerabilities and responses to HIV/AIDS in different communities and neighborhoods, appear to have been instrumental in the geographic distribution of infection and its impacts in rural communities, an area requiring further study. The finding that the impacts of the epidemic vary among neighborhoods and communities suggests that responses need to be directed to households and livelihoods (Muller 2004; UNAIDS 2010). Considering that individual and group behavior is influenced by multiple personal, sociocultural, economic, and structural/environmental factors, further research is required to identify linkages and responses amenable to prevention and mitigation strategies.

As mentioned previously, some evidence suggests that households in Sub-Saharan Africa that experience the death of income earners are increasingly relying on community-owned natural resources for subsistence and to generate revenue, particularly fuel wood, wild food, and medicinal plants and water. The intensified use of scarce natural resources may exacerbate their degradation and destruction, deemphasize stewardship, and further jeopardize the livelihood of populations (Hunter et al. 2011; Oromasionwu et al. 2011, see also Lopez 2008). This under-researched problem demands further study to enable planners and affected communities to develop appropriate and effective remedial measures.

Community and workplace responses

Collective actions are increasingly being taken by community-based organizations, businesses, and volunteers to help the increasing number of PLWHA, AIDS orphans, widows, and elderly cope with the socioeconomic and cultural impacts of the disease. In addition to efforts to mitigate impacts on the infected and affected, mobilization of collective resources for HIV prevention is an important community response. Educational campaigns to create awareness about various aspects of HIV/AIDS, condom distribution, and the promotion of voluntary VCT are the main efforts in the community and workplace environments, although new prevention approaches are widening the choices available to health authorities and companies (see Chapters 8 and 9).

Some traditional self-help and support groups, particularly traditional funeral associations (*iddirs*) in Ethiopia, are playing an active role as entry points to community mobilization against the spread of HIV/AIDS and its impacts. With a view to responding more effectively to the emerging challenges of the pandemic, these grassroots institutions have been undergoing changes. *Iddirs* have been revising their customary objectives, by-laws, and scope of activities; they try to expand their networks to cooperate with other *iddirs*, government organizations, and NGOs toward more effective preventive and mitigation responses. Hence, *iddirs* currently operate beyond their traditional mandates of providing burial services and payouts on death to their members; a number of them now participate in the delivery of care and support services to PLWHA and AIDS orphans. Specifically, *iddirs* now offer psychosocial counseling, cash payments, nutritional support, and education assistance for the infected and affected (Pankhurst et al. 2008).

HIV/AIDS has become a major threat to the work environment and is becoming an acute workplace and community issue in most Sub-Saharan African countries (ILO 2001). Workplace HIV/AIDS policies are increasingly considered to be central to developing and implementing HIV/AIDS prevention, care, and support programs for workers and their families. Interventions are most difficult to implement in small businesses in the informal sector because of lack of capacity. Studies in Botswana (Kapunda 2007) and Kenya (Muiruri 2008) found that collective responses for preventing the spread of HIV and mitigating its impacts are generally weaker at small-scale industrial enterprises than at medium and large manufacturing firms. Kapunda (2007) noted that none of the rural microenterprises he studied in Botswana had any AIDS-related policies or educational pro-grams in place, indicating that the mobilization of collective action to mitigate impacts and prevent HIV/AIDS has been inadequate at small firms. But Muiruri's (2008) study of the food, beverage, and tobacco manufac-turing sectors in Nairobi reveals that education and awareness creation programs were well established in most of the manufacturing firms studied, although they had weak policy frameworks and institutional mechanisms for combating HIV/AIDS. Muiruri (2008) reported that medium and large-scale enterprises, mostly multinational manufacturing firms, implemented workplace HIV/AIDS programs and strategies to prevent the spread of HIV and mitigate its impact. The major response strategies adopted were the formulation of workplace HIV/AIDS policies; awareness; education and pre-vention programs; and the provision of treatment, care, and support services to HIV-positive workers.

Government responses

The multidimensional impacts of HIV/AIDS on individuals, households, and communities have cumulative economic, political, and security effects at the national level, exacerbating existing problems of capacity, sustainability, and vulnerability. Countrywide collective interventions are essential in mobilizing and coordinating efforts to stem the epidemic. The political commitment of governments has become an overriding factor in the mobi-lization of available social and material resources to control the epidemic and mitigate its effects (McKee et al. 2004).

The Sub-Saharan-wide analysis by Robinson (2011) shows that the orga-nizational and structural context of individual countries dating back to the 1980s and 1990s strongly predicted HIV prevalence and incidence at the national level between 2001 and 2009. Countries that forged population policies in the aftermath of the postcolonial era, particularly Senegal and Uganda, were able to promote reproductive health infrastructure and sexual behavior change. Such efforts, or lack thereof, in conjunction with political and cultural factors, impacted condom use, number of sexual partners, and age at first sex and drove overall HIV outcomes.

In the course of HIV/AIDS response, the limited government interven-tions initially consisted of health sector-specific activities and programs that considered HIV/AIDS as a mere public health problem. As the challenges of controlling and preventing the epidemic proved to be complex, and when it became clear that HIV/AIDS affected all aspects of human life, governments gradually mounted multisectoral responses (McKee et al. 2004).

The impacts of the AIDS epidemic in Sub-Saharan Africa have extended far beyond households and communities; they affect whole societies, not sparing institutions at higher levels of social organization. In response, the commitment of national governments, supported technically and finan-cially by international organizations, has played a pivotal role in curbing the spread of the virus and mitigating the consequences with the objective of providing universal access to treatment, care and support by 2015 (UNAIDS 2010; WHO 2010). HIV prevalence rates have significantly declined where there has been the political will to make multisectoral efforts to mobilize resources and coordinate actions, an issue further addressed below and in subsequent chapters. The major contributions of committed political leadership have been in the areas of policy formulation on HIV/AIDS prevention, care and support, impact mitigation, mobilization and coordination of various stakeholders, and the creation of enabling environments for strategic interventions.

Government shortcomings in achieving stated national HIV/AIDS goals are inevitably associated with lack of resources and experience in dealing with an epidemic of unprecedented proportions but in some cases also with deficiencies in organization and the politicization of HIV/AIDS, as in South Africa and Zimbabwe. In South Africa, the current HIV/AIDS program was implemented only after long confrontations between AIDS activists and the central government (Grebe 2008), and in Zimbabwe the government's response to the epidemic has been compromised by several political and social crises (AVERT 2011c). Although South Africa has made great progress in recent years in rolling out antiretroviral therapy (ART) and reducing the incidence of HIV infection, it has encountered problems of cost containment; financing; and replacing its hospital-based, staff-intensive model of ART services delivery with an alternative, community-based model (Navarro et al. 2010).

The case of Uganda, widely praised for its ability to reduce HIV prevalence from 15% in 1991 to 5% in 2001 through the mobilization and coordination of sociocultural and religious leadership, civil society, NGOs, and government institutions (Hogle 2002, in McKee et al. 2004; Opio et al. 2008), highlights the role of outside stakeholders and the unexpected effects of the ART rollout. The government's shift in prevention policy away from the ABC (abstinence, be faithful, condoms) approach to the US-backed abstinence program and the availability of free ART since 2004 have been associated by several investigators with increased HIV risk behavior and a slight increase in prevalence in recent years (AVERT 2011d). Moreover, limited access to ART in South Africa has recently been associated by the public with a lack of political will (Muula 2008). These examples of government shortcomings in HIV/AIDS programs indicate the need for further research to identify underlying bottlenecks and examine possible avenues for effective, equitable, and sustainable prevention, mitigation, and control approaches.

These various scenarios indicate that the state has a vital role to play as a principal actor at a high level of social organization. The mobilization of local stakeholders, including businesses, public service institutions, and community-based organizations, as part of decentralization drives and up-scaling of HIV prevention and AIDS treatment programs has been the major intervention strategy of most governments. Indigenous and international NGOs and donors are also playing major roles in assisting states and communities in supporting this multisectoral effort.

Conclusion

The socioeconomic and cultural challenges of HIV/AIDS experienced at the individual, household, workplace, and community levels as well as at higher levels of social organization have generated a wide range of responses in Sub-Saharan Africa. The major hardships experienced by infected individuals are stigmatization and discrimination; death of spouses, mostly husbands; and the burden of assisting and supporting sick partners and paternal or maternal orphans. Fear and prejudice caused by stigma from within the family or the community and self-stigmatization, or felt stigma, are other consequences to which PLWHA are subjected. Families of PLWHA have been adversely affected by the sociocultural and psychological problems caused by HIV/AIDS of infected household members. The problems have altered inter- and intra-household relationships, transforming the socio-demographic structure of affected households and resulting in the real-location of roles and identities as well as new forms of intra-household interactions. Consequently, the formation of orphan-dominated households and the emergence of households headed by widows, widowers, orphaned children, and elderly family members constitute important changes in household socio-demographic structure.

In the area of socialization processes, newly emerging social and economic relationships have come into being by which AIDS-affected households are forced to interact with nonaffected households and the community. Due to the presence of HIV-infected members in the family, interhousehold social relations of affected families have become constrained. Thus, affected households have experienced prejudice, social distance and 'courtesy' stigma from neighbors. This often means that uninfected family members are stigmatized as well. These changes are bound to have far-reaching implications for existing cultural norms, customs, and traditions of local communities.

Although the least researched of the socioeconomic entities examined in this chapter is the business firm, it is becoming increasingly clear that the epidemic exerts a profound impact in the workplace. Existing information indicates that HIV impacts include increased costs and reduced productivity, which in turn severely affect the profitability and competitiveness of firms. These and other issues needing urgent attention are examined further in Chapter 7.

The role of governments in anti-HIV/AIDS programs, essential as it is, is being modified and reduced as decentralization of governance proceeds and HIV/AIDS services using the primary health care approach are brought closer to and involve the participation of users, further discussed in Chapter 8.

Lastly, certain socioeconomic and cultural aspects of HIV/AIDS require further study; some existing theories, models, and assumptions need revisiting in light of emerging issues, new developments, and evolving government commitments and capabilities.

References

Alonzo, A.A. and Reynolds, N.R. 1995. Stigma, HIV and AIDS: An exploration and elaboration of stigma trajectory. *Social Science and Medicine* 30:303–315.

AVERT. 2011a. *The Impact of HIV & AIDS in Africa.* www.avert.org/aids-impact-africa. htm (accessed 12 December 2011).

AVERT. 2011b. *HIV and AIDS in South Africa.* http://www.avert.org/aidssouthafrica.htm (accessed 12 December 2011).

AVERT. 2011c. *HIV and AIDS in Zimbabwe.* http:///www.avert.org/aids-zimbabwe.htm (accessed 11 December 2011).

AVERT. 2011d. *HIV and AIDS in Uganda.* www.avert.org/aids-uganda.htm (accessed 11 December 2011).

Barnett, T. and Whiteside, A. 2006. *AIDS in the Twenty-First Century: Disease and Globalization.* 2nd ed. New York: Palgrave Macmillan.

Chiu, J., Grobbelaar, J., Sikkema, K. et al. 2008. HIV-related stigma and social capital in South Africa. *AIDS Education and Prevention* 20:519–530.

Clarke, A. 2001. *The Sociology of Healthcare.* Harlow, UK: Prentice Hall.

Collins, D.L. and Leibbrandt, M. 2007. The financial impact of HIV/AIDS on poor households in South Africa. *AIDS* 21(Suppl. 7):S75–S81.

ECA (Economic Commission for Africa). n.d. *Africa: The Socioeconomic Impact of HIV/AIDS.* Addis Ababa: ECA, Commission on HIV/AIDS and Governance in Africa.

Grebe, E. 2008. *Transitional Networks of Influence in South African Treatment Activities.* AIDS2031 Working Paper No. 5.Cape Town: Center for Social Science Research.

Hunter, L.M., Twine, W. and Johnson, A. 2011. Adult mortality and natural resource use in rural South Africa: Evidence from the Agincourt health and demographic surveillance site. *Society & Natural Resources* 24:256–275.

ILO. 2001. *An ILO Code of Practice on HIV/AIDS and the World of Work. Global Program on HIV/AIDS and the World of Work.* Geneva: International Labor Office.

Kapunda, S.M. 2007. Socioeconomic impact of HIV/AIDS on rural small-scale industrial sub-sector: The case of selected villages in Botswana. In OSSREA (ed.), *The HIV/AIDS Challenge in Africa, an Impact and Response Assessment: The Case of Botswana,* pp. 93–165. Addis Ababa: OSSREA.

Lopez, P. 2008. The subversive links between HIV/AIDS and the forest sector. In Colver, C.J.P. (ed.), *Human Health and Forests: A Global Overview of Issues, Practice and Policy,* pp. 221–238. London: Earthscan.

Mangoma, J., Chimbari, M. and Dhlomo, E. 2008. An enumeration of orphans and analysis of the problem and wishes of orphans: The case of Kariba, Zimbabwe. *Journal of Social Aspects of HIV/AIDS* 5(3):120–128.

McKee, N., Bertrand J. and Becker-Benton, A. 2004. *Strategic Communication in the HIV/AIDS Epidemic.* New Delhi: Sage Publications.

Mhloyi, M.M. 2008. Report on the social and economic impact of HIV/AIDS on rural households in Masvingo Province: The case of Gutu district. In OSSREA (ed.), *The HIV/AIDS Challenge in Africa, an Impact and Response Assessment: The Case of Zimbabwe,* pp. 43–109. Addis Ababa, OSSREA.

Moime, W.M. 2009. The effect of orphanhood on the psychological development of pre-primary and primary school children. PhD dissertation, University of South Africa, Cape Town.

Mojola, S.A. 2010. Fishing in dangerous waters: Ecology, gender and economy in HIV risk. *Social Science and Medicine* 72:149–156.

Mugabe, R. 2005. The impact of HIV/AIDS on rural household welfare in Rukungiri District. Unpublished paper, CODESRIA HIV/AIDS Program, Addis Ababa University, Addis Ababa.

Muiruri, P. 2008. A situational analysis on responses to HIV/AIDS challenges in the food, beverages and tobacco manufacturing sectors in Nairobi City, Kenya. In OSSREA (ed.), *The HIV/AIDS Challenge in Africa, an Impact and Response Assessment: The Case of Kenya*, pp.191–245. Addis Ababa: OSSREA.

Muller, T.R. 2004. *HIV/AIDS and Agriculture in Sub-Saharan Africa: Impacts on Farming Systems, Agricultural Practices and Rural Livelihoods: An Overview and Annotated Bibliography*. Wageningen, The Netherlands: Academic Publishers.

Muula, A. 2008. South Africa's national response to HIV and AIDS treatment: Popular media's perspective. *Croatian Medical Journal* 49:114–119.

Nattrass, N. 2004. *The Moral Economy of AIDS in South Africa*. Cambridge, MA: Cambridge University Press.

Navarro, P., Bekker, L.-G., Blecher, M. et al. 2010. Special report on the state of HIV/AIDS in South Africa. *Global Health Magazine* 16 July. http://www.globalhealthmagazine.com

Nuwagaba, A. 2008. HIV and AIDS in armed conflict situation in northern Uganda. In OSSREA (ed.), *The HIV/AIDS Challenge in Africa, an Impact and Response Assessment: The Case of Uganda*, pp. 1–45. Addis Ababa: OSSREA.

Nyanzi, S. 2011. Ambivalence surrounding elderly widows' sexuality in urban Uganda. *Ageing International* 36:378–400.

Opio, A., Mishra,V., Hong, R. et al. 2008. Trends in HIV-related behaviors and knowledge in Uganda, 1989–2005: Evidence of a shift toward more risk-taking behaviors. *Journal of Acquired Immune Deficiency Syndromes* 49:320–326.

Oromasionwu, C.U., Daniels, K.R., Labrechte, M.J. and Frei, C.R. 2011. The environmental and social influences of HIV/AIDS in sub-Saharan Africa: A focus on rural communities. *International Journal of Environmental Research and Public Health* 8:2967–2979.

Pankhurst, A. and Haile Mariam, D. 2004. The *Iddir* in Ethiopia: Historical development, social functions, and potential role in HIV/AIDS prevention and control. *Northeast African Studies* 7:35–57.

Pankhurst, A., Tesfaye, A., Gebre, A. et al. 2008. Social responses to HIV/AIDS in Addis Ababa, Ethiopia with reference to commercial sex workers, people living with HIV/AIDS and community-based funeral associations in Addis Ababa. In OSSREA (ed.), *The HIV/AIDS Challenge in Africa, an Impact and Response Assessment: The Case of Ethiopia*, pp. 141–309. Addis Ababa: OSSREA.

Robinson, R.S. 2011. From population to HIV: The organizational and structural determinants of HIV outcomes in sub-Saharan Africa. *Journal of the International AIDS Society* 14(Suppl. 2):S6.

Scambler, G. 1984. Perceiving and coping with stigmatizing illness. In Fitzpatrick, R., Kinton, J., Newman, S. et al. (eds.), *The Experience of Illness*, pp. 203–226. London: Tavistok.

Shiferaw, T. 2002. Civil society organizations in poverty alleviation, change and development: The role of iddirs in collaboration with government organizations: The cases of Akaki, Nazareth and Kolfe areas of Addis Ababa (1996–2002). MA thesis, Department of Sociology and Anthropology, Addis Ababa University, Addis Ababa.

Skovdal, M. 2011. Examining the trajectories of children providing care for adults in rural Kenya: Implications for service delivery. *Children and Youth Services Review* 33:1262–1269.

Sory, S., Gyapong, J., Ocran, B. et al. 2011. Economic impact of ARV treatment on persons living with AIDS and their household members. *Abstracts of the International Conference on AIDS and STIs in Africa*, Addis Ababa, Abstract MOPE002.

Taylor, S.E. 1999. *Health Psychology*, 4th ed. Boston: McGraw-Hill.

UNAIDS. 2006. *Report on the Global AIDS Epidemic*, Chapter 4. Geneva: UNAIDS.

UNAIDS. 2009. *AIDS Epidemic Update*. Geneva: UNAIDS.

UNAIDS. 2010. *Report on the Global AIDS Epidemic*. Geneva: UNAIDS.

Wegelin-Schuringa, M. 2006. Local responses to HIV/AIDS from a gender perspective. In van der Kwaak, A. and Wegelin-Schuringa, M. (eds.), *Gender, Society, and Development: A Global Source Book*, pp. 95–108. Amsterdam: Royal Tropical Institute.

WHO. 2010. *Towards Universal Access: Scaling up Priority HIV/AIDS Interventions in the Health Sector: Progress Report 2010*. Geneva: WHO.

Books, papers, websites, and other useful resources for further reading

Lomborg, B. (ed.). 2012. *Rethinking HIV/AIDS Priorities: A Cost-Benefit Analysis.* Cambridge: Cambridge University Press.

Mbonu, N.C., van den Borne, B. and De Vries, N.K. 2009. Stigma of people with HIV/AIDS in Sub-Saharan Africa: A literature review. *Journal of Tropical Medicine* 16 August. doi:10.155/2009/145891

Website for publications by ILO (International Labor Organization). http://www.portal.unesco.org/aids

Website for publications on HIV/AIDS by UNDP. http://www.undp.org/hiv

7

HIV/AIDS and the Mining and Commercial Agricultural Sectors in Southern Africa

Charles Hongoro, Getnet Tadele, and Helmut Kloos

Introduction

The United Nations has reported that 5% of adults in their prime working years (ages 15–49) in Sub-Saharan Africa were infected with HIV in 2009 but between 11% and 26% in the nine continental southern African countries (UNAIDS 2010, p. 181). Although HIV-related incidence, prevalence, and mortality have decreased in recent years, rates are still extraordinarily high in the region, and while the number of people dying from AIDS in southern Africa decreased from 740,000 in 2004 to 610,000 in 2009 (UNAIDS 2010, p. 185), the continuing increase in the number of infected people surviving on antiretroviral therapy (ART) increases costs for many businesses. The impacts of HIV/AIDS on businesses are particularly severe in southern Africa because the region's economies depend on labor-intensive industries that are extremely vulnerable to endogenous factors such as human capital and external shocks, particularly changes in commodity prices and international trade. Impact studies indicate that businesses in the region have been significantly affected by these and other factors (Casale and Whiteside 2006; ILO 2004, p. 18; SABCOHA 2004).

Epidemiological data and information from several studies of HIV infection among the labor forces in mines and commercial farms reveal that migrant workers are particularly vulnerable (Campbell 2003; Corno and de Walque 2012). In the southern African context, there is a need to consider the spatial dynamics of HIV/AIDS linked to the various extensive population movements in the region. The International Organization for Migration (IOM) suggested that vulnerabilities in southern African migrant-dependent businesses, particularly commercial farms, stem not only from individuals' risky behaviors, but also from numerous socioeconomic, demographic, and structural factors. Conceptually the relationship between these factors and vulnerability to HIV/AIDS lends itself to advocacy for structural changes and the implementation of prevention and impact mitigation policies and programs in the mining and agricultural sectors in this region (IOM 2010a; Moreriane 2011).

This chapter describes the context of high HIV vulnerabilities among migrant laborers in mines and on commercial farms in southern Africa, briefly summarizes the policy environment bearing on migrant labor, highlights major impacts on businesses, and summarizes a firm's responses to the epidemic in these workplaces. The chapter ends with recommendations for reducing and mitigating HIV/AIDS impacts at the sectoral and company levels. The mining and commercial agricultural sectors were selected because of the high HIV prevalence in these sectors and their dependence on migrant laborers, whose health and social problems are demanding more attention from governments and companies (ILO 2003).

Labor migration to the mines and commercial farms

Labor migration in southern Africa dates from the middle of the nineteenth century and has been a major factor in the economic development and social dynamics of the region. The volume and complexity of labor migration increased sharply after the collapse of apartheid in South Africa in 1990, after the wars in Mozambique and Angola, and as a result of the turbulent political economy of Zimbabwe. There are no reliable statistics on the volume of different types of migration in the region, and the UN figure of 3.5 million migrants living in the southern African countries in 2000 is probably an underestimate (Crush and Williams 2010) because millions of unregistered migrants tend to avoid immigration and other recording establishments of the government (Crush and Williams 2002).

A survey by the Southern African Migration Program showed that 29% of all migrants entering South Africa in the late 1990s from the main originating countries – Botswana, Lesotho, Mozambique, Namibia, and Zimbabwe – were labor migrants (Crush and Williams 2010). The proportion of foreign-born gold miners increased to 59% of all gold miners in South Africa in 1997 but declined to 38% by 2006 in the wake of the downsizing of mines due to mechanization and declines in gold prices. The motivations for migrating varied greatly, with 67% of the Mozambicans and only 10% of the Botswanans who entered South Africa doing so to work or look for work. Mozambican laborers in the South African gold mines had overtaken laborers from Lesotho as the largest transborder migrant group of gold miners by 2006; Mozambique was the only nation reporting an increase in the number migrating to the mines during the 1990–2006 period. The reasons the number of miners from Mozambique rose during that period of worker layoffs were rumored to be a greater willingness of Mozambican laborers to accept poor working conditions in the mines and the lower HIV rates in Mozambique in the 1990s (Crush and Williams 2010, pp. 8, 10). The latter reason corroborates the widespread sentiment in southern Africa that miners are prone to become HIV-infected (IOM and SAMP 2005). The mining sector is a major source of employment and foreign exchange earnings in southern Africa, where most national economies rely heavily on the extraction of primary commodities such as gold, platinum, copper, diamonds, coal, and other minerals. These primary products support vertical linkages and supply manufacturing industries with raw materials for products destined for local and international markets. Although most countries in southern Africa have large mining sectors, only South Africa currently depends on neighboring countries for laborers. Mines in the other countries employ mostly nationals, including migrants from other regions within the same country (Schachter 2009). In Botswana, for instance, mines employ workers from different parts of the country and house them in company-owned single-sex villages; workers therefore live away from home for lengthy periods and send remittances to their families (Campbell 2008). In Zimbabwe, nearly all of the estimated 100,000 to 300,000 miners working in small- to medium-sized mines are natives living with their families in mining villages (IOM n.d.). Larger numbers of Zimbabweans (1.5–2 million) emigrated to other countries, especially South Africa, but relatively few of them work in mines (IOM 2010c).

Labor migration in southern Africa traditionally involved both formal, or legal, migration – through the recruitment of miners in their home countries by mostly South African corporations – and informal, or illegal, migration across porous borders, mostly by refugees escaping political turmoil and economic instability. While formal migrations have leveled off or even decreased since the enactment of post-apartheid laws that make it more difficult for mining companies to recruit migrant laborers, informal migrations, which meet mainly the demands of the commercial agricultural sector, have increased. South Africa, the major receiving nation for migrants, is estimated to have between 1 and 8 million undocumented migrants (Schachter 2009).

Most migrant mine workers periodically return home to visit their families, with implications for HIV/AIDS, as discussed later in this chapter. Family Health International reported that 11,317 Basotho miners working in South Africa visited their homes in Lesotho on a weekly basis, 60% of the miners from Lesotho returned home monthly, and another 25% returned at least once every three months, mostly to visit families (IOM 2002). While migrant remittances have had a positive impact on the economy of Lesotho and have contributed significantly to the income of rural households there, migrant labor is the key driver of the HIV/AIDS epidemic in Lesotho (IOM 2002).

Agriculture has traditionally been the economic mainstay in most southern African countries where, on average, more than two-thirds of the populations depend on the sector for their livelihood: food, employment, and income (Southern African Development Community 2008). In the countries with few mining and manufacturing firms (Malawi, Angola, Mozambique, and Madagascar), agricultural employment accounts for about three-quarters of all jobs, a significantly larger proportion than in countries with large mining/manufacturing sectors (Draper et al. 2009, p. 9).

Subsistence and commercial farming, although structurally and operationally different, are interdependent in southern Africa because overpopulated and food-insecure subsistence farming areas generate migrant laborers who leave the areas and send remittances home to meet costs of living and farming expenses. Jayne et al. (2006) suggested that high AIDS mortality may reduce land pressure in parts of eastern and southern Africa and thus reduce international migration. Although comprehensive cause-specific mortality and disability data do not exist for agricultural laborers in southern Africa (ILO 2004), the high HIV infection rates in that region may be another factor in migration dynamics, an issue that needs further research.

Most information on migration to commercial farms comes from South Africa. South African commercial farms, mostly in Limpopo, Mpumalanga, Free State, and Northern provinces, employ large numbers of migrant workers from neighboring countries, particularly Lesotho, Mozambique, and Zimbabwe (Crush and Williams 2010; Krieger 2006). South African farmers along these borders prefer to employ female migrants in the canning factories and fields (Ulicki and Crush 2007). In Zimbabwe, a large proportion of the labor force of commercial farms came from Malawi, Zambia, and Mozambique before the collapse of the Zimbabwean economy (IOM and SAMP 2005).

The policy environment

Labor migrants in southern Africa have always been denied the same basic rights as local workers, and several recent changes in labor policies and regulations have further affected migrant laborers negatively (Crush and Williams 2010, p. 35). The downsizing of the mining industry reversed trade union gains that had been made in the 1980s following the 1987 mineworkers' strike by increasing subcontracting of production and nonproduction functions. Subcontracting companies have been hiring more groups vulnerable to exploitation, and the decline of unions associated with this restructuring resulted in a decline in wages, poorer working conditions, less safety, and less job security.

Some governments, large companies, employers' and workers' organizations, and the International Labor Organization have implemented workplace policies aimed at creating conditions amenable to improving the workplace environment for HIV-infected people (AGOA Forum 2001; ILO 2011; IOM 2010c; Rampersad 2010). Key elements of these policies in southern African countries address stigma, employee rights (including nondiscrimination and confidentiality), medical care and treatment, and other management responses (AGOA Forum 2001). However, many workplace policies fall short of adequately covering the rights of migrant workers, particularly in the commercial agricultural sector workforce in southern Africa (ILO 2003; IOM n.d.). Half of 200 companies in the Sub-Saharan region, many in southern Africa, especially smaller and less profitable companies, made no mention of HIV/AIDS in their annual online reports for 2006 (Barako et al. 2010). Even in corporate organizations with workplace policies in place, the issue to what extent they should address HIV/AIDS and disclose its impact on their business as dictated by good corporate governance and shareholder interests has been contentious (Rampersad 2010). Moreover, companies do not always institutionalize workplace policies and translate them into good practice at every level (Kundecha et al. 2011).

HIV/AIDS in the mining sector

A number of epidemiological studies summarized by IOM and SAMP (South African Migration Project) (2005) and Campbell and Williams (1999) reported high HIV infection rates and high-risk living conditions around the mines. Many miners are migrants from poor, distant, rural areas. Most workers employed in this sector are classified as marginalized, with little chance of obtaining formal employment elsewhere due to either lack of proper education or limited job opportunities in other sectors. The living and working conditions for South African miners were described in detail by Campbell (2003), whose situational analysis of a gold mining community portrayed an environment that is highly conducive to HIV transmission. Campbell's and other studies link vulnerability of migrants to HIV/AIDS to elements of their lifestyle – accommodation in company-owned, single-sex hostels and working long periods of time away from their families – together with a thriving sex industry within the vicinity of the mines. Lack of knowledge about HIV/AIDS prevention and transmission and lack of resources facilitate the rapid spread of HIV in mining towns and throughout southern Africa. Mine workers transmit HIV to their spouses and thus to their communities when they return home on vacation or when they get ill from AIDS (Brummer 2002; IOM and SAMP 2005; UNAIDS 2002). A number of studies in different mines, particularly in the Carletonville gold mining complex and in the town of Summertown near Johannesburg, have described the sexual networks and vulnerability contexts in mining towns that render both miners and nearby communities vulnerable to HIV infection. These studies show that not only the miners themselves, but also all members of the wider mining community are at risk (Campbell 2003; IOM and SAMP 2005).

In South Africa, HIV prevalence among gold miners increased from 1.3% in 1990 to 20–30% by 1998 (Sonnenberg et al. 2011). The company-owned mining villages in Zimbabwe, described as a 'colonial legacy' in that they reflected capitalistic methods of labor and cost control, were also highly

conducive to the spread of HIV in the 1990s (Matangi 2006). A 1995 seroprevalence study by ILO (in Matangi 2006) in 18 mining-related firms in
Zimbabwe reported 36.8% HIV positivity among general workers, a rate three
times that of Zimbabwean men aged 15–24 in the general population in 1999
(UNAIDS 2000b). The fact that miners had disposable incomes and the presence of sexual networks created conditions conducive to HIV transmission
and high infection rates in Zimbabwean mining towns at that time (Ndlovu
2011). HIV vulnerability in Zimbabwe dropped after the mining companies
stopped employing migrant workers.

Migrant miners working in South Africa have for many years been thought
responsible for increasing HIV rates in their home countries. This hypothesis was strengthened by the recent study by Corno and de Walque (2012),
which found higher infection rates among migrating miners than nonminers in Lesotho and Swaziland, with higher likelihood of extramarital sex and
less frequent condom use among miners than nonminers. Equally important, the researchers described a parallel effect of migration to the mines on
the wives of miners, who engaged in high-risk sexual behavior while their
husbands were away.

The high HIV rates among migrant laborers and the prevailing perception
among indigenous populations that the migrant laborers are foreigners who
should not be accorded the same rights as local workers have resulted in
poor social relations. In spite of their HIV vulnerability, very few small and
medium-sized mining (and agricultural) companies in the southern African
countries provide HIV services to seasonal workers, and most large corporations restrict their services to permanent employees. Xenophobic attitudes
toward migrant workers, widespread in the general population, sometimes
permeate even government decision-making, as in South Africa, where
Malawian miners were wrongly accused in 1988 of being responsible for the
spread of HIV in South Africa and expelled from the country (Crush 1997).

HIV/AIDS in the agriculture sector

A number of publications describe the living conditions and HIV vulnerability of farm workers, particularly migrant laborers, on commercial farms.
The pattern of farm labor migration has been described as seasonal movements between urban and rural areas and within rural areas (many of them
across international borders) that involve large numbers of poor, undereducated, and undocumented 'illegal' males and females. Farms employ these
workers for low pay, often under exploitive working conditions, and provide them with overcrowded accommodations with poor sanitation and
scarce health services. Access to information and health services is poor and
misconceptions about HIV/AIDS are widespread. Workers rarely get time
off to go to clinics, which are far from their work sites, causing them to
access health services only at advanced stages of their illness. Migrant farm

laborers, many of them lacking the security of tenure and many of them females, have been identified as one of the most vulnerable groups. Many are discriminated against by local communities, adding to their precarious living conditions on the farms (IOM 2010a, 2010c; IOM and SAMP 2005).

Some of the highest HIV infection rates (39.5%) of any occupational group have been recorded among farm workers on 23 farms in Limpopo Province in South Africa, with even higher rates among female workers, who represented 54% of the study population (IOM 2010b). In the Mpumalanga farming area, where 65% of the workforce is female and three-quarters of them are seasonal workers in the 18- to 39-year-old age group, 41% of the seasonal workers aged 30–34 years and 33% of the female workers but only 21% of males were HIV-infected in 2010 (IOM 2010a). In a sugar cane farm in Zimbabwe, 35% of the workers were infected before the company implemented a comprehensive prevention and treatment program that reduced prevalence by nearly half (IOM 2010a). One of the few studies of mortality in commercial farms found that the death rate from AIDS more than tripled between 1995 and 1999 (USAID 2009).

The increasing mobility of females in southern Africa, not only as seasonal farm workers but also as sex workers, traders, and refugees, was labeled by Dodson (2001) the 'feminization' of migration to South Africa. Dodson attributed the rising mobility to political factors, changing sociocultural traditions, and increasing poverty. Imbalanced power and sexual relations between older males obtaining higher salaries and young females are major causes of the higher HIV risk for females. Females are often taken advantage of through promises of work opportunities and shelter.

Another factor in the high vulnerability to HIV/AIDS in the agriculture sector is the fact that the multiethnic and multinational workforces on the farms foster sexual activities that are riskier than the types of activities in which men and women engage in their home areas (IOM 2010a). The vulnerabilities that prevail on commercial farms for which information is available have resulted in HIV rates among migrants working on commercial farms in South Africa that are significantly higher than in the migrants' home areas. The International Organization for Migration, which conducted much of the research on commercial farms in South Africa, therefore labeled the farms (and mines) 'spaces of vulnerability' based on the linkage between HIV vulnerability and various environmental factors specific to given locations (IOM 2010a).

Impacts of HIV/AIDS on the business sector

HIV/AIDS impacts companies in the business sector primarily through increased medical costs and lost productivity due to worker sickness, increased worker turnover, and increased recruitment and training costs (Casale and Whiteside 2006, pp. 262–288; ILO 2004; Rosen et al. 2003).

A study of over 1,000 companies in different sectors in southern Africa found that 9% had been significantly affected by AIDS. In areas hit hardest by the epidemic, up to 40% of the companies reported that HIV and AIDS had reduced profit levels (SABCOHA 2004). On the demand side, HIV/AIDS can change the consumption needs and priorities of people affected by the epidemic for goods and services that businesses produce, market, and distribute (Casale and Whiteside 2006). Although there is no comprehensive study of the magnitude of these various costs, existing information indicates that this burden may be heavy enough to discourage investment in the region. Rosen et al. (2004, cited in Casale and Whiteside 2006) estimated that the cost of HIV/AIDS to businesses in Africa adds between 0.4% and 5.9% to the cost of annual salaries and wages.

UNAIDS (2000a) developed a cause and effect model that is applicable to different sectors of the economy experiencing aggregated impacts at the company and community levels. The model links impacts not only to the company environment, but also to the wider community due to the connectedness of communities and businesses. In addition to declining morale, mental health impacts need to be specified in this model. Mental health impacts of the epidemic have received relatively little attention in southern Africa and in resource-poor areas in general due to the difficulty of measuring the impacts of depression, compromised cooperation, lower worker productivity, fear, discrimination, and stigmatization (Freeman et al. 2005; Rohleder et al. 2009). Comprehensive assessment of these and other costs are needed to address HIV/AIDS impacts holistically and ameliorate those impacts.

The degree of impact of the epidemic on business profits is still inadequately understood in the absence of recent detailed studies. In the pre-ART era, projections of the impacts of HIV/AIDS on businesses presented a grim picture. Research in several southern African countries estimated that the combined impacts of AIDS-related absenteeism, productivity declines, health-care expenditures, and recruitment and training expenses could cut profits by at least 6–8%; absenteeism alone could contribute 25–54% to business losses (UNAIDS 2003). A study by Roberts et al. (1996) of several larger companies revealed the following breakdown of their costs of HIV- and AIDS-related absenteeism: 52% labor costs, 16% burial benefits, 21% labor turnover and recruitment and training of replacement workers, 6% funeral attendance, and 5% health care. Rosen and colleagues (2006) studied 14 large companies and found that heavily impacted companies reported a doubling of labor costs associated with HIV/AIDS. Companies in countries with mature epidemics, including Botswana and Zambia, had particularly high AIDS-related mortality.

Replacing professional staff poses a major challenge for most companies because it takes time to train new workers to the level of the deceased or retiring workers who had accumulated considerable skills and knowledge. The South African Business Coalition reported in 2004 that 30% of firms had higher workforce turnover rates and 24% experienced increased recruitment and training costs due to the disease (SABCOHA 2004, p. 34). These and other estimates need to be revised in view of recent health initiatives taken by southern African companies, described later. Moreover, although scholars generally accept that HIV and AIDS can significantly impact businesses, there is considerable evidence that actual and potential impacts vary considerably among sectors (UNAIDS 2000a).

In order to obtain information of a quality sufficient to promote effective HIV/AIDS prevention and amelioration interventions, policy makers need impact studies that involve the companies that are affected. The lack of company-based information on the impacts of HIV/AIDS, the use of flawed methodologies, and inadequate analysis of data in many publications have hindered comprehensive and objective assessments of the impacts of this disease on businesses. Although the epidemic has far-reaching social and economic implications, most studies have examined primarily short-term impacts. Impacts need to be more thoroughly analyzed and research results need to be shared with managers, business leaders, and policy makers as part of an effort to strengthen multisectoral responses to HIV/AIDS at the national and lowers levels.

The impact of different HIV/AIDS stages on businesses and workers' behavior

HIV/AIDS affects business in stages as different cohorts of workers, if untreated, experience different levels of illness. The four stages of HIV/AIDS recognized by WHO (2007) contribute differently and progressively to escalating the cost and production losses of businesses. These four stages indicate the large window of uncertainty workers in the mining and agricultural sectors have to deal with prior to the appearance of HIV/AIDS symptoms in an environment of scarce HIV/AIDS services, lack of information, and precarious socioeconomic conditions.

Stage 1: Early, asymptomatic stage

Although the early stage of infection with HIV has no external symptoms, infected workers may take more sick days and visit health care providers more frequently, and employers reimburse many of these expenses (Sonnenberg et al. 2011). The productivity of workers may start to decline, depending on how work teams function and how team members compensate for coworker absences. These data about employees are usually available from company clinic patient records and routine HIV test results for certain time periods (Dorrington et al. 2004).

Stage 2: Minor HIV/AIDS manifestations and opportunistic infections

As the diseases progresses, minor manifestations of upper respiratory tract infection and opportunistic infections (such as tuberculosis, sexually transmitted infections, skin rashes, and diarrhea) become more common (WHO 2007). Health care costs and sick days tend to increase and infected employees may be made to leave or moved to less demanding positions. During this stage, the economic impact of HIV/AIDS to businesses starts to increase if people are not put on treatment in time (Dorrington et al. 2004; ILO 2007).

Stage 3: HIV cases become AIDS patients

The cumulative total of AIDS cases rises as HIV infections progress to full-blown AIDS. Early investigators estimated that companies would not notice the impact of HIV for five to ten years after initial infection due to the latency period between infection and the onset of symptoms (Rosen et al. 2003). The largest proportion of the HIV-infected workforce could be in Stages 1 and 2 of their illness, at which points employees generally continue to hold their jobs. However, Sonnenberg et al. (2011) recently documented that absenteeism among miners in four gold mines in South Africa increased in the first two years after sero-conversion, long before the recommendation for the commencement of ART, pointing to a larger disease burden for both companies and individuals than previously thought. Firms may start experiencing the full economic impact of HIV/AIDS as existing HIV cases progress to AIDS and infected workers take leaves due to illness (Dorrington et al. 2004; WHO 2007).

Stage 4: The final stage of the disease

Employees sick with AIDS use health services more frequently and work on an irregular basis, and many leave the workforce when they qualify for disability benefits. Deaths among employees rise rapidly after they become sick with the disease (Dorrington et al. 2004). Sonnenberg et al. (2011) found miners to be off work nearly 40% of the time during the year of their death. Costs for business firms increase substantially at this stage, incomes fall, and skills shortages can become acute in the most affected job categories. The heavy work of mining and some agricultural activities make employment at this stage unlikely (UNAIDS 2000a). In workplaces where discrimination prevails, workers tend to delay HIV testing and seek medical help only after symptoms appear. In a mine in Botswana, for instance, Mukumbira (2003) found that only 10% of HIV-positive employees sought medical services at Stage 1 but over 50% at Stage 4.

This discussion indicates that the traditional competitive advantage of the southern African mining industry deriving from the abundance of cheap labor and large-scale mining operations is now being challenged by a less available, less productive, higher-cost workforce and higher company costs and lower profitability associated with HIV/AIDS. It also shows that the impacts of HIV infection affect the workforce much earlier than previously thought. There is an urgent need to document the experiences of individual firms and sectors of the mining and associated manufacturing industries as well as agrobusiness impacted variously by the disease and guide national, community, and company efforts directed at preventing infection, treating and caring for AIDS patients, and minimizing repercussions on companies.

Interventions at the workplace and migrant workers' health issues

After years of hesitation by many companies in southern Africa and procrastination in responding to the HIV/AIDS threat (Maphosa 2005), companies are beginning to address the epidemic. Their actions were likely prompted by the mounting costs and declining productivity many businesses experienced during the last two decades as a result of HIV/AIDS. Among mining companies, the recognition that the nature of the work poses high HIV risk appears to have been a decisive factor (EIRIS 2008). A measure of moral responsibility also may have given companies a greater resolve to respond to the epidemic.

There is increasing evidence that providing health services is in the best interest of companies because it is profitable. Results from mathematical modeling show that companies are likely to benefit from investing in HIV/AIDS control programs; they can reduce South Africa's 'AIDS tax' by as much as 40.4% if they provided antiretroviral drugs, among other measures (Rosen et al. 2003). Other studies show cost savings from preventing HIV/AIDS as high as 3.5–7.5 times the cost of intervention (Bolton 2008). The Gold Fields Corporation estimated that the cost of an ounce of gold it produced would increase by $10 in the absence of interventions but only $4 with interventions (EIRIS 2008). In a diamond mine in Botswana, company provision of ART to employees and their spouses reduced sick leave and mortality by about 20% (Mukumbira 2003). Matangi (2006), concerned about declining productivity of Zimbabwean mines due to declining skills levels caused by high AIDS-related mortality, recommended that companies utilize infected workers to minimize recruitment and training costs, suggesting that maintaining their health through ART is preferable to hiring new workers.

Companies that provide HIV/AIDS services for their workforces use various means to deliver and pay for these services. Surveys of seven labor sectors, including mining and agriculture, in Angola, Lesotho, Malawi, Mozambique, Namibia, South Africa, Swaziland, and Zambia found that companies invest mostly in education and condom distribution and, to a smaller but increasing extent, also in ART and care and support; their service provision and payment arrangements include on-site services, referrals to other clinics, financing arrangements, and health insurance. The corporations that provided health services were primarily large, multinational companies; more than 60% of the companies studied did not have formal HIV/AIDS policies, illustrating the need to reach many small and middle-sized firms (IOM 2010c; Zellner and Ron 2008). A study of the largest 40 corporations in South Africa revealed that all 11 mining companies surveyed had HIV/AIDS policies and offered the full complement of prevention, treatment, care and support services (EIRIS 2008).

Bloom et al. (2006) and Bolton (2008) described the range of health services provided by manufacturing firms in southern Africa (mostly in South Africa); they included voluntary HIV counseling and testing (VCT), wellness clinics, and ART in line with national HIV/AIDS policies and in partnership with global initiatives such as President's Emergency Plan For AIDS Relief (PEPFAR) and the Global Fund to Fight AIDS, TB and Malaria. The researchers concluded that most companies implementing interventions have benefited in terms of reduced absenteeism and lower health care costs as well as increased productivity. Furthermore, the integration of many HIV prevention, care, and support programs into screening and treatment programs for TB and other occupational diseases as part of comprehensive occupational disease and safety strategies, particularly in the mining sector, makes the programs more cost-effective and sustainable.

On the other hand, some interventions have been ineffective or are controversial, especially in the agricultural sector. Verheijen and Minde (2007) pointed out that most interventions aimed at mitigating the effects of HIV/AIDS in the subsistence agricultural sector of South Africa have benefited men only because they provide extension services and new technologies mainly to men. This situation has exacerbated gender inequality by further eroding women's social status. This and other sector-specific information points to the relatively greater difficulty of implementing viable anti-HIV/AIDS programs in agriculture than in mining in southern Africa, although cost–benefit studies need to be carried out in commercial farms.

Conclusion

This examination of HIV vulnerabilities and impacts and responses to HIV/AIDS among laborers in mines and commercial farms in southern Africa reveals extremely high infection rates due to largely preventable conditions and human rights dilemmas. Major drivers of worker vulnerabilities are poverty, gender, and laborer inequalities and discrimination, inadequate health and social services, and a weak policy environment, although the latter two factors are currently receiving attention from policy makers and companies.

The dynamics of HIV infection among multiethnic, impoverished, and socially peripheralized migrant populations requires innovative and proactive interventions and activities in at least two areas: (1) the provision of different combinations of HIV prevention, treatment, care, and support programs to meet local needs and (2) structural and environmental changes at the workplace that ensure the rights, safety, and well-being of all workers. Integration of structural and environmental changes may remove underlying vulnerabilities in the communities in which businesses exist, requiring community-based programs and participation to define health agendas and support company and government efforts. The encouraging effects of various workplace and collaborative interventions in southern Africa addressing absenteeism, morbidity, and mortality, particularly the effects on the profitability of different types of businesses, bode well for mining corporations and commercial farms. Company investments in the well-being of workers therefore need to be seen as investments in the future productivity and financial stability of mines and commercial farms.

Changes in corporate culture, policies, and practices, which are underway in some companies, may result in increased employee access to health services and to relevant company information on the workforce that will, in turn, encourage multiinstitutional research. Reliable and comprehensive information may give managers insights into the nature of key drivers of the epidemic and HIV-related costs at the company level and thus guide the development of cost-effective and appropriate interventions. Empirical evidence of the impact of HIV and AIDS on business is critical if policy makers at the government and company levels are to develop comprehensive policies and effective programmatic interventions. General modeling and interdisciplinary case studies of individual companies examining vulnerabilities in the workforce, above all among migrant laborers and females, and access to treatment, support, and care services may guide the design and implementation of interventions. Rapid increases in costs of medical and human resources and production give urgency to the need for research of individual businesses and industrial complexes. The recent adoption by several southern African governments of HIV/AIDS prevention strategies that address issues of HIV/AIDS in the workforce, together with continuation of decentralization of health services as specified in their national UNGASS reports for 2010 (see Chapter 11), may facilitate these research efforts. Lastly, there is also a need for policy makers and companies to address the toxic combination of nationalism and fear of the disease that drive discrimination against migrant workers and increasing their vulnerability.

References

AGOA Forum. 2001. *Plenary Session on HIV/AIDS*. Chapter 4. Washington, DC: African Growth and Opportunities Act Forum.

Barako, D.G., Taplin, R.H. and Brown, A.M. 2010. HIV/AIDS information by African companies: An empirical analysis. *Journal of Asian and African Studies* 45:387–405.

Bloom, D.E., Bloom, L.R., Steven, D. and Weston, M. 2006. *Business and HIV/AIDS: A Healthier Partnership? A Global Review of the Business Response to HIV/AIDS 2005–2006*. Geneva: World Economic Forum.

Bolton, P.L. 2008. Corporate responses to HIV/AIDS: Experience and leadership from South Africa. *Business and Society Review* 113: 277–300.

Brummer, D. 2002. *Labour Migration and HIV and AIDS in Southern Africa.* Pretoria: International Organisation for Migration, Regional Office for Southern Africa.

Campbell, E.K. 2008. Moderating poverty: The role of remittances from migration in Botswana. *African Development* 33:91–115.

Campbell, S. 2003. *'Letting them Die': Why HIV/AIDS Prevention Programs Fail.* Oxford: International African Institute in Association with James Currey.

Campbell, C. and Williams, B. 1999. Beyond the biomedical and behavioural: Towards an integrated approach to HIV prevention in the southern African mining industry. *Social Science and Medicine* 48:1625–1639.

Casale, M. and Whiteside, A. 2006. *The Impact of HIV/AIDS on Poverty, Inequality and Economic Growth.* IDRC Working Papers on Globalization, Growth and Poverty, Paper No. 3. Ottawa: IDRC.

Corno, L. and de Walque, D. 2012. *Mines, Migration and HIV/AIDS in Southern Africa.* Policy Research Working Paper No. 5966. Washington, DC: World Bank.

Crush, J. 1997. Contract migration to South Africa: Past, present and future. Briefing for the Green Paper Task Team on International Migration, Pretoria. Unpublished.

Crush, J. and Williams, V. 2002. *Making up the Numbers: Measuring Undocumented Migration in Southern Africa.* Cape Town: Southern African Migration Program.

Crush, J. and Williams, V. 2010. *Labour Migration Trends and Policies in Southern Africa.* SAMP Policy Brief No. 23. Cape Town: Southern African Migration Programme.

Dodson, B. 2001. Discrimination by default?: *Gender concern in South African migration policy. Africa Today* 48:73–90.

Dorrington, R., Johnson, L. and Budlender, D. 2004. *ASSA 2002 AIDS and Demographic Models: User Guide.* Cape Town: Center for Actuarial Research, University of Cape Town.

Draper, O., Kiratu, S. and Hichert, T. 2009. *How Might Agriculture Develop in Southern Africa?* Winnipeg: International Institute for Sustainable Development.

EIRIS. 2008. *Positive Corporate Responses to HIV/AIDS: A Snapshot of Large-cap South African Companies.* www.eiris.org/files/research%20publications/hivaidsbriefingnov08.pdf

Freeman, M., Patel, V., Collins, P.A. and Bertolote, J. 2005. Integration of mental health in global initiatives for HIV/AIDS. *British Journal of Psychiatry* 187:1–3.

ILO. 2003. *ILO Activities in Africa 2000–2003.* Geneva: International Labour Organization.

ILO. 2004. *HIV/AIDS and Work: Global Estimates, Impact and Response.* Geneva: International Labour Organization.

ILO. 2007. *Positive Corporate Responses to HIV/AIDS: A Snapshot of Large-cap South African Companies.* Geneva: International Labour Organization.

ILO. 2011. HIV/AIDS Prevention in Africa. Project documentation, 23 February. Geneva: International Labour Organization.

IOM. n.d. *Briefing Note on HIV and Labour Migration in Zimbabwe.* Geneva: International Organization on Migration.

IOM. 2002. *Briefing Note on HIV and Labour Migration in Lesotho.* Pretoria, South Africa: IOM Regional Office for Southern Africa.

IOM. 2010a. *Commercial Agriculture Sector Report.* Geneva: International Organization for Migration. Geneva: International Organization for Migration.

IOM. 2010b. *Integrated Biological and Behavioural Surveillance Survey (IBBSS).* Geneva: International Organization for Migration.

IOM. 2010c. *Regional Assessment on HIV-Prevention Needs of Migrants and Mobile Populations in Southern Africa*. Geneva: International Organization for Migration.

IOM and SAMP. 2005. *HIV/AIDS, Population Mobility and Migration in Southern Africa: Defining a Research and Policy Agenda*. Cape Town: International Organization for Migration and South African Migration Project.

Jayne, S.J., Villareal, M., Pingali, P. and Hemrich, G. 2006. HIV/AIDS and the agricultural sector in Eastern and Southern Africa: Anticipating the consequences. In Gillespie, S. (ed.), *AIDS, Poverty, and Hunger*, Chapter 8. Washington, DC: IFPRI.

Krieger, N. 2006. *Unprotected Migrants: Zimbabweans in South Africa's Limpopo Province*. New York: Human Rights Watch.

Kundecha, R., Ungile, M., Osborne, K. et al. 2011. Making the workplace work for HIV. *Abstracts of the International Conference on AIDS and STIs in Africa*, Addis Ababa. Abstract MOAD0402.

Maphosa, F., 2005. HIV/AIDS at the workplace: A study of corporate responses to the HIV/AIDS pandemic in Zimbabwe. Unpublished report to OSSREA.

Matangi, C.N. 2006. Skills under threat: The case of HIV/AIDS in the mining industry in Zimbabwe. *Journal of International Development* 18:599–628.

Moreriane, M. 2011. A comprehensive multi-level approach to address health vulnerabilities in migration-affected communities. *Abstracts of the International Conference on AIDS and STIs in Africa*. Addis Ababa, Abstract MOPE138.

Mukumbira, R. 2003. Botswana: Mining giant fights workplace HIV/AIDS. *News from Africa*, August 2003. http://www.newsfromafrica.org/newsfromafrica/articles/art_1252.html

Ndlovu, P. 2011. HIV rate soars in mining towns. *The Zimbabwean*, 25 July. http://www.thezimbabwean.co.uk/news/zimbabwe/51188/hiv-rate-soars-in-mining.html

Rampersad, R. 2010. An assessment of corporate governance and HIV/AIDS in the South African corporate sector. *African Journal of Business Management* 4:2269–2276.

Roberts, M., Rau, B. and Emery, A. 1996. *Private Sector AIDS Policy: Business Managing AIDS – A Guide for Managers*. Arlington, VA: Family Health International AIDSCAP.

Rohleder, P., Swartz, L., Kalichman, S.C. and Simbayi, L.C. 2009. *HIV/AIDS in South Africa: 25 Year on Psychological Perspectives*. New York: Springer.

Rosen, S., Feeley, F., Connelly, P. and Simon, J. 2006. *The Private Sector and HIV and AIDS in Africa: Taking Stock of Six Years of Applied Research*. Boston: Boston University, Center for International Health and Development.

Rosen, S., Simon, J., Vincent, J.R. et al. 2003. AIDS is your business. *Harvard Business Review* 81:80–87.

SABCOHA. 2004. *The Economic Impact of HIV/AIDS on Business in South Africa, 2003*. Johannesburg: South African Business Coalition on HIV/AIDS.

Schachter, J.P. 2009. Data assessment of labour migration statistics in the SADC Region: South Africa, Zambia and Zimbabwe. Report prepared for the International Organization for Migration. Unpublished.

Sonnenberg, P., Copas, A., Glynn, J.R. et al. 2011. The effect of HIV conversion on time off work in a large cohort of gold miners with known dates of seroconversion. *Occupational and Environmental Medicine* 68:647–652.

Southern African Development Community. 2008. *Strengthening the Role of Agriculture in Poverty Reduction*. Gaborone, Botswana: SADC Secretariat.

Ulicki, T. and Crush, J. 2007. Poverty, gender and migrancy: Lesotho's migrant farmworkers in South Africa. *Development Southern Africa* 24:155–172.

UNAIDS. 2000a. *The Business Response to HIV/AIDS: Impact and Lessons Learned*. Geneva: UNAIDS.

UNAIDS. 2000b. *Report on the Global HIV/AIDS Epidemic.* Geneva: UNAIDS.
UNAIDS. 2002. *Report on the Global HIV/AIDS Epidemic – 2002.* Geneva: UNAIDS.
UNAIDS. 2003. *HIV/AIDS: It's Your Business.* Geneva: UNAIDS.
UNAIDS. 2010. *Report on the Global AIDS Epidemic.* Geneva: UNAIDS.
USAID. 2009. *How Does HIV/AIDS Affect African Businesses?* Washington, DC: USAID.
Verheijen, J. and Minde, I. 2007. Agricultural innovations: A potential tool to HIV mitigation. *Journal of SAT Agricultural Research* 5:1–8.
WHO. 2007. *WHO Case Definitions for Surveillance and Revised Clinical Staging and Immunological Classification of HIV-related Disease in Adults and Children.* Geneva: WHO.
Zellner, S. and Ron, I. 2008. *HIV/AIDS Services through the Workplace: A Survey in Four Sub-Saharan Africa Countries.* Bethesda, MD: Private Sector Partnership-One project, Abt Associates Inc.

Books, papers, and other resources for further reading

Abdool Karim, S.S. and Abdool Karim, A.K. 2005. *HIV/AIDS in South Africa.* Cambridge: Cambridge University Press.
Crush, J. 2008. *South Africa: Policy in the Face of Xenophobia.* Washington, DC: Migration Information Source.
Hunter, M. 2010. *Love in the Time of AIDS: Inequality, Gender, and Rights in South Africa.* Bloomington: Indiana University Press.
Squire, C. 2007. *HIV in South Africa: Talking about the Big Thing.* Oxford: Routledge.
Thomas, F., Haour-Knipe, M. and Aggleton, P. 2010. *Dangerous Liaisons? Mobility, Sexuality and AIDS.* London: Routledge.

8
Access to Treatment, Care, Support, and Prevention Services

Getnet Tadele, Woldekidan Amde, and Helmut Kloos

Introduction

In 2006, all UN member states made a commitment at the United Nations General Assembly Special Session on HIV/AIDS to sharply scale up their HIV/AIDS responses and provide universal access to HIV prevention, treatment, care, and support services by 2010 (WHO 2007). Largely due to the subsequent massive rollout of antiretroviral treatment (ART), the total number of deaths from AIDS declined from 2.2 million in 2005 to 1.8 million in 2010, and 2.5 million deaths were averted between 1995 and 2010. By the end of 2010, an estimated 6.6 million of the 14.2 million people (47%) eligible for treatment in low- and middle-income countries received ART (UNAIDS 2011a, pp. 6, 19). In Sub-Saharan Africa, 56% of people needing treatment in 2011 were receiving it, 19% more than in 2010 – more than in any other region (UNAIDS 2012, p. 19); the total number of new infections decreased from 2.6 million in 1997, when the epidemic peaked, to 1.8 million in 2010, and in 22 countries HIV incidence fell more than 25% between 2001 and 2009 (UNAIDS 2011a, p. 7). A recent study in Uganda estimated that life expectancy of people living with HIV/AIDS (PLWHA) taking ART increased to nearly normal levels (Mills et al. 2012).

The rapid increase in the availability and use of ART in Sub-Saharan Africa has contributed significantly to increasing the life expectancy of PLWHA, reducing suffering, easing long-term care, promoting the use of HIV testing services, providing hope to infected people living with HIV/AIDS, reducing the number of AIDS orphans, and generating socioeconomic benefits at all levels of society. Prevention, care, and support services have been strengthened and gender and human rights issues addressed parallel with implementation of treatment programs as part of a mutually reinforcing continuum (UNAIDS 2010a), a prerequisite for an effective international response. Nearly 37% of those eligible for treatment in Sub-Saharan Africa were able to access ART in 2009, a sharp increase since 2003, when a mere 2% of all PLWHA received treatment (UNAIDS 2008, 2010a).

ART coverage varies across Sub-Saharan Africa, with 48% of PLWHA in need of treatment covered in eastern and southern African countries and 30% in West and Central Africa in 2009. Even greater variations in coverage have been reported for infected children across subregions, with only 15% in West and Central Africa receiving ART in 2008 (UNAIDS 2009a, p. 25). Botswana achieved universal access (above 80% coverage; see below) to ART for children, and Botswana, Namibia, Zambia, and South Africa for HIV testing in 2009 (UNAIDS 2010a, pp. 97, 98, 248, 249). By 2010, Botswana, Namibia, and Rwanda had achieved universal access to ART for adults (UNAIDS 2011a, p. 19).

HIV prevention, a key component of comprehensive control programs, dates to the beginning of the HIV epidemic. Programs have evolved from health education/behavior change approaches, including the ABC approach (abstinence, being faithful, using condoms), to combination and integrated HIV prevention, including biomedical, behavioral, and structural strategies (UNAIDS 2010b).

This chapter explores progress and constraints in HIV/AIDS treatment and prevention and AIDS care and support services in Sub-Saharan Africa from a social science perspective. We examine different aspects of the development, access, and utilization of ART, including the change from therapeutic to preventive use of antiretrovirals, as in the prophylactic treatment of pregnant women to curb mother-to-child transmission of HIV, and other combination prevention approaches; the recent change from hospital-based to decentralized and home-based treatment, care, and support; strengthening of mother and child health services and community-based interventions; persisting challenges such as inequitable access to treatment and care for some high-risk groups; and the role of socioeconomic, political, and cultural constraints in upscaling programs. Several areas of HIV prevention, including health education, condom use, and food security, are discussed in different chapters, particularly in Chapters 2, 4, 5, 6, and 10.

Discourse about the development of and access to HIV/AIDS services

This section examines a wide range of issues, including traditional medicine, biomedical prevention research, structural interventions, and upgrading of health services and community-based initiatives, all of which must be considered in the context of HIV/AIDS prevention, care, and treatment (MacQueen 2011).

Universal access to treatment

Universal access to ART is guided by core ideals of equity, accessibility, affordability, adequate large-scale financial backing, and international commitment to sustainability (UNAIDS 2009b). Universal access is generally defined as access to HIV/AIDS services to 80% or more of people in need of accessing a given service or intervention. The 80% cut-off was decided upon in 2005 by the Group of Eight (G8) nations because even where services are provided for the total population it is unlikely that more than 80% of people will use them (IAS 2009; UNAIDS 2005). The treatment guidelines issued by WHO in 2010 recommending that antiretroviral therapy be started at CD4 count of <350 cells/mm³ increased the number of PLWHA medically eligible for ART by 50% worldwide. The guidelines increased the size of the eligible population and raised the bar for achieving universal access (UNAIDS 2010a, p. 96).

ART coverage varies considerably among Sub-Saharan African countries, ranging from 88% of adults in Rwanda to 20% in Burundi in 2009. In the 15–24 years age group, coverage was higher in all countries among females than males. Among children below 15 years, treatment rates varied between 91% in Botswana and 14% in Burundi and coverage was lower than for adults in all but four countries (Table 8.1). It is encouraging that the high-HIV prevalence countries Botswana, Lesotho, Namibia, South Africa, and Swaziland achieved universal access of pregnant women living with HIV to ART in 2010.

ART coverage is generally related to annual spending per person living with HIV, reflecting heavy infusion of external funding in poor countries such as Rwanda, Mozambique, and Malawi. Whereas 95–100% of all spending on care and treatment in Rwanda, Madagascar, Gambia, Democratic Republic of the Congo, Equatorial Guinea Mozambique, Malawi, Central African Republic, and Niger was from international sources in 2009, about 75% came from public sources in Botswana and South Africa. Spending on prevention followed a similar pattern. These differences reflect the national economic levels and political will of these countries and the commitment of the international community to assist the poorest countries (UNAIDS 2010a).

The statistics in Table 8.1, while providing useful information on coverage, do not illustrate persisting inequities in access among subgroups. In particular, the scarcity of data on marginalized populations such as commercial sex workers, men having sex with men (MSM), people who inject drugs, prison populations, and refugees renders assessments of these groups' access to ART extremely difficult. There are indications that these groups are being neglected and discriminated against, even though some countries have begun to provide ART services to them (UNAIDS 2010a; see also Chapter 11). The hesitance of governments to take proactive stands on being all inclusive is also indicated by the fact that although Sub-Saharan Africa faces increasing illicit drug use, particularly in a number of cities in eastern Africa, it has the lowest rate of needle-syringe distribution through intervention programs (Beckerleg et al. 2005; Kloos and Haile Mariam 2008; Mathers et al. 2010).

Table 8.1 ART coverage of adults and children under 15 years in 18 Sub-Saharan African countries (December 2009)

Country	No. of HIV-positive people	No. of people receiving ART	Adult ART coverage (%)[a]	Child ART coverage (%)[b]
Rwanda	170,000	76,726	88	60
Botswana	320,000	145,190	83	91
Namibia	180,000	59,376	76	77
Zambia	980,000	283,863	68	31
Ethiopia[c]	1,116,216	176,632	53	19
Kenya	1,500,000	336,980	50	31
Lesotho	290,000	61,736	50	25
Malawi	920,000	198,846	48	29
Uganda	1,200,000	200,413	43	21
South Africa	5,600,000	971,556	36	58
Zimbabwe	1,200,000	218,589	34	37
Mozambique	1,400,000	170,198	32	20
Tanzania	1,400,000	199,413	32	14
Cameroon	610,000	76,228	30	14
Côte d'Ivoire	450,000	72,011	29	15
Ghana	260,000	30,265	25	14
Nigeria	3,300,000	302,973	23	13
Burundi	180,000	17,661	20	14

[a] Based on Table 4.2 and the graph on page 116.
[b] Approximated from the graph on page 116.
[c] Based on FDRE (2010).
Sources: UNAIDS (2010a, pp. 110, 111, 116, 248–252; 2012, p. 123; FDRE (2010).

Contrary to the expectation that the massive ART rollout would reduce stigma, recent studies show that this is not the case. For example, Maughan-Brown (2010) demonstrated an increase in stigma in different groups in South Africa after the commencement of ART. Similarly, in camps of displaced people in northern Uganda, the availability of ART contributed to reducing only the stigma linked to the visible signs of AIDS but not new forms of stigma associated with the invisibility of the illness within the social context and disease trajectory (Wilhelm-Solomon 2010). Examination of the impact of ART on the various types of stigma in different socioeconomic and cultural settings may guide the development of antistigma programs.

Issues in prevention

Combination prevention approach

The HIV prevention programs employed in the early stage of the epidemic, many of them unsuccessful in making significant inroads on HIV transmission (Campbell 2003), are increasingly being replaced by integrated interventions with continuing rollout of ART due to the realization that fundamental issues in vulnerability to infection must be addressed to control the epidemic (Merson et al. 2008). The integrated interventions include the combination of behavioral and biomedical approaches – delay in sexual debut, reduction in multiple sexual partners, condom use, voluntary HIV counseling and testing (VCT), AIDS treatment of the general and high-risk populations, antiretroviral prophylaxis to prevent mother-to-child transmission, and male circumcision – with structural approaches, and possibly the still experimental ARV-based microbicides and oral preexposure (PrEP) drugs (Gupta et al. 2008; Kalibala and Littlefield 2010; UNAIDS 2011a) and simple, low-cost, home-based HIV testing (Walensky and Basset 2011). One study in South Africa found that the use of PrEP by uninfected individuals in relationship with HIV-infected partners and sex workers reduced the risk of infection by about half. However, cost-effectiveness of these expensive ARVs and possible changes in sexual behavior in response to perceived lowering of risk need to be determined (Okwundu et al. 2012).

While few data are available on the effectiveness of most combined prevention approaches, the rapid decline in new HIV infections in young people worldwide has been associated with behavioral changes, particularly reductions in the number of multiple sexual partners, delay in sexual debut, and condom use (International Group 2010). A number of Sub-Saharan countries that implemented combination HIV prevention programs have reported sharp decreases in HIV infection since the end of the 1990s. In Namibia, which was able to achieve both significant reduction in risk behavior and increases in ART, new infections had declined by 60% by 2010; in Botswana, Zimbabwe, and Lesotho, declines in infections were associated with improvements in their combined prevention programs. Although significant increases in condom use were associated with the drop in HIV rates in Namibia (UNAIDS 2011a), South Africa, and several other countries (Johnson et al. 2012), condom use is not the reliable HIV prevention method it is often portrayed to be, as indicated by widespread resistance to its use among married couples (see Chapter 2) and youth (Chapter 4) and recent reports of its improper use in Africa and elsewhere (Improper 2012). The use of female condoms, potentially effective in HIV prevention and found to be used by females where they cannot negotiate male condom use, is expected to increase as prices decline (Republic of South Africa 2010; USAID 2011a), but their use will also depend on cultural perceptions of sexuality as discussed elsewhere in this volume.

In spite of this and other evidence of the effectiveness of the combination prevention approach, particularly when the prevention program includes ABC, male circumcision, and ART of PLWHA and pregnant women, scarcity of evaluations still precludes a thorough assessment of the relative effectiveness of combination approaches in different intervention contexts (Bärnighausen et al. 2012), and a number of barriers make their uptake difficult, particularly for women. Moreover, stigma and disclosure issues may impede the effective use of some of the tools in combination approaches, and researchers need to study the effect of home testing on unprotected sex and legal aspects of the use of rapid antibody tests in households and wider community settings (UNAIDS 2011a; Walensky and Bassett 2011). Similarly, although the CDC (2011) has labeled the proposed use of vaginal microbiocides a 'game changer' because it enables women to control their HIV risk, prospects for the widespread use of microbiocides (and of PrEPs) in the near term are questionable because men tend to control sexual relations, as described in Chapters 1–4 in this volume. The social science approach, although largely neglected in the past, may, according to MacQueen (2011), enhances the success of biomedical HIV prevention research if social scientists move beyond the social science versus biomedical debate and address issues of the relationship between biomedical dynamics and social change.

Prevention of mother-to-child transmission of HIV (PMTCT) through antiretroviral prophylaxis is vital in prolonging the lives of mothers and preventing children from becoming infected. Of the nearly half a million children who contracted HIV in 2008, nine out of ten were living in Sub-Saharan Africa. There is growing recognition of the need to reduce MTCT in this region, where women aged 19–49 account for about three-fifths of all infected people. In South Africa, nearly one-third of all pregnant women who visited health centers in 2008 were HIV-positive (UNAIDS 2009b). With the possibility of three out of ten children born to infected women likely to become positive, PMTCT holds great promise of significantly reducing the number of new HIV infections.

PMTCT coverage among pregnant women in eastern and southern Africa increased from 15% in 2005 to 68% in 2009 (UNAIDS 2010a) and reached the universal access target by 2010 in Botswana, Lesotho, Namibia, South Africa, and Swaziland. In Malawi and Angola, as well as in a number of other countries in Sub-Saharan countries, coverage remained low (UNAIDS 2011a, p. 40). In Ethiopia, for example, only 18% of pregnant women and 15% of infants born to HIV-infected mothers received ART in 2008. Low accessibility rates in Sub-Saharan Africa are due to a combination of scarce family planning services for HIV-positive women and poor access to antenatal care and PMTCT services. A study in a hospital in Uganda, for example, where adherence to the postnatal PMTCT program was 38%, identified social, logistic, and treatment-related factors during the two-month period after delivery as major factors in low uptake of PMTCT (Nassali et al. 2009). Other challenges facing Sub-Saharan countries are lack of resources necessary to develop adequate preventive health services, social problems restricting women's choice and access to mother and child health services, and the integration of HIV prevention and treatment programs in antenatal care, postpartum care, and other maternal and child services (see UNAIDS 2011a, p. 41).

The potential usefulness of male circumcision in preventing HIV transmission was first indicated by higher HIV prevalence among some populations in the traditional African noncircumcision belt (Kloos and Haile Mariam 2008). A number of recent randomized trials in Sub-Saharan Africa have demonstrated the effectiveness of male circumcision in reducing the transmission of HIV and some sexually transmitted infections (STIs) that increase the risk of HIV infection. These include papillomavirus infection, trichomoniasis, syphilis, and genital ulcer disease (Weiss et al. 2010). However, although male circumcision is cost-effective (Uthman et al. 2011) and large numbers of uninfected males in Sub-Saharan Africa are undergoing this procedure, there is concern that male circumcision may promote unsafe sex practices fostered by the wrong belief that it confers full protection. This may compromise women's ability to negotiate safer sex, requiring awareness raising and additional research on the sociocultural context of male circumcision (Andersson and Cockcroft 2012).

Structural approaches to HIV prevention

Structural approaches to HIV prevention, designed to reduce individuals' vulnerability by creating the social, economic, cultural, and political conditions in which people can adopt safer behaviors, have been used since the early stage of the epidemic and are now recognized as an important, distinct area of HIV prevention. The health sector has often neglected structural approaches to addressing the economic, environmental, and political factors underlying HIV risk and vulnerabilities as too broad and difficult to integrate into interventions (Gupta et al. 2008). Policy makers increasingly recognize, however, that social and economic changes will be required to ensure effective upgrading and sustainability of both prevention and control programs. The pathways leading to various types of risk must be understood to visualize the points of maximum effect for a given intervention or organization (Gupta et al. 2008).

Several structural intervention trials combining microfinance, gender equity, and HIV education have been implemented in South Africa since 2006. One contributed to a 55% decrease in the incidence of intimate partner violence and improved household well-being, empowerment, and social capital (Pronyk et al. 2006); another increased communication about HIV and sexuality within the household (Pronyk et al. 2008). A microfinance program in rural villages in Côte d'Ivoire raised the economic status of PLWHA and increased access to ART and psychosocial support while reducing AIDS stigma (Holmes et al. 2011). In addition, in Ethiopia people in the community saw PLWHA actively engaged in work, earning their living, improving their own lives, taking better care of their children, and in some cases even creating wealth through microfinance and other income-generating activities run by government and nongovernment organizations (NGOs). This view of PLWHA was credited with contributing to a decrease in the level of stigma and discrimination against PLWHA by members of their own family as well as the general community (Tadele et al. 2011).

Education for girls constitutes a structural intervention that is beginning to improve the livelihood of females, give them greater independence, and reduce their risk of HIV infection. Girls' participation in school and school-based HIV programs, briefly discussed in Chapter 3, has resulted in postponement of sexual debut and reduction in high-risk behavior and HIV infection among female students. The Demographic and Health Survey (DHS) reports from eight Sub-Saharan countries show that girls attending secondary schools consistently initiated sex later than out-of-school girls (Gupta and Mahy 2003). Moreover, study results from other Sub-Saharan countries reveal that girls enrolled in school had fewer sexual partners (Wambe et al. 2005), strong evidence that education is a powerful HIV prevention tool. Cash transfers to the families of students mitigated social and economic drivers of HIV vulnerability and resulted in increased school attendance among beneficiaries (Leclerc-Madlala 2008) and later marriage and reduced pregnancy and sexual activity among girls (Baird et al. 2009). They also resulted in a halving of the HIV prevalence among school girls in targeted communities in Malawi (World Bank 2010a). A multicountry workplace peer education HIV prevention program for male and female workers resulted in significant improvements in knowledge and attitude indicators (Richter et al. 2011).

The effectiveness of some of these interventions, particularly microcredit, appears partly due to the fact that they were tailored to local social, political, economic, and epidemic contexts (USAID 2011b). These small-scale interventions need to be up-scaled, and operational issues such as linkages between economic empowerment and HIV infection and ways to integrate structural approaches into comprehensive HIV prevention need to be addressed to reduce vulnerability to HIV on a broad front (Kim et al. 2008; USAID 2011b). The consistently positive effect of education on sexual behavior and risk of girls, on the other hand, indicates the powerful influence of knowledge on self-confidence and female autonomy that bodes well for further improvements with continuing school enrolment.

Community participation and ownership of programs

In efforts to decentralize HIV/AIDS programs and render them more cost-effective, some governments have begun to promote community-based initiatives and interventions. Rosen and Fox (2012) reported very high ART adherence (97.5%) achieved by the employment of community groups in Mozambique. In South Africa, May and Ingle (2011) concluded that PLWHA receiving support from community health workers had better treatment outcomes than those using the clinical services. The utilization of family members, treatment partners (HIV-positive family members, friends or neighbors who assist, encourage, and socialize with PLWHA during ART), and community health workers in home-based care of PLWHA and orphan care is discussed below and in Chapters 6 and 9. Prospects and experiences of community-based prevention, care, and support programs using *iddir* burial associations in Ethiopia are examined below and in Chapter 6.

Holding community conversations is another approach to grassroots interventions initiated and implemented by communities. Community conversations can raise the capacity of HIV-affected communities to create an enabling environment conducive to learning, changing behavior, and identifying community needs and concerns. This approach stands in contrast to the awareness-raising approach characterized by prescriptive messages that tended to overwhelm communities with outsider-provided information to which community members rarely can relate. Community conversations give participants the benefit of dialogue and broad-based, spontaneous community participation, advocacy, and ownership (UNDP 2005).

The informal, interpersonal communications within communities are generally well accepted and have been associated with significant increases in VCT in Tanzania, Zimbabwe, and South Africa (Hendriksen et al. 2009). In Ethiopia they were instrumental in discontinuing widow inheritance, female genital cutting, domestic violence, and sexual abuse (Chege et al. 2011), and they also decreased misconceptions and discriminatory behavior and increased HIV/AIDS knowledge (Gedefaw et al. 2011), school enrolment, age at marriage of girls, reproductive knowledge, and contraceptive use (Erulkar and Muthengi 2009). In Lesotho, community conversations facilitated the formation of support groups (UNDP 2011). The success of the community conversation approach and its application to HIV prevention in sectors other than health has made it a useful tool in community development. Several countries, including Ethiopia, have adopted community conversations as a priority strategy for community mobilization nationwide (UNAIDS 2009c). In Uganda, the Traditional and Modern Health Practitioners Together Against AIDS and Other Diseases (THETA) identified and trained *sengas* (paternal aunts) and *kojjas* (maternal uncles) to engage communities in discussing HIV prevention and mitigation of sociocultural factors such as polygamy, social pressure to have children, widow inheritance, early marriage, and multiple sexual partners (Government of Uganda 2010). This program is grounded in the traditional community dialogues and couple discussions *sengas* and *kojjas* held with couples and young people on the subjects of relationships, marriage strengthening, sexuality, reproductive health services, and promoting traditional cultural values (Wabwire-Mangen et al. 2008). There is a need for further studies of the adaptability and effectiveness of community conversations in different socioeconomic, cultural, and intervention contexts in different countries and communities to more fully evaluate their potential contribution to prevention, care, and support efforts.

Moreover, African traditional institutions of governance, many of which have proven to be influential in peoples' lives, may contribute to community-based prevention and advocacy programs (ECA 2007). This issue has been neglected in the HIV/AIDS discourse and there is clearly a need to advocate for greater global international support for community-based strategies (Kesby 2004). There is evidence that traditional political leaders can provide much needed community leadership in HIV/AIDS programs. Collaboration between health officials and leaders of the traditional *Gada* organization, an egalitarian social system in Ethiopia, facilitated HIV prevention programs in Ethiopia (Elemo 2005). In Ghana, Queen Mothers and *Magajias*, both traditional female community leaders, were trained to advocate on female issues and develop plans to support PLWHA in their respective districts (Farorsey and Amolo n.d.).

Patient care and support

The provision of long-term perpetual care and support of PLWHA, an increasingly important component of integrated HIV/AIDS services, presents tremendous challenges to Sub-Saharan countries, all of which lack sufficient resources to deal with large patient populations. Moreover, the great majority of patients and their families prefer home treatment over inadequate care in overcrowded public hospitals and unaffordable private clinics (Dilger 2010). The needs of homebound and bedridden AIDS patients go far beyond treatment; they include psychosocial, physical, socioeconomic, and legal support. The high cost and limited capacity of hospital facilities coupled with sociocultural preferences for home-based palliative care means that the overwhelming numbers of AIDS patients in Sub-Saharan Africa are cared for in the home environment.

Many experts consider home-based care ideal for the provision of quality physical care and psychosocial support for PLWHA and their families (Van Dyk 2008). Home-based care teams ideally consist of primary caregivers (patients' next of kin, partner, friend, or a foster or adoptive parent); community caregivers helping the primary caregiver; a professional person (nurse, social worker, or community health worker); and trained volunteers from religious organizations, NGOs, or youth groups (Van Dyk 2008). This home-based model has not been achieved in Sub-Saharan Africa. The services provided by primary caregivers, predominantly women, tend to be inadequately recognized, and the caregivers often have difficulty obtaining the resources, training, and support necessary to provide life-saving responses (UNAIDS 2010a).

There is increasing evidence that drug adherence, a major factor in the success of ART, may be improved by treatment partnering in the home setting. In this intervention, a PLWHA selects a family member, friend, or neighbor as a treatment partner who supports him or her in adhering to treatment, reporting and managing side effects, and assisting with clinic appointments and pharmacy refills. Based on traditional African values of social responsibility and social capital preservation, treatment partnerships can also benefit patients' social and psychological well-being by helping to restore social connections and reduce their isolation (O'Laughlin et al. 2012).

Community-based groups in various African countries are attempting to meet the rapidly rising demand for care and support. One of the most successful groups is the burial association (*iddir*) in Ethiopia, described by Ayalew Gebre et al., as a progressive and innovative institution in Chapter 6. *Iddirs* now also provide, in addition to burial assistance, palliative care for PLWHA in collaboration with health services and financial support for affected families. Wube et al. (2010) reported that *iddir*-supported services in 14 towns reduced stigma and discrimination of PLWHA and vulnerable children, increased the use of VCT, and improved the economic stability of affected families.

The socioeconomic impacts of HIV/AIDS on orphans and affected family members, particularly females, together with the coping behaviors of those affected, are described in Chapter 6 and in greater detail in the institutional context in Chapter 9. Aspects of food security and nutritional management of patients, important factors in treatment outcomes (Afoakwa et al. 2004), are discussed in Chapter 5, and the provision of psychosocial services, a largely neglected issue (Shacham et al. 2008), is briefly examined in Chapter 6. Integration of these and other community-based resources into care and support structures requires research and community initiatives in traditional and popular social networks and institutions.

Donor-driven policies and programs: Prevention versus treatment

The early HIV/AIDS programs characteristically compartmentalized prevention and treatment as separate entities. They are rapidly giving way to programs integrating the two approaches because of the multiple secondary benefits of ART and the need to consider prevention and treatment as a continuum in comprehensive HIV/AIDS programs. Treatment is being used in PMTCT in two ways: to provide postexposure prophylaxis and to reduce viral load at the individual and population levels. These benefits may be fully realized in communities that provide ART access to everyone in need of treatment and communities that employ people-empowered prevention programs (Cohen 2010; UNAIDS 2010b).

The ART rollout constituted a major departure from the earlier development discourse, which tended to favor prevention and tacitly ignored care and treatment, leaving an immense unfilled need for HIV/AIDS care and treatment services. The call to feature care and treatment in the development discourse and donor policies has been well heeded. It is now generally recognized that any successful plan of action to fight the epidemic has to follow a multipronged approach. Countries committed themselves at the United Nation's Declaration of Commitment on HIV/AIDS in 2001 and the

Political Declaration on HIV/AIDS in 2006 to provide universal access to HIV prevention, treatment, care and support services to those in need by 2015, thereby also supporting the Millennium Development Goals (MDGs; UNAIDS 2011b).

However, recent concerns over sustainability of donor funding have created an environment of uncertainty as enrolling new patients for treatment jeopardizes the supply of ARVs. Moreover, donors have started to divert funds to other health issues in spite of the rising cost of increasingly comprehensive HIV/AIDS packages (MSF 2010; Sherr 2008). UNAIDS (2010a) reported that international investments, representing about half of all resources available for HIV/AIDS, are not increasing; they declined from $7.8 billion in 2008 to $7.7 billion in 2009. MSF (2010) conducted an investigation of donor commitment toward scaling up ART in eight countries (Malawi, Mozambique, Zimbabwe, South Africa, Lesotho, Kenya, Uganda, and the Democratic Republic of the Congo) and found that donors have started to shun their commitment to support expansion of HIV care and treatment, affecting the availability and quality of these services. This has brought to memory the dreadful reality of a decade ago when few HIV-infected persons could afford ART. Raising the funds necessary to meet national targets of universal access is becoming a daunting task for countries in Sub-Saharan Africa.

The recent change from ART as a kind of 'magic bullet' to structural and other preventive approaches may inadvertently be facilitated by the world economic crisis and the rising cost of ART caused by the growing need for more costly second-line antiretroviral drugs due to evolving drug resistance (see, for example, Aghokeng et al. 2011). UNAIDS does not report levels of ARV resistance or side effects in individual countries, impeding the monitoring of these two parameters. The Center for Global Development estimated that 22% of AIDS patients switch to second-line therapies after an average of 20 months on first-line therapy (Norris 2011), making treatment less cost-effective. In addition to economic constraints, interest of donors in the application of new prevention tools (Over 2010; UNAIDS 2010a) may increasingly favor prevention approaches in the search for cost-effective anti-AIDS programs.

Centralized versus decentralized service delivery systems

The debate over centralized (hospital-based) care versus decentralized diagnostic and treatment services and home-based care continues in many Sub-Saharan countries. While the centralized approach is still used in most countries and offers PLWHA the benefit of treatment by a highly trained health workforce, resource-poor countries are increasingly adopting the decentralized approach. Often labeled 'task shifting', decentralization is more feasible with limited resources and is more cost-effective (Assefa et al. 2010; Hermann et al. 2009). UN member states agreed at the 2006 High-Level

Meeting on HIV/AIDS to use the task-shifting approach to achieve universal access to comprehensive HIV treatment, care, and support. This approach of delegating tasks previously carried out by doctors to less specialized health workers, including nurses (Callaghan et al. 2010; Lehmann et al. 2009), has a number of positive outcomes, including greater access to life-saving treatment; improvement of workforce skills and health system efficiency; strengthening of community participation; and reducing of costs, attrition, and international 'brain drain' (Zachariah et al. 2009). Scholars note that this strategy will bear fruit only with strong political will, sustained financial support, and establishment of standards of safety and quality that address challenges inherent in the application of approaches involving nonhealth personnel, many of them volunteers (Lehmann et al. 2009; Zachariah et al. 2009).

The support for decentralized services is gaining momentum, with WHO at the forefront promoting the use of less skilled health workers to expand ART in light of the shortage of physicians at hospitals (Gilks et al. 2006). WHO promotes a model that delegates most ART activities to nurses, with doctors providing only supervision and offering solutions when cases have complications. The evidence for the success of this model is scant but positive results have been observed in Botswana, Mozambique, and Malawi (Zachariah et al. 2009). Zambia also successfully implemented this approach (Lehmann et al. 2009). In Ethiopia, Uganda, Malawi, Namibia, and Mozambique, the employment of community health workers with mandates to serve as counselors, educators, treatment providers, and advocates is increasing the accessibility and acceptability of ART (Assefa et al. 2011; Celletti et al. 2010; Simon et al. 2009). Part of the growing momentum for the adoption of task-shifting strategies is coming from community health workers; they are playing a crucial role in increasing the rollout of ART since they can execute many of the tasks that conventionally were carried out by health professionals. A growing body of evidence suggests that with close quality supervision and better remuneration and training, community health workers can play a vital role in HIV/AIDS services scale-up in Sub-Saharan Africa (Assefa et al. 2011; Hermann et al. 2009).

A study in a rural community in South Africa (Tsai et al. 2009) strengthened the case for expansion of services to marginalized people. The researchers reported that PLWHA who visited hospitals fared better than the average person in the community in terms of education and employment. Tsai et al. (2009) argued for a supplementary approach to improving access to HIV/AIDS care and treatment that addresses the shortcomings of clinic-based intervention in under-resourced areas. Other researchers call for closer scrutiny of the cost-effectiveness and sustainability of home-based care. Akintola (2008) noted that policies and programs promoting home-based care tend to ignore the contributions nonremunerated women make as caregivers.

A key objective of decentralization is improvement in accessibility of services. Earlier concerns that quality of health services may suffer due to the low level of skill used to drive this process (Gilks et al. 2006) have increasingly been proven to be unwarranted. The installation of quality and safety standards can facilitate the effective up-scaling of ART (Gilks et al 2006; Lehmann et al. 2009). Researchers in Zambia, examining the feasibility and effectiveness of primary care facilities in expanding access to ART, asserted that effective service delivery in settings such as Sub-Saharan Africa is possible. Expanding accessibility through decentralization promises to be effective since it can result in early detection and treatment and thus contribute to reducing mortality rates (Stringer et al. 2006). Gilks et al. (2006) suggested that larger numbers of PLWHA can be treated through public and private health facilities using standardized simplified treatment protocols and decentralized service delivery. They proposed simplified tools and approaches to clinical decision-making, centered on the 'four Ss': starting drug treatment, substituting for toxicity, switching after treatment failure, and stopping treatment.

Integrated vs. specialized programs and services: HIV/AIDS and TB

Integration of HIV/AIDS programs and services is becoming the order of the day in two areas: multidisease control and linkage with and strengthening of primary health care services. At the United Nations Millennium Summit in 2000, the international community targeted the three major killing diseases in developing countries – AIDS, tuberculosis, and malaria – in its Millennium Development Goals. This step and the subsequent commitment of governments to develop and implement a package for HIV prevention, treatment, and care with the aim of achieving the goals by 2015 prompted governments, development agencies, and financial institutions, particularly the Global Fund, to fight these three diseases by allocating resources and scaling up interventions.

The integration of services for HIV/AIDS and TB, two highly prevalent diseases in Sub-Saharan Africa that require similar case findings and chronic care procedures, has been essential to improving their diagnosis, treatment, and outcomes (Howard and El-Sadr 2010) and increasing the cost-effectiveness of programs that address them. There is considerable demand for these services in southern Africa (UNAIDS 2009b), and the high percentages of adult-incident tuberculosis cases infected with HIV in all eastern African countries, ranging from 17% in Ethiopia to 59% in Uganda (USAID 2010), suggests that integration of services would be useful. A qualitative study in South Africa about PLWHA's perceptions of HIV/AIDS care and treatment services concluded that the more integrated the services, the less the stigmatization (Orner et al. 2008). Nevertheless, major challenges remain, including assuring the financial sustainability of these integrated programs (Katz et al. 2010; Komatsu et al. 2010; World Bank 2010b).

The urgent need to integrate HIV/AIDS services into primary health care stems from the current diversion of scarce resources from other urgent sexual, reproductive, and maternal health services, particularly services dealing with other STIs, family planning, and mother and child health. Public health departments in many Sub-Saharan countries are responding to a potentially imbalanced health development scenario by using AIDS treatment and care resources to strengthen their primary health care systems, thereby also improving HIV/AIDS services (Pfeiffer et al. 2010). At least two countries – Ethiopia and Malawi – successfully met this challenge by revising their human resource policies and strengthening their health manpower at the community and facility levels, which strengthened not only ART services, but also general curative, mother and child health services and improved overall health outcomes (Rasschaert et al. 2011).

Although governments are interested in providing health services equitably, inadequately trained staff and the absence of laws protecting the rights of all PLWHA or failure to enforce such laws may add to the stigma and discrimination problem. For example, UNAIDS (2009b) suggested that the health needs of MSM be met by establishing clinics for men only where they can access VCT, referral, and treatment services. Men-only clinics could lessen the stigma and other complications MSM face in a homophobic context and an environment in which homosexuality is considered criminal.

The importance of properly training health staff in centers where integrated services are offered cannot be overstated. Reis et al. (2003, in UNAIDS 2007) reported the existence of stigma and discrimination against PLWHA among health professionals in Nigeria, where 430 of 1,000 health professionals interviewed claimed to have witnessed colleagues engaged in discriminatory practices. Several forms of stigma and discrimination by health workers have been reported from Ethiopia. For example, two-thirds of 30 traditional birth attendants interviewed wanted AIDS patients to be isolated because they thought the patients could infect others through hand shaking (Negassa et al. 2001), and many death certificates did not state that patients had died of AIDS (Lindtjørn 2001).

Constraints in scaling up access to treatment, care, and support

Notwithstanding the progress made so far in expanding HIV services, numerous factors constrain universal access to ART treatment, care, and support (UNAIDS 2010a). These include weak health systems (lack of doctors and nurses), the prohibitive cost of drugs or lack of appropriate drugs, CD4 and viral load tests, urban-biased health services, staggering deficits in funding, delays in patients reporting and starting treatment, poor treatment adherence, a large population unaware of their sero-status or the availability of treatment services, lack of coordination and collaboration among different stakeholders, and pervasive stigma against PLWHA.

Funding shortfalls and health manpower shortage

The rapid scale-up of ART services in Sub-Saharan countries has been hampered by inadequate health personnel and insufficient funding of programs in highly affected and resource-poor areas (Uebel et al. 2007). Despite the rapid increase on ART coverage and the strengthening of health services made possible through increased government and donor spending, the expansion of treatment programs has added to the burdens on health systems in many countries that were already under-resourced. The daunting disease burden, the exodus of high-level health manpower, and a demotivating working environment have exacerbated the health worker shortage throughout Sub-Saharan Africa (Lehmann et al. 2008, 2009; WHO 2006; Zachariah et al. 2009). AIDS-related diseases that claim the lives of many health professionals have amplified the manpower shortage. In Zambia, for instance, two-fifths of nurse attritions in the public sector have been attributed to deaths (MSF 2010). In South Africa, Malawi, Mozambique, and Swaziland, the shortage of human resources, exacerbated by high mortality among health workers (Bemelmans et al. 2011a), staff resignations, and migration, is a major obstacle to expanding HIV/AIDS services.

The trend of dwindling or diverted funding has manifested itself in various ways. The ITPC (2006) explained how a budget shift from AIDS treatment services to food emergencies in some rural parts of Kenya led to a decline in AIDS services, which aggravated the lack of health workers. Rural–urban funding differences and better living conditions for health workers in towns contributed to these disparities (Lehmann et al. 2008). Implementation of the 2009 WHO treatment guidelines, which provide for earlier and safer ART and put additional demands on health services, had to be modified or delayed in over half of the countries with the highest HIV prevalence (Bemelmans et al. 2011b). One of the hardest hit countries is the Democratic Republic of the Congo, where drastic cutbacks in funding required health facilities to charge for diagnostic and treatment services, resulting in significant reductions in new patient intakes, increased loss to follow-up and, thus apparently to increased pre-ART mortality and poor treatment outcomes (Phillips et al. 2011).

Many HIV/AIDS program managers are in the process of dealing with he discrepancy between funding and increased demand for services by developing innovative, more cost-effective interventions and management skills, by increasing domestic spending, and by exploring innovative funding schemes. A more targeted and strategic approach to investment in HIV/AIDS promises to increase the cost-effectiveness of programs by incorporating efficiency gains from community participation, synergies between program activities, and benefits of the extension of ART for prevention of HIV transmission (Schwartländer et al. 2011; UNAIDS 2020, p. 53). The challenges of this and other interventions integrating combinations of biomedical, behavioral, and structural approaches are significantly greater than those of single interventions, particularly in regard to the evaluation of component strategies, the place-specific nature of intervention outcomes, and the general lack of information regarding contextual factors (Gupta et al. 2008; Padian et al. 2011). Additional cost savings may be possible through further progress in ART administration using task shifting and simpler and less expensive HIV testing (UNAIDS 2012, p. 53).

Increased national ownership of programs and innovative funding are similarly promising to meet funding shortfalls. South Africa, for example, increased funding for HIV/AIDS five-fold between 2007 and 2011, spending an estimated $2 billion in 2011, more than any other low- and middle-income country. At least another dozen Sub-Saharan countries are exploring innovative ways to expand domestic funding of programs. They include an AIDS levy charged as a portion of personal and corporate income tax (Zimbabwe), establishment of an AIDS trust fund financed from various sources (Kenya and Zambia), levies in the mobile phone industry (Rwanda and Uganda), and a levy on airline travel (various countries) (UNAIDS 2012, pp. 104–107).

Stigma and discrimination

Being pervasive, instances of stigma in Sub-Saharan Africa are not always easy to discern (Greeff et al. 2008; Mbonu et al. 2009; Ncama et al. 2008). When stigma causes covering up and inability to admit one's status, it undermines the uptake of HIV/AIDS-related services, including treatment, care, and support. For example, a recent study by Tadele (2012) revealed that stigma and discrimination compromised uptake of and adherence to PMTCT-related services. The growing body of literature on stigma in the region recognizes the need to consider the role of the socio-cultural environment in addressing the treatment, care, and support needs of PLWHA (Mbonu et al. 2009).

The intricate social reality of AIDS impacts and discrimination in the public sphere and in all walks of life makes many PLWHA shun diagnostic and treatment services; many would rather turn to a diverse range of unconventional but culturally acceptable care, such as seeking the help of traditional healers, to avoid stigma. Even when people do start ART, they often discontinue treatment when they feel better. Many PLWHA either resort to indigenous medicines exclusively or combine them with manufactured drugs, as reported from Tanzania and Ethiopia (Berhanu 2010; Mbonu et al. 2009).

A study in Ethiopia showed that stigma associated with HIV/AIDS inhibits many PLWHA from accessing or adhering to ART. This problem is particularly serious among persons who have not disclosed their infection status. They find themselves in challenging scenarios, such as during fasting season when they abstain from specific foods or have no food at all for a certain period during the day, or when they visit holy water sites where the use of these drugs may be considered weakness of faith. Hence, they suspend taking their drugs for some time or try to take them clandestinely. This makes adhering to schedules difficult and emphasizes the role of contextual factors in ART access and adherence (Bezabih 2007).

Mills's (2006, in UNAIDS 2007) description of the responses by PLWHA in South Africa illustrates the stigmatizing context well. He noted that many PLWHA jeopardize drug adherence by postponing or rejecting services or trying to conceal medicines by travelling to other communities for care because of fear of breaches of confidentiality. A better understanding of adherence is needed toward meeting the goal of universal access to ART. Skovdal et al. (2011a) developed a broadly based framework for ART program planners and implementers in rural Zimbabwe that considers a number of contextual and psychosocial factors in ART adherence, which may be applied in other resource-poor areas.

Political will

Many studies have addressed the issue of central governments' 'commitment' to mounting effective responses to HIV, but the concept of political commitment is ill-defined. It does not, for example, allow distinctions between the relative impacts of government initiatives and systemic social and behavioral factors on recent declines in HIV prevalence (Fox et al. 2011). The most widely researched stance of any government in confronting the HIV/AIDS epidemic is that of South Africa, which has struggled in recent years, especially during the presidency of Thabo Mbeki, with lack of political will, denial of AIDS, and constraining the involvement of civil society and affected communities in HIV/AIDS interventions (ITPC 2006). In countries manifesting strong political will, by contrast, progress has been much faster. For example, ART coverage is at least twice as high in Botswana, Namibia, and even poorer Rwanda than in South Africa (Table 8.1).

Political will is important because interventions against HIV/AIDS in resource-poor areas need to be broad-based to achieve optimum results, involving partnerships and networks among stakeholders (UNAIDS 2010a). A partnership involving academic, government, and nongovernment institutions in KwaZulu-Natal, for example, improved visibility, relevance, pace, and effectiveness of programs (Pawinski and Lalloo 2006). Maher and Harries (2010) envisioned improvements in the standard of HIV/AIDS-related services as an entry point for collaboration of clinicians and public health workers. The massive ART rollout and the implementation of the combination HIV prevention approach, both of which require expanded testing, treatment, and care in conjunction with various evidence-based prevention approaches, make the mobilization of political will all the more important (Mayer and Krakower 2012).

Disability

Many interventions against HIV/AIDS in Sub-Saharan Africa neglect the needs of disabled people, leaving them at risk of HIV infection. This appears to be due to the erroneous perception that disabled people are not sexually active. In South Africa, 14% of people with disabilities studied in a 2008 national HIV survey were HIV-positive, a higher prevalence than reported for MSM and recreational drug users (Republic of South Africa 2010, p. 25). The stigma and discrimination attached to their disability undermines their access to HIV/AIDS care and treatment. Medical personnel often focus on the disabilities, leaving the sexual health needs of disabled people unattended. Many disabled persons in Sub-Saharan Africa live in poverty, further undermining their access to AIDS treatment, care, and support (Hanass-Hancock et al. 2011). A study in Zambia identified several factors undermining the access of disabled HIV-infected women to health facilities, including shortage of appropriate means of transport, lack of access to supportive equipment, and prejudice among health professionals. The situation of disabled PLWHA may therefore be more complicated than described in the literature (Rohleder et al. 2009).

Gendered access

Three in five PLWHA 15 years and older in Sub-Saharan Africa are women (UNAIDS 2010a), and women may be less able than men to access ART services in the predominantly patriarchal societies of this region, where social, cultural, economic, and other structural factors undermine their social rights (Cornell et al. 2009; Onyango 2008). Lower ART utilization rates in Malawi and South Africa (ITPC 2006) among women than men were associated with sociocultural disadvantages of women during the early stage of the ART roll-out. However, recent statistics across the subregion show that the proportion of females and males on ART mirrors the gendered infection rates: 55–70% of all people receiving treatment are women (UNAIDS 2010a).

Surprisingly, the relatively large number of females receiving treatment is due in part to better health-seeking behavior of women and the tendency of men to initiate ART at more advanced disease states than women (Bassett et al. 2010; Chen et al. 2008; Muula et al. 2007), which Skovdal et al. (2011b) attributed to the 'masculinity barrier' to use HIV services. This contrasts with the situation in Latin America and much of Asia, where concentrated epidemics put more males at HIV risk (UNAIDS 2010a, Annex 2). Cornell et al. (2011) noted that most ART-related policies in Africa neglect men's treatment needs, rendering assessment of equitable access to treatment services difficult. Amuron et al. (2007) found that men in Uganda were less interested in accessing care services than women, raising the question whether women, as child bearers and mothers, are more likely to seek treatment towards protecting their children. The relatively high access of women to ART and delays in male ART initiation are in stark contrast to the great disadvantages women face in sexual and social relations and underscore the importance of promoting communication between sexual partners and their joint use of ART services.

Although women have relatively good access to ART, female youth who were raped and sex workers face difficulties in accessing health services similar to those of MSM and other high-risk male groups in much of Sub-Saharan Africa. Females in South Africa under 18 years of age represent about 40% of all rapes and other forms of sexual assault but face numerous barriers in seeking medical and psychological assistance (Smith et al. 2010).

Poverty

Although the provision of free antiretroviral treatment in most Sub-Saharan countries has greatly reduced the cost of accessing treatment, poorer people in many communities continue to be vulnerable to HIV infection and its impacts. PLWHA have difficulty covering expenses for transportation and drugs for opportunistic diseases, further undermining access to treatment. In the Democratic Republic of the Congo, PLWHA visited health facilities in the late stage of their illness due to lack of money for prerequisite CD4 testing to start ART (MSF 2010), and at a South African AIDS clinic, 17.3% of delays in ART initiation by children were due to socioeconomic obstacles (Feucht et al. 2007). Tsai et al. (2009) found socioeconomic disparities in access to hospital-based HIV/AIDS treatment programs in a rural community in South Africa, with poorer PLWHA being underrepresented. Many PLWHA in Sub-Saharan Africa who are able to access ART experience food insecurity, a major factor in poor ART adherence, treatment outcomes, and patient survival (Anema et al. 2009; Weisser et al. 2010).

These deficiencies highlight the need for improved access to HIV/AIDS care and treatment without the shortcomings of clinic-based intervention in under-resourced areas. Home-based care is clearly increasing the affordability and sustainability of patient care because it is largely provided by family members in Sub-Saharan African communities. The variable findings and particularly the complex and often counterintuitive pathways described elsewhere in this volume indicate that poverty is multidimensional and interacts with numerous other socioeconomic factors in creating vulnerability to HIV, further requiring that interventions are place- and context- specific, as has been noted by a number of researchers (Gupta et al. 2008; Kim et al. 2008).

Religion and cultural tradition

Since the mid-1990s, different religious traditions in Sub-Saharan Africa have developed their own distinctive responses to the HIV/AIDS epidemic. Religious convictions and ideologies in churches in Botswana and Islamic centers in Nigeria, for example, govern institutional and practical relations that have evolved around the ART rollout. Religious institutions have mobilized antiretroviral drives in Zambia and other southern African countries, and faith-based therapies are widely used by some populations (Dilger et al. 2010). In Ethiopia, visits of PLWHA belonging to the Orthodox Church to holy water sites in search of healing from HIV have greatly increased in recent years. At one holy water site in the vicinity of Addis Ababa, the number of PLWHA increased from 192 in 1998/99 to 3,680 in 2003/04. Bezabih (2007) attributed this increase to individuals' claims of being cured by treatment with holy water. There is no clear consensus among religious followers and leaders whether people turning to spiritual healing can also make effective use of ART. Doing so is considered by devout believers as questioning the healing power of faith. Out of 120 PLWHA studied at a holy water site outside of Addis Ababa in 2006, 36% were against taking ARV drugs (Berhanu 2010).

Belief in witchcraft and the widespread use of traditional medicines also influence the health-seeking behavior of PLWHA in parts of Sub-Saharan Africa. According to Kwena et al. (2011), in a rural Kenyan community, rapid and persistent weight loss was labelled 'witchcraft-disease'. In Ghana, traditional healing and faith camps have been set up for PLWHA who believe AIDS is caused by the supernatural (Benefour et al. 2011). In a rural village in South Africa, half of the people who had missed appointments for ART allegedly took alternative medicines, mostly traditional remedies (Mpufo et al. 2011). These and other findings indicate that despite greatly improved access to ART, widespread belief in spiritual causation of AIDS has prevented many individuals from seeking diagnosis and treatment. Notwithstanding these and other facets of traditional medical systems that impede the health-seeking behavior of PLWHA, some positive aspects of traditional healing, such as the active participation of healers in prevention programs, have been recognized; these are described in Chapter 2.

Although studies on these and other intervention issues indicate the need to contextualize HIV/AIDS interventions by considering socioeconomic, cultural, political, and institutional factors, few studies have been carried out. After reviewing the literature on ART adherence in southern Africa, Kagee et al. (2011) recommended that new approaches be developed for the ART delivery system that better meet local needs and capacities at the individual, community, and national levels. They called for multipronged research agendas and strong collaboration among researchers, clinicians, policy makers, funding agencies, and community groups to develop effective programs that are achievable and sustainable in different settings. Ouma and van der Kwaak (2009) evaluated the content, accessibility, and quality of sexuality counseling services provided by an NGO at Nairobi and Kisumu youth centers. They reported a number of encouraging characteristics of the youth-friendly services and recommended follow-up studies to determine their impact on behavior change and other positive health outcomes.

Conclusion

This chapter highlighted prominent issues related to the development of and access to HIV/AIDS treatment, prevention, care, and support services. The call for implementation of treatment policies and programs has been receiving growing support from governments, donors, and other national and international stake holders, with the aims of providing universal access to treatment, recognizing the rights of PLWHA, and addressing issues of equity. The sharp increase in the provision of and access to HIV/AIDS treatment, prevention, care, and support services in Sub-Saharan Africa during the first decade of the twenty-first century is evidence of political will and collaboration among government, civil society, and NGOs.

But there is danger that further up-scaling of anti-HIV/AIDS programs may become jeopardized by priority shifts initiated by donors and the worldwide economic recession. This is cause for great concern in the face of the increasing numbers of people needing treatment, care, and support. Solutions require both innovative funding approaches and cost-effective, sustainable treatment and prevention programs that harness community resources and build new coalitions. In response to recent funding cuts and lack of resources globally, some African governments are starting to mobilize more internal resources for HIV/AIDS prevention, treatment, care, and support, although these efforts are still sporadic and not fully integrated into national HIV/AIDS programs.

In addition to the macroeconomic issues, a number of socioeconomic, psychological, and infrastructural constraints and human rights issues need to be addressed to ensure greater accessibility and utilization of preventive, treatment, care, and support services. The level of access to services tends to reflect existing socioeconomic hierarchies at the community level, where poor people have far less access than wealthier groups. Nevertheless, persisting low access by marginalized groups, including rural dwellers, disabled persons, youth, and other groups at high risk requires changes in social policy and structural approaches that strengthen stigma and discrimination reduction programs. Despite having access to HIV-related services, many PLWHA struggle to adhere to ART due to stigma and discrimination coupled with lack of emotional and financial support.

The massive rollout of ART needs to consider the broad range of social, economic, and psychological needs of PLWHA as well as health infrastructure capacity if recent progress is to be maintained. Greater efforts must be made to reach individuals in vulnerable groups, particularly orphans and children in general, married or cohabiting partners, MSM, and sex workers, considering that they account for a significant proportion of new HIV cases in urban communities.

Evidence is rapidly accumulating that acute shortages of health workers and health services in Sub-Saharan Africa can be overcome through new approaches. The shift from hospital-based care to community- and home-based care may reduce and ameliorate shortages and facilitate the scaling up of programs, particularly those using comprehensive and integrated prevention/treatment strategies. Possibilities of enlisting well-accepted community-based institutions such as the *iddir* need to be explored and psychosocial services extended to provide wider coverage of care and support needs. Multidisease platforms for service delivery, especially those encompassing HIV/AIDS, reproductive health, tuberculosis, and STI services, increase the prospects of better identifying, monitoring, and serving HIV/AIDS cases. Interventions benefiting from harmonization of government, community-based, civil society, and NGOs stand to accomplish the most.

References

Afoakwa, E.O., Owusu, W.B. and Adjei, M.R. 2004. Nutritional management, care and support for people living with HIV/AIDS in sub-Saharan Africa. *Abstracts, 15th International AIDS Conference*, Bangkok. Abstract D10071.

Aghokeng, A.F., Kouanfack, C., Laurent, C. et al. 2011. Scale-up of antiretroviral treatment in sub-Saharan Africa is accompanied by increasing HIV-1 drug resistance mutations in drug-naïve patients. *AIDS* 13:2183–2188.

Akintola, O. 2008. Unpaid HIV/AIDS care in Southern Africa: Forms, context, and implications. *Feminist Economics* 14:117–147.

Amuron, B., Coutinho, A. and Grosskurth, H. 2007. A cluster-randomised trial to compare home-based with health facility-based antiretroviral treatment in Uganda: Study design and baseline findings. *Open AIDS Journal* 1:21–27.

Andersson, N. and Cockcroft, A. 2012. Male circumcision, attitudes to HIV prevention and HIV status: A cross-sectional study in Botswana, Namibia and Swaziland. *AIDS Care* 24:301–309.

Anema, A., Vogelthaler, N., Frongilo, F.A. et al. 2009. Food insecurity and HIV/AIDS: Current knowledge, gaps, and research priorities. *Current HIV/AIDS Reports* 6:224–231.

Assefa, Y., Kiflie, A., Tesfaye, D. et al. 2011. Outcomes of antiretroviral treatment program in Ethiopia: Retention of patients in care is a major challenge and varies across health facilities. *BMC Health Services Research* 11:81. doi: 101186/1472-6963-11-81

Assefa, Y., Van Damme, W., Haile Mariam, D. and Kloos, H. 2010. Toward universal access to HIV counselling and testing and antiviral treatment in Ethiopia: Looking beyond HIV testing and ART initiation. *AIDS Patient Care and STDs* 24: 521–525.

Baird, S., Chirwa, E., McIntosh, C. and Ötzler, B. 2009. *The Short-Term Impacts of a Schooling Conditional Cash Transfer Programme on the Sexual Behaviour of Young Women*. Policy Research Working Paper. Washington, DC: World Bank.

Bärnighausen, T., Tanser, F., Dabis, F. and Newell, M.L. 2012. Interventions to improve the performance of HIV systems for treatment-as-prevention in sub-Saharan Africa: The experimental evidence. *Current Opinions in HIV and AIDS* 7:140–150.

Bassett I.V., Regan S., Chetty S. et al. 2010. Who starts antiretroviral therapy in Durban, South Africa?... Not everyone who should. *AIDS* 24(Suppl.)1:S37–S44.

Beckerleg, S., Telfer, M. and Hundt, G.L. 2005. The rise of injecting drug use in East Africa: A case study from Kenya. *Harm Reduction Journal* 2:12.

Bemelmans, M., Lynch, S., Woods, S. et al. 2011a. Countries forced to phased or partial implementation of WHO guidelines due to funding shortfalls. *Abstracts of the International Conference of AIDS and STDs in Africa*, Addis Ababa. Abstract WEA0405.

Bemelmans, M., van der Akker, T., Pasulani, O. et al. 2011b. Keeping health staff healthy: Evaluation of a workplace initiative to reduce morbidity and mortality from HIV/AIDS in Malawi. *Journal of the International AIDS Society* 14:1.

Benefour, S., Duodu, J., Nana Fosua, C. et al. 2011. Engaging traditional health practitioners to improve access to antiretroviral therapy in Ghana. *Abstracts of the International Conference on AIDS and Sexually Transmitted Diseases*, Addis Ababa. Abstract WEPE147.

Berhanu, Z. 2010. Holy water as an intervention for HIV/AIDS in Ethiopia. *Journal of HIV/AIDS & Social Services* 9:240–260.

Bezabih, E. 2007. Antiretroviral treatment – its social and religious challenges: The experience of 32 members from two associations – Tesfa Setechign Mariam and Mekdim Ethiopia. Master's thesis, Addis Ababa University, Graduate School of Social Work.

Callaghan, M., Ford, N. and Schneider, H. 2010. A systematic review of task-shifting for HIV treatment and care in Africa. *Human Resources for Health* 8:8. http://www.human-resources-health.com/content/8/1/8

Campbell, C. 2003. Why HIV prevention programs fail. *British Medical Journal* 11:437–480.

CDC. 2011. CDC trial and another major study find PrEP can reduce risk of HIV infection among heterosexuals. Press release. Atlanta: Centers for Disease Control and Prevention. http://www.cdc.gov/nchhstp/newsroom/PrePHeterosexuals.html

Celletti, F., Wright, A., Palen, J. et al. 2010. Can the deployment of community health workers for the delivery of HIV services represent an effective and sustainable response to health workforce shortages? Results of a multicountry study. *AIDS* 24(Suppl. 1):S45–S57.

Chege, J., Meassick, E., Afework, S. et al. 2011. Can communities be agents of their own change through addressing social norms that increase girls' and womens' vulnerability to HIV infection risk behavior? *Abstracts of the International Conference on AIDS and STI in Africa*, Addis Ababa. Abstract MOPE144.

Chen, S.C., Yu, J.K., Harries, A.D. et al. 2008. Increased mortality of male adults with AIDS related to poor compliance to antiretroviral therapy in Malawi. *Tropical Medicine and International Health* 13:513–519.

Cohen, M. 2010. HIV treatment as prevention: To be or not to be? *Journal of Aquired Immune Deficinecy Syndromes* 55:137–138.

Cornell, M., McIntyre, J. and Myer, L. 2011. Men and antiretroviral therapy in Africa: Our blind spot. *Tropical Medicine and International Health* 21:828–829.

Cornell, M., Myer, L., Kaplan, R., et al. 2009. The impact of gender and income on survival and retention in a South African antiretroviral therapy programme. *Tropical Medicine and International Health* 14:722–731.

Dilger, H. 2010. Morality, hope and grief: Anthropologies of AIDS in Africa. In Dilger, H. and Ute Luig, U. (eds.), *Morality, Hope and Grief: Anthropologies of AIDS in Africa*, pp. 102–126. New York: Berghahn Books.

Dilger, H., Burchard, M. and van Dijk, R. 2010. Introduction: The redemptive moment, HIV treatment and the production of new religious spaces. *African Journal of AIDS Research* 9:373–383.

ECA. 2007. *Relevance of African Traditional Institutions of Governance*. Addis Ababa: Economic Commission for Africa.

Elemo, I.A. 2005. HIV/AIDS, gender and reproductive health promotion: The role of traditional institutions among Borana Oromo, southern Ethiopia. Unpublished.

Erulkar, A.S. and Muthengi, E. 2009. Evaluation of Berhane Hewan: A program to delay child marriage in rural Ethiopia. *International Perspectives on Sexual and Reproductive Health* 35:6–10.

Farorsey, C.K. and Amolo, R.K. n.d. *Empowering Queeen Mothers and Magajias in the Fight against HIV/AIDS*. Washington, DC: CEDPLA.

FDRE (Federal Democratic Republic of Ethiopia). 2010. *Report on Progress towards Implementation of the UN Declaration of Commitment on HIV/AIDS 2010*. Addis Ababa: Federal HIV/AIDS Prevention and Control Office.

Feucht, U.D., Kinzer, M. and Kruger, M. 2007. Reasons for delay in initiation of antiretroviral therapy in a population of HIV-infected South African children. *Journal of Tropical Pediatrics* 53:398–402.

Fox, A.M., Goldberg, A.B., Gore, R.J. and Bärninghausen, T. 2011. Conceptual and methodological challenges to measuring political commitment to respond to HIV. *Journal of the International AIDS Society* 14(Suppl. 2):S5.

Gedefaw, M., Endawoke, Y., Mekonnen, D. et al. 2011. Outcome and challenges of community conversations on HIV/AIDS prevention and control in Amhara National Regional State, Ethiopia. *Abstracts of the 16th International Conference on AIDS and STIs in Africa*, Addis Ababa. Abstract TUAD0804.

Gilks, C. F., Crowley, S. and Ekpini, R. 2006. *The WHO Public-health Approach to Antiretroviral Treatment Against HIV in Resource-limited Settings*. Geneva: WHO.

Government of Uganda. 2010. *UNGASS Country Progress Report Uganda*, January 2008–December 2009. http//:data.unaids.org/pub/Report/2010/Uganda_2010_country_progress-report-en.pdf

Greeff, M., Phetlhu, R., Makoae, L. N. et al. 2008. Disclosure of HIV status: Experiences and perceptions of persons living with HIV/AIDS and nurses involved in their care in Africa. *Qualitative Health Research* 18:311–324.

Gupta, N. and Mahy, M. 2003. Sexual initiation among adolescent girls and boys: Trends and differentials in sub-Saharan Africa. *Archives of Sexual Behavior* 32:41–53.

Gupta, G.R., Parkhurst, J.O., Ogden, J.A. et al. 2008. Structural approaches to HIV prevention. *Lancet* 372:764–775.

Hanass-Hancock, J., Strode, A. and Grant, C. 2011. Inclusion of disability within national strategic responses to HIV and AIDS in Eastern and Southern Africa. *Disability and Rehabilitation* 33:2389–2396.

Hermann, K., Van Damme, W., Pariyo, G.W. et al. 2009. Community health workers for ART in sub-Saharan Africa: Learning from experience – capitalizing on new opportunities. *Human Resources for Health* 7:31.

Holmes, K., Winskell, K., Hennink, M. and Chidiac, S. 2011. Microfinance and HIV mitigation among people living with HIV in the era of anti-retroviral therapy: Emerging lessons from Côte d'Ivoire. *Global Public Health* 6:447–461.

Howard, A.A. and El-Sadr, W.W. 2010. Integration of tuberculosis and HIV services in sub-Saharan Africa: Lessons learned. *Clinical Infectious Diseases* 50(Suppl.): S238–S244.

IAS (International AIDS Society). 2009. Reaffirming the G8 commitment to universal access: Gleneagles + five. 19 November.

Improper. 2012. Improper condom use a public health issue worldwide. *Medical News Today*, 23 February. http://www.medicalnewstoday.com/release/241999.php

International Group (International Group on Analysis of Trends in HIV Prevalence and Behaviours in Young People in Countries Most Affected by HIV). 2010. Trends in HIV prevalence and sexual behaviour among young people aged 15–24 years in countries most affected by HIV. *Sexually Transmitted Infections* 96(Suppl. 2):ii72–ii83.

ITPC (International Preparedness Coalition). 2006. *Missing the Target, Off Target for 2010: How to Avoid Breaking the Promise of Universal Access.* http://www.hivpolicy.org/Library/HPP001360.pdf

Johnson, L.F., Hallett, T.B., Rehle, T.M. and Dorrrington, R.E. 2012. The effect of changes in condom usage and antiretroviral treatment coverage on human immunodeficiency virus incidence in South Africa: A model-based analysis. *Journal of the Royal Society Interface* January 18:1444–1554. doi: 10.1098/rsif.2011.0826

Kagee, A., Remien, R.H., Berkman, A. et al. 2011. Structural barriers to ART adherence in Southern Africa: Challenges and potential ways forward. *Global Public Health* 6:83–97.

Kalibala, S. and Littlefield, A. 2010. The role of ARVs in HIV prevention: Microbicides and PrEP. *GMHC Treatment Issues.* http://www.gmhc.org/files/editor/file/r_ti_1210.pdf2

Katz, I., Komatsu, R., Low-Beer, D. and Atun, R. 2010. Scaling up towards international targets for AIDS, tuberculosis, and malaria: Contribution of Global Fund-supported programs in 2011–2015. *PLoS ONE* 6(2):e17166.

Kesby M. 2004. Participatory diagraming and the ethical and practical challenges of helping Africans themselves to move HIV work 'beyond epidemiology.' In Kalipeni E, Craddock S, Oppong J, Gosh J (eds.), *HIV & AIDS in Africa: Beyond Epidemiology*, pp. 217–239. Oxford: Blackwell.

Kim, J., Pronyk, P., Barnett, T. and Watts, C. 2008. Exploring the role of economic empowerment in HIV prevention. *AIDS* (Suppl. 4):S57–S71.

Kloos, H. and Haile Mariam, D. 2008. Some neglected and emerging factors in HIV transmission in Ethiopia. *Ethiopian Medical Journal* 45:103–108.

Komatsu, R., Korenromp, E.L., Watt, C. et al. 2010. Lives saved by Global Fund-supported HIV/AIDS, tuberculosis and malaria programs: Estimation approach and results between 2003 and end-2007. *BMC Infectious Diseases* 10:109.

Kwena, Z., Manyasa, E., and Mwanzo, I. 2011. The care provider's perspectives on effect of witchcraft beliefs on the management of AIDS patients. *Abstracts of the International Conference on AIDS and Sexually Transmitted Disease*, Addis Ababa. Abstract CD172.

Leclerc-Madlala, S. 2008. Intergenerational/age-disparate sex: Policy and programme action brief. Technical Meeting on Young Women in HIV Hyper-endemic Countries in Southern Africa. Sunninghill, South Africa: UNAIDS Regional Support Team for West and Central Africa. http://www.unaidsrstesa.org/usefiles/file/womenGirls_AgeDisparate.pdf

Lehmann, U., Dieleman, M. and Martineau, T. 2008. Staffing remote rural areas in middle- and low-income countries: A literature review of attraction and retention. *BMC Health Services Research* 23(8):19.

Lehmann, U., Van Damme, W., Barten, F. and Sanders, D. 2009. Task shifting: The answer to the human resources crisis in Africa? *Human Resources for Health* 7:49.

Lindtjørn, B. 2001. Letter in response to 'Words that are not spoken: An inside look at the African AIDS crisis.' *MedGenMed* 29 January:E8–E9.

MacQueen, K. 2011. Global HIV prevention research: biomedical, social and ethical crossroads. Unpublished paper. www.youtube.com/watch?v=hUAQJ5Dky00

Maher, D. and Harries, A.D. 2010. Quality care: A link between clinical and public health approaches to HIV infection in developing countries. *Tropical Medicine and International Health* 15:391–395.

Mathers, B.M., Degenhardt, L., Ali, H. et al. 2010. HIV prevention, treatment, and care services for people who inject drugs: A systematic review of global, regional, and national coverage. *Lancet* 22(375):961–963.

Maughan-Brown, B. 2010. Stigma rises despite antiretroviral rollout: A longitudinal analysis in South Africa. *Social Science and Medicine* 70:368–374.

May, M.T. and Ingle, S.M. 2011. Life expectancy of HIV-positive adults: A review. *Sexual Health* 8:526–533.

Mayer, K.H. and Krakower, D. 2012. Antiretroviral medication and HIV prevention: New steps foward and new questions. *Annals of Internal Medicine* January 156:312–314.

Mbonu, N.C., van den Borne, B. and De Vries, N.K. 2009. Stigma of people with HIV/AIDS in Sub-Saharan Africa: A literature review. *Journal of Tropical Medicine* epub 16 Aug, doi: 10.55/2009/145891.

Merson, M.H., O'Malley, J., Serwadda, D. and Apisuk, C. 2008. The history and challenge of HIV prevention. *Lancet* 372(9637):475–488.

Mills, E.J., Bakanda, C., Birungi, J. et al. 2012. Life expectancy of persons receiving combination antiretroviral theraphy in low-income countries: A cohort analysis from Uganda. *Annals of Internal Medicine* 155:209–216.

MSF (Médecins Sans Frontières). 2010. *No Time to Quit: HIV/AIDS Treatment Gap Widening in Africa*. Special Report, 26 May. http://www.doctorswithoutborders.org/publications/article.cfm?cat=special-report&id=4492

Mpufo, D., Shilagu, T. and Adoons, D. 2011. Engaging traditional health practitioners in HIV treatment, care and support in South Africa. *Abstracts of the International Conference on AIDS and Sexually Transmitted Diseases*, Addis Ababa. Abstract WEPE146.

Muula, A.S., Ngulube, T.J., Siziya, S. et al. 2007. Gender distribution of adult patients on highly active antiretroviral therapy (HAART) in Southern Africa: A systematic review. *BMC Public Health* 7:63. http://www.biomedcentral.com/1471-2458/7/63

Nassali, M., Nakanjako, D., Kyabayinze, D. et al. 2009. Access to HIV/AIDS care for mothers and children in sub-Saharan Africa: Adherence to the postnatal PMTCT program. *AIDS Care* 21:1121–1131.

Ncama, B. P., McInerney, P.A., Bhengu, B.R. et al. 2008. Social support and medication adherence in HIV disease in KwaZulu-Natal, South Africa. *International Journal of Nursing Studies* 45:1757–1763.

Negassa, A., Wold, Michael K. and Negassa, A. 2001. Knowledge, attitude and practices of traditional birth attendants on HIV/AIDS in Jimma town, southwest Ethiopia. *Ethiopian Journal of Health Science* 1:123–129.

Norris, J. 2011. *Global UNAIDS Report: All the Good Done Can Be Undone*. Washington, DC: Center for Global Prosperity, Hudson Institute.

Okwundu, C.I., Uthman, O.A. and Okoramah, C.A.N. 2012. Antiretroviral pre-exposure prophylaxis (PrEP) for preventing HIV in high-risk individuals. *Cochrane Database of Systematic Reviews* 7. doi: 10.1002/14651858.CD007189.pub3.

O'Laughlin, K.N., Wyatt, M.A., Kaaya, S. et al. 2012. How treatment partners help: Social analysis of an African adherence support initiation. *AIDS and Behavior* 16:1308–1315.

Onyango, D. 2008. Great challenges to PMTCT in the South: The role of the developed nations in supporting strategies that work. *Retrovirology* 5(Suppl. 1):1–2.

Orner, P., Cooper, D., Myer, L. et al. 2008. Clients' perspectives on HIV/AIDS care and treatment and reproductive health services in South Africa. *AIDS Care* 20: 1217–1223.

Ouma, A.J. and van der Kwaak, A. 2009. *Promotion of Sexual Health for Young People in Kenya*. Amsterdam: KIT.

Over, M. 2010. A refreshingly open debate on the values of universal access to AIDS treatment for U.S. foreign policy. Center for Global Development. http://cgdev.org/global health/2010/08/a-refreshingly-open-debate-on-the-value-of-universal-access-to-aids-treatment-on-u-s-foreign policy.php/

Padian, N.S., McCoy, S.I., Mania, S. et al. 2011. Evaluation of large-scale combination HIV prevention programs essential issues. *Journal of Acquired Immune Deficiency Syndromes* 58(2):e23–e28.

Pawinski, R.A. and Lalloo, U.G. 2006. Multisectoral responses to HIV/AIDS: Applying research to policy and practice. *American Journal of Public Health* 96: 1189–1191.

Pfeiffer, J., Montaya, P., Baptista, A.J. et al. 2010. Integration of HIV/AIDS services into African primary health care: Lessons learned for health system strengthening in Mozambique – a case study. *Journal of the International AIDS Society* 13:3.

Phillips, M., Benazeh, C., Camara, M. et al. 2011. Rationing HIV treatment in real life: Funding shortfall causes a widening, deadly treatment gap in Democratic Republic of the Congo (DRC). *Abstracts of the International Conference on AIDS and STDs in Africa*. Addis Ababa. Abstract MOPE294.

Pronyk, P.M., Hargreaves, J.R., Kim, J.C. et al. 2006. Effect of a structural intervention for the prevention of intimate partner violence and HIV in rural South Africa: Results of a cluster randomized trial. *Lancet* 368:1973–1983.

Pronyk, P.M., Kim, J.C., Abramsky, T. et al. 2008. A combined microfinance and training intervention can reduce HIV risk behaviour in young female participants. *AIDS* 22:1659–1665.

Rasschaert, F., Pirard, M., Philips, M.P. et al. 2011. Positive spill-over effect of ART scale up on wider health systems development: Evidence from Ethiopia and Malawi. *Journal of the International AIDS Society* 14(Suppl. 1):S3.

Republic of South Africa. 2010. *Country Progress Report on the Declaration of Commitment on HIV/AIDS 2010*. Final Report. Submitted to UNAIDS, Geneva.

Richter, K., Phillips, S.C., McInnis, A.M. and Rice, D.A. 2011. Effectiveness of a multi-country workplace intervention in sub-Saharan Africa. *AIDS Care* 13(Suppl. 2):S1.

Rohleder, P. Braathen, S.H., Swartz, L. and Eide, A.H. 2009. HIV/AIDS and disability in Southern Africa: A review of relevant literature. *Disability & Rehabilitation* 31: 51–59.

Rosen, S. and Fox, M.P. 2012. Retention in HIV care between testing and treatment in sub-Saharan Africa: A systematic review. *Public Library of Science Medicine* S:e 1001056.

Schwartländer, B., Stover, J., Hallet, T. et al. 2011. Towards an improved investment approach for an effective response to HIV/AIDS. *Lancet* 377(9782): 2031–2041.

Shacham, E., Reece, M., Ong'or, W.O. et al. 2008. Characteristics of psychosocial support seeking during HIV-related treatment in western Kenya. *AIDS Patient Care* 22:595–601.

Sherr, L. 2008. Strengthening families through HIV/AIDS prevention, treatment, care and support-a review of the literature. Paper prepared for the Joint Learning Initiative on Children and HIV/AIDS (JLICA), Royal Free and University College Medical School, London.

Simon, S., Chu, K., Frieden, M. et al. 2009. An integrated approach of community health worker support for HIV/AIDS and TB care in Angonia district, Mozambique. *BMC International Health and Human Rights* 9:13.

Skovdal, M., Campbell, C., Madanhire, C. et al. 2011a. Masculinity as a barrier to men's use of HIV services in Zimbabwe. *Globalization and Health* 7:13.

Skovdal, M., Campbell, C., Nhongo, K. et al. 2011b. Contextual and psychosocial influences on antiretroviral therapy adherence in rural Zimbabwe: Towards a systematic framework for programme planners. *International Journal of Health Panning and Management* 26:296–316.

Smith, K., Bryant-Davis, T., Tillman, S. and Marks, A. 2010. Stifled voices: Barriers to help-seeking behavior for South African childhood sexual assault survivors. *Journal of Child Sexual Abuse* 19:255–274.

Stringer, J.S.A., Zulu, I. and Levy, J. 2006. Rapid scale-up of antiretroviral therapy at primary care sites in Zambia: Feasibility and early outcomes. *Journal of the American Medical Association* 296:782–793.

Tadele, G. 2012. Gender-related barriers to services to prevent vertical transmission of HIV in high-burden countries: The case of Ethiopia. Report submitted to UNAIDS Ethiopia. Unpublished.

Tadele, G., Loevinsohn, M., Ayalew, A. and Fleming, V. 2011. Strengthening livelihoods in communities confronting HIV: An exploratory study in Ethiopia: Report submitted to STOP AIDS NOW, Amsterdam. Unpublished.

Tsai, A.C., Chopra, M., Pronyk, P.M. and Martinson, N.A. 2009. Socioeconomic disparities in access to HIV/AIDS treatment programs in resource-limited settings. *AIDS Care* 21:59–63.

Uebel, K.E., Nash, J. and Avalos, A. 2007. Caring for the caregivers: Models of HIV/AIDS care and treatment provision for health care workers in Southern Africa. *Journal of Infectious Diseases* 196(Special Issue 3):S500–S504.

UNAIDS. 2005. *Resource Needs for an Expanded Response to AIDS in Low- and Middle-Income Countries.* Geneva. http://data.unaids.org/pub/Report/2005/jc1255_resource_needs_en.pdf

UNAIDS. 2007. *Reducing HIV Stigma and Discrimination: A Critical Part of National AIDS Programmes.* Geneva: UNAIDS. http://data.unaids.org/pub/Report/2008/jc1521_stigmatisation_en.pdf

UNAIDS. 2008. *AIDS Epidemic Update, 2008.* Geneva. http://data.unaids.org/pub/EPIslides/2007/2007_epiupdate_en.pdf

UNAIDS. 2009a. *AIDS Epidemic Update.* http://data.unaids.org/pub/Report/2009/jc1700_epi_update_2009_en.pdf

UNAIDS. 2009b. *Annual Report 2009.* http://data.unaids.org/pub/Report/2010/2009_annual_report_en.pdf

UNAIDS. 2009c. AIDS responses and action in rural Ethiopia. *Feature Story* 22 April. http://www.unaids.org/en/resources/presscentre/featurstories/2009/april/20090422ruralethiopia/

UNAIDS. 2010a. *Report of the Global AIDS Epidemic 2010.* Geneva: UNAIDS.

UNAIDS. 2010b. *Combination HIV Prevention: Tailoring and Coordinating Biomedical, Behavioural and Structural Strategies to Reduce New HIV Infections.* Geneva: UNAIDS.

UNAIDS. 2011a. *World AIDS Day Report 2011.* Geneva: UNAIDS.

UNAIDS. 2011b. *Universal Access to HIV Prevention, Treatment, Care and support: From Countries to Regions to the High Level Meeting on AIDS and Beyond, 2011 Road Map.* Geneva: UNAIDS.

UNAIDS. 2012. *Together We Will End AIDS.* Geneva: UNAIDS.

UNDP. 2005. *Community Capacity Enhancement Handbook.* www.undp.og/hiv/docs/progr_guides/cce_handbook.pdf

UNDP. 2011. Community conversations' success celebrated in Leribe. *News release*, 17 December. http://www.undp.org.ls/newsCCLE_2011

USAID. 2010. *HIV Profile: East Africa*. Nairobi: USAID.

USAID. 2011a. The Female Condom. http://www.usaid.gov/our_work/global_health/aids/TechAreas/prevention/femalecondom.hlml

USAID. 2011b. *Structural Interventions: An Overview of Structural Approaches to HIV Prevention*. Washington, DC: USAID. http://www.aidstar-one.com/focus_areas/prevention/pkb/structural_interventions/overview_structural_approaches_hiv_prevention

Uthman, O.A., Popoola, T.A., Yahaya, I. et al. 2011. The cost-utility analysis of adult male circumcision for prevention of heterosexual acquisition of HIV in men in sub-Saharan Africa: A probabilistic decision model. *Value Health* 14:70–79.

Van Dyk, A. 2008. *Caring and Counselling: A Multidisciplinary Approach*. Sandton, Gautend, South Africa: Pearson South Africa.

Wabwire-Mangen, F., Odiit, M., Kirungi W. et al. 2008. *Analysis of HIV Prevention Response and Modes of HIV Transmission: The Uganda Country Synthesis Report*. Kampala: UGANDA AIDS Commission and UNAIDS.

Walensky, R.P. and Bassett, I.V. 2011. HIV self-testing and the missing linkage. *PLoS Medicine* 8(10):e1001101.

Wambe, M., Gregson, S., Nyamupapa, C.A. et al. 2005. HIV infection and reproductive health in teenage women orphaned and made vulnerable by AIDS in eastern Zimbabwe. *Abstracts of the 15th International AIDS Conference*, Bangkok. Abstract TUORCI153.

Weiss, H.A., Dickson, K.E., Agot, K. and Hankins, C.A. 2010. Male circumcision for HIV prevention: Current research and programmatic issues. *AIDS* 24(Suppl. 4):S61–S69.

Weisser, S.D., Tuller, D.M., Frongillo, F.A. et al. 2010. Food insecurity as a barrier to sustainable antiretroviral therapy adherence in Uganda. *PLoS One* 5(4):e10340.

WHO. 2006. *The World Health Report 2006: Working together for Health*. Geneva: WHO.

WHO. 2007. *Task Shifting to Tackle Health Worker Shortage*. Geneva: World Health Organization.

Wilhelm-Solomon, M. 2010. *Stigmatization, Disclosure and the Social Space of the Camp: Reflections on ART Provision to the Displaced in Northern Uganda*. Center for Social Science Research, Working Paper No. 267. Cape Town: Center for Social Science Research.

World Bank. 2010a. *A Cash Transfer Program Reduces HIV Infections among Adolescent Girls*. Washington, DC: World Bank.

World Bank. 2010b. *Southern Africa: HIV/AIDS and Tuberculosis Plan of Action, 2010–2011 for Botswana, Lesotho, South Africa and Swaziland*. Washington, DC: World Bank.

Wube, M., Horne, C.J. and Stuer, F. 2010. Building a palliative care program in Ethiopia: The impact on HIV and AIDS patients and their families. *Journal of Pain and Symptom Management* 40:6–8.

Zachariah, R., Ford, N., Philips, M. et al. 2009. Task shifting in HIV/AIDS: Opportunities, challenges and proposed actions for sub-Saharan Africa. *Transactions of the Royal Society of Tropical Medicine and Hygiene* 103(6):549–558.

Books, papers, websites, and other resources for further reading

Bello, G., Ndhlovu, T. and Hallett, T.B. Evidence for changes in behaviour leading to reductions in HIV prevalence in urban Malawi. *Sexually Transmitted Infections* 87:296–300.

Braitstein, P., Boulle, A., Nash, D., et al. 2008. Gender and the use of antiretroviral treatment in resource-constrained settings: Findings from a multicenter collaboration. *Journal of Women's Health (Larchmt)* 17:47–55.

Lomborg, B. (ed.). 2012. *Rethinking HIV/AIDS Priorities in Africa: A Cost-Benefit Analysis.* Cambridge: Cambridge University Press.

Lule, E. and Haaker, M. 2012. *The Fiscal Dimension of HIV/AIDS in Botswana, South Africa, Swaziland, and Uganda.* Washington, DC: World Bank.

Poku, N.K. n.d. *HIV/AIDS and Governance in Africa.* ECSP Population, Health, Environment, and Conflict Report, issue 12. http://www.wilsoncenter.org/topics/pubs/Poku12.pdf

Poku, N.K. and Sandkjaer, B. 2007. Meeting the challenges to scaling up HIV/AIDS treatment in Africa. *Development in Practice* 17:279–290.

Website of UNIFAB: http://www.unfap.org/aids/index.htm

Website of the United Nations Office on Drugs and Crime Prevention: http://www1.unodc.org/odccp/drug_demand_hiv_aids.html

9
Care and Support for AIDS Orphans

Woldekidan Amde and Getnet Tadele

Introduction

There were 14.8 million children orphaned by AIDS living in Sub-Saharan Africa in 2009, an increase from 8.9 million in 2001. Nearly 60% of these orphans lived in the high-prevalence countries of South Africa, Zimbabwe, Malawi, Mozambique, Tanzania, Kenya, Uganda, and Zambia (UNAIDS 2010, p. 186). The surge in the number of children who lost either one or both parents is putting great strains on the welfare and development of children and the overall socioeconomic development of countries. Children orphaned by AIDS suffer not only from lack of parental love and care but also from stigma and discrimination by the community at large. A study of 1,480 community-based and 192 institution-based caregivers in five countries including Tanzania, Ethiopia, and Kenya found that 25% of the caregivers harbored feelings of stigma regarding AIDS, which in turn may affect their relations with the orphans for whom they care (Messer et al. 2010). These findings indicate that the willingness of extended families to care for and support AIDS orphans is highly complicated, often resulting in child mobility, exploitation, and neglect. The welfare and livelihood of orphaned children are further jeopardized by stigma and discrimination that discourage them from accessing basic services such as health care and welfare services (Richter 2010; Smart 2003).

Care for AIDS orphans consists of a continuum of formal and informal care provided by institutions (including medical institutions), families, friends, relatives, and communities. This chapter focuses on the care provided by institutions and extended families to children orphaned by AIDS. It aims to contribute to an understanding of issues regarding different forms of child care for AIDS orphans in Sub-Saharan Africa. We focus on recurring and overarching themes covered in seminal studies conducted in the region. We give particular attention to issues surrounding disparities in terminology, contentions regarding vulnerability of orphans, debates over interventions for AIDS orphans, and arguments for and against the various approaches in regard to quality of care and impact on the children.

While numerous investigators have studied the care of orphans by extended families, little information is available about alternative forms of community-based child care (such as care by guardians, reunification, and group homes). The contention that the issue of AIDS orphans has its own nuances also needs more study. Some strongly advocate against treating AIDS orphans separately as separate treatment exposes them to discrimination and stigma. Besides, parents die for any number of reasons, and stigma may keep children from admitting or knowing how they lost their parents. These issues and the fact that AIDS orphans and other vulnerable children face similar problems (Akwara et al. 2010) point to the need to treat orphans the same as other groups of vulnerable children. Therefore, this chapter addresses not only the issue of care for AIDS orphans but also alternative forms of child care in general.

Competing terminologies: Who are the orphans?

Different usages of the term 'orphan' are common and bewilderment abounds regarding which groups of children fall into this category. The terms 'maternal orphan', 'paternal orphan', and 'double orphan' denote which parent is deceased. Different researchers do not use these terms consistently, hampering comparative understanding. The disparity in conceptualizing the term orphan is of far greater significance than lack of uniformity and ineptitude in comparing studies or making broad generalizations. The way we choose to understand the term also impacts policies and programs dealing with the issue, as some programs address double orphans only while others embrace single orphans as well (Kareithi et al. 2008; Skinner et al. 2004; Subbarao et al. 2001; World Vision 2008).

Many scholars adopt a narrow understanding of the term orphan, using it only for those children who have lost both parents (double orphans) or those who have lost their mother (maternal orphans). The argument over definition does not end in identifying which parent has died, but also includes the issue of age. Scholars differ regarding threshold age, some choosing 15 and others 18 years. UNAIDS (2010, p. 112) considers an orphan to be someone below the age of 18 years who is bereft of one or both parents. This definition addresses concerns that the previous 15-year age limit excludes many vulnerable children (Skinner et al. 2004; Subbarao et al. 2001).

A look into the way the term 'orphan' is conceptualized in the literature reviewed in this chapter reveals wide discrepancies in its use. Kareithi et al. (2008) adopted a more comprehensive definition whereas Kodero (2008) used the 'double orphan' definition, claiming that this narrower definition captures to a great extent the reality on the ground. He argued that because heterosexual intercourse is the main cause of the disease, AIDS is bound to claim the lives of both parents. Kodero also suggested the narrower definition differentiates between children in extended families and those in orphanages, who mostly happen to be double orphans. The current use of the comprehensive definition of the term by UNAIDS and many other organizations recognizes that the loss of even one parent often results in the breakup of the family and a change in living situation for the child (World Vision 2008, p. 1).

The appropriateness of the term 'orphan' has been questioned in the African context, in which members of the extended family readily look after these children. Historically, the term has been difficult to define in a typical African setting because the extended family system ensured protection of children even after the death of their biological parents. Bledsoe and Brandon (1987) reported that for a long time in much of Sub-Saharan Africa, the need for adoption in the formal administrative sense was preempted by extended family systems taking in the offspring of kin who died. Even today, HIV-infected parents assume that the extended family will care for their children after they die. Kodero (2008) found that 96.8% of deceased parents sampled in the Kisumu district of Kenya had not contacted caregivers about placement and custody of their children. They had apparently assumed that their blood relatives would informally adopt their children.

The forgoing discussion suggests that various researchers and organizations define the term 'orphan' to suit different methodological and programmatic needs. Thus, the concept remains poorly understood and individuals and organizations use it without fully understanding its implications for public policy and programs. This makes it difficult for researchers, program planners, and implementers to communicate with one another and agree on priorities and responses.

Vulnerability: Impact of HIV/AIDS on orphans

Vulnerable children are defined by Children, Youth and Family Affairs Organization (CYFO) and The Italian Corporation (1995) as children receiving little care from their families, specifically children deprived of adequate affection, protection, and support. Many studies question the vulnerability of AIDS orphans, emphasizing the fact that they may not be in any worse situation than children from economically disadvantaged families or those orphaned by other causes. Unlike other orphaned children, however, children orphaned by HIV/AIDS experience discrimination emanating from the fact that people tend to pass moral judgment on the HIV-infected because of the association of the infection with infidelity/promiscuity, and they tend to look on the surviving children with the same disdain. This attitude results in discrimination and a disregard for the situation of orphans (NASCP 1996, in Kodero 2008). According to UNICEF (2006, p.7), stigma can expose children who lost their parents to even greater difficulties, often limiting their access to health care and schooling and subjecting them to rejection by family, friends, and the community.

AIDS orphans endure a plethora of discriminating treatment and stigma following the death of their parents. The loss of parents makes them vulnerable to starvation, stigma and discrimination, abuse, and exploitation; it also bars or hinders their access to basic services such as health and education (de Wagt and Connolly 2005; Matshalaga and Powell 2002; Nyambedha et al. 2003; Richter 2010). The plight of orphans is further increased when they head a household or live in child-headed households, live with a sick parent, live outside family care, or are HIV-infected or disabled (Malinga and Ntshwarang 2011). The negative consequences vary according to whether the child lost one or two parents, the age of the child, whether he/she receives support, and the quality of the substitute family environment (Pharoah 2005). Although the quality of foster homes varies considerably, they are generally disadvantaged because of a high dependency ratio and their relatively low socioeconomic status related to the fact that most households are headed by females or older people (Miller 2007).

Measurement of impact

How to measure the impact of AIDS orphanhood is one of the recurring controversies in the research on child orphans. The many impacts of the epidemic on orphans unfold over several years and without any discernible pattern, rendering them too intricate to fully capture through many of the research tools in the social sciences (UNAIDS 2008). Similarly, the obscurity of impacts at the national level may conceal severe social stresses and burdens experienced by severely affected subpopulations that tend to increase HIV/AIDS-related inequalities (UNAIDS 2008).

One of the much-researched aspects of the impact of AIDS-caused orphanhood on children is education, which is instrumental for socialization, development of a healthy sense of self, financial independence, and reducing vulnerability to exploitation and HIV/AIDS infection (Matshalaga and Powell 2002). Results from studies on the topic are not always in harmony, apparently due to disparities in study contexts and the use of different methodologies. In assessing the impact of the loss of parents on school attendance, for example, some researchers purport the mere presence of children in school/class is an index while others draw attention to the ultimate academic achievement of the children as the most pertinent indicator.

Household surveys from 56 countries show that school attendance was on average 12% lower for orphans in highly affected countries than for orphans in countries with less than 5% HIV prevalence; school attendance was 4% lower for orphans than nonorphans (Birdsall and Hamoudi 2004, in UNAIDS 2008). Sengendo and Nambi (1997, in de Wagt and Connolly 2005) examined the impact of orphanhood on education of Ugandan children between 15 and 19 years of age and found that following the death of parents, one in four children missed classes and 45% quit school. Children taken in by their grandparents were the most affected. According to the 2003/2004 South Africa DHS (Demographic and Health Survey), 20% of 5,562 orphans and children not living with their parents aged 8–14 were behind in public school (Chuong and Operario 2012). In a rural community in Kenya, where one-third of children under the age of 18 were orphans, families found it increasingly difficult to cover school fees (Nyambedha et al. 2003).

School attendance among orphans in countries most affected by HIV/AIDS has risen in recent years due to increasing support from families, communities, and national and international organizations. A study in rural Uganda identified no significant differences in school participation of orphan and nonorphan children between the ages of 7 and 14 (Yamano et al. 2005). In a few instances school participation rates were even higher among orphans than nonorphans, owing much to the success of programs targeting the former in Côte d'Ivoire, Gabon, Tanzania, and Zambia (UNAIDS 2008). Nonetheless, the level of support available to orphans is far from adequate: In 11 Sub-Saharan countries with HIV prevalence of 5% or higher, only 15% of households with orphans received any form of assistance in 2007 (UNAIDS 2008). Low educational achievement of orphans in hyperendemic HIV/AIDS countries will most likely undermine the socioeconomic well-being of affected nations for many years.

Analysis of DHS data from Cameroon, Côte d'Ivoire, Kenya, Lesotho, Malawi, Tanzania, Uganda, and Zimbabwe found few differences in nutritional status and access to health care between OVC and non-OVC, although the few parameters studied render these results rather inconclusive. However, orphans experienced higher malaria risk because of lower mosquito-net use and they became sexually active at an earlier age, reemphasizing the need for continuing schooling (Mishra and Bignami-Van Assche 2008).

Factors affecting level of impact

The well-being of orphaned children due to AIDS and their developmental needs vary depending on whether they have lost just their mothers, their fathers, or both (UNICEF 2006). A study by Young Lives (2009) in Ethiopia identified the two most important factors determining the well-being of orphans. These are the age of the child and whether the deceased parent was the mother or the father. Losing a parent when a child is younger than six years seems to have far less impact on the child's well-being than by the age of 12 years. This is perhaps because immediate kin tend to embrace younger children more readily. Conversely, if the child is between age 7 and 12 when losing a parent, especially the mother, regardless of the child's sex, the child's academic and psychosocial development will probably be hindered (Case et al. 2004; Young Lives 2009).

According to some studies, the impact of AIDS orphanhood on children is worse on female children, who usually shoulder the burden of managing the dwindling economic resources in the aftermath of the death of parents. Increasing numbers of children, especially girls, drop out of school to care for sick family members and help with household chores. In Swaziland, over one-third of students (36%) – primarily girls – drop out of school, due mainly to HIV/AIDS (Desmond et al. 2000, in Ssamula 2008). Among orphans heading households in a community in Uganda, females were more susceptible to survival and transactional sex associated with impaired social connectedness and drug use than boys (Ntaganira et al. 2011).

A study conducted in rural Uganda found that female orphans who lost both parents or who were not living with their surviving parent were more likely to be out of school (Yamano et al. 2005). Similarly, a UNICEF study in Burundi on 10,000 children found that significantly fewer double orphans were enrolled in school than children with both living parents. That research also confirmed that children who lost their mothers were more affected than those who lost their fathers, and female orphan children were worse off than their male peers (Subbarao et al. 2001). Most studies on orphanhood and education found that maternal death affected children's education significantly more than the death of their fathers (Mishra and Bignami-Van Assche 2008, p. 3).

The gender differences are due to the attendants of HIV-related orphanhood, including declining financial well-being, lack of support, and discrimination. The ensuing abject poverty, coupled with girls' involvement in unhealthy practices to sustain themselves in their desperate attempt to eke out a living, make it ever more difficult for children, especially females, to continue their education (UNAIDS 2008).

Cultural factors influence the fate of orphan children to a large extent. For instance, the probability of single orphans living with the surviving parent tends to depend on whether the surviving parent is the mother or the father. In Malawi, three out of four orphan children live with their mothers and one in four with their fathers (UNAIDS and WHO 2005, in UNICEF 2006). In Ethiopia, the loss of mothers appears to result in a drastic change in living arrangement. Most Ethiopian children without mothers end up under the care of someone other than their fathers, and someone who is not a close relative cares for over two-fifths. Poor academic performance and intermittent school attendance among such children are mainly attributed to this drastic change in caretakers and place of residence. Paternal orphans, conversely, appear not to be perturbed to the same extent; nine-tenths of them continue to live with their mothers and they decline far less in educational performance (Young Lives 2009).

The situation of paternal orphans is complicated in Sub-Saharan Africa, mainly due to practices inherent in patrilineal societies, which deprive widows of resources after the death of their husbands. Widowed women are very vulnerable economically since they are not allowed to either access or use the property their husbands left behind, and their lack of education and employment skills further reduce their options for improving their situation. To deal with this misfortune, many poor single mothers resort to selling whatever resources they have at their disposal to make ends meet (Ssamula 2008). In Uganda, the burden of the socioeconomic impact of HIV and AIDS disproportionately affects rural women. Widows lose access to land, labor inputs, credit, and support services. HIV and AIDS stigmatization severs assistance from the extended family and the community (MAAIF Report 2002, in Ssamula 2008, p. 56). On the other hand, Kodero (2008) found that female AIDS orphans in Kenya were more likely to receive better quality of emotional care regardless of whether the child care alternative was extended family, guardian, or orphanage.

In addition to issues of measurement, the extent to which gender differences could be influenced by cultural contexts in which girls and women are not expected to express their needs and problems is worth taking into account. In one Kenyan community, stigma, discrimination, and isolation of orphans were rare and orphans were generally regarded and treated in the same way as the biological offspring of foster families (Kareithi et al. 2008).

Separation of siblings in the aftermath of the death of parents is one of the repercussions of AIDS orphanhood. Many have advocated keeping siblings together to protect them from further trauma/inconvenience and to ensure that they are able to cope with their loss. This option has been promoted as a minimum standard (Gilborn 2002, in Kodero 2008). However, Kodero highlighted the impractical nature of keeping siblings together after the death of their parents and when they are taken in by foster families, considering that host families may not have the resources to care for siblings. Keeping siblings together is particularly difficult in the face of a growing number of orphan children and a declining number of foster families willing to care or capable of caring for them and where existing social networks are stretched beyond the limit. Regardless of their host destiny, no significant difference has been reported in the quality of emotional care separated and nonseparated orphans receive (Kodero 2008).

By various measures, orphanhood exacts a great socioeconomic toll on households. A UNICEF/UNAIDS/USAID survey in Blantyre in Malawi found that multiple-orphan households and households caring for at least one foster child were between two and six times more food insecure than nonorphan households (Rivers et al. 2010).

Whether AIDS orphans are particularly exposed to conflict with the law is another subject of interest, and existing studies in Sub-Saharan Africa are not conclusive (Marcus 1999, in Pharoah 2005). The issue is usually shunned in public discourse because it exacerbates existing discrimination and stigma against this group of children (Pharoah 2005).

Contentions surrounding intervention approaches for HIV/AIDS orphans

Caring for orphan children by extended families

Diverse conceptions of the extended family prevail in Sub-Saharan Africa. The characteristic features of most definitions are that it is based on lineage (blood relation transcending generations) and serves as a form of social safety net involving a set of norms outlining a sense of responsibility toward members of the family (UNICEF 2004, in Kodero 2008). The practice of extended family members caring for one another is embedded in most Sub-Saharan African cultures and is executed with little formal arrangement. When parents pass away, close or relatively well-off relatives take over their responsibilities (Kareithi et al. 2008).

Of the different alternative forms of orphan care, the extended family is the most popular in Sub-Saharan Africa and tends to reduce the number of child-headed families (Kareithi et al. 2008). The proportion of orphans who remain in their parents' house after the death of their parents is far lower than that of those who move away from their house to be cared for through alternative arrangements. Only three out of ten children remain in the house in which they lived with their mother before her death; seven leave the home for alternative residential arrangements (Mutangadura 2001, in Ssamula 2008). Most extended families in Sub-Saharan Africa exert great effort to care for orphans; an estimated 90% of orphans in Sub-Saharan Africa are taken in by extended families (Miller et al. 2006). The significance of extended families in the care for orphan children is likely to remain strong. This is not just because of a lack of alternative care arrangements, but also due to a move away from small-scale government and nongovernment interventions in the area of institutional care as a result of the increasing negative perception of such alternatives coupled with a rise in the number of orphans (Kodero 2008).

However, the place of the extended family as an alternative child care approach has been increasingly undermined by the rapidly growing numbers of AIDS orphans, the stigma attached to AIDS orphans, the economic pressure of caring for these children (Kareithi et al. 2008), and broader socioeconomic changes predating the arrival of HIV. Extended families have become increasingly challenged to care for kin with the spread of urbanization, labor migration, the cash economy, and increased life expectancy and family size, all of which weakened extended families (Malinga and Ntshwarang 2011). Also, many studies show that extended family members are often needy and aged (Kodero 2008; Saoke and Mutemi 1994, in Kareithi et al. 2008; Ssamula 2008). In more than one-third of 400 female-headed households in two districts in Kenya, orphans were living with grandparents, and over a quarter of the families remained in the same child-headed households following the death of parents (Ayieko 1997). Some researchers dubbed this situation in Kenya a 'grandmother crisis' (Alipui 2002, in Kodero 2008, p. 92). Similarly, in Namibian communities three out of five children are looked after by their grandparents (Foster and Williamson 2000, in Kodero 2008).

In other cases, relatives who know or suspect that parents of a child are deceased due to AIDS-related causes may not wish to foster orphan children for fear of infection to themselves or their children. Such fear and discrimination related to the epidemic further drive people away from assuming the responsibility of caring for children, as reported from Addis Ababa (MOWA 2009).

On the other hand, extended families hosting orphan children may be neither capable nor willing to look after them but do so because of societal expectations and pressures. As a result, many host families resent the cultural arrangement, the obligation it entails, and lack of support in caring for children from other members of the extended family (Kareithi et al. 2008). Ayieko (1997) estimated that in two districts in western Kenya, three-fifths of those who looked after orphan children found themselves in that position because of their lineage obligations.

Families generally agree that whoever comes forward in orphan child care will carry almost all the burden with little support from other extended family members. Orphans become the responsibility of the host family exclusively, as not many relatives extend support. In a Kalenjin community, a staggering 60% of foster families received no support whatsoever from extended families (Kareithi et al. 2008).

Paternal relatives are usually more likely to assume a direct or indirect role in caring for the orphan child. In Kalenjin society, this may reflect patrilineal norms (Kareithi et al. 2008). In some cases, foster parents, particularly if they are women or relatives of the mother, are subject to culturally condoned discrimination by relatives from the father's side when it comes to having custody of the property the children inherited from their parents due to widely prevailing patriarchal inheritance practices (Kareithi et al. 2008).

Perceptions about hosting orphan children by extended family: Responsibility, burden, or opportunity for self-improvement?

The practice of taking in orphan children is to a large extent rooted in the cultural norms and values of communities and is one of the prevailing social expectations in Africa. Describing this tradition of caring for orphans among the Kalenjin, Kareithi et al. (2008) concluded that it is a moral obligation rather than an act of kindness. Similarly, caring for orphaned, abandoned, and vulnerable children is considered by most ethnic groups in Ethiopia as a cultural requirement and a dictate of religion (Assefa 1995, in MOWA 2009).

The motive for extended families hosting orphans is often complicated. Foster parents' willingness to care for orphan children by no means can be considered a reflection of their capacity, as they may be poor, aged, or ill themselves and not in a position to care for others. They may assume the responsibility only out of moral obligation or adherence to cultural norms. A growing number of foster parents are single females and grandparents with few resources at their disposal owing to the declining portion of people in the extended family with the capacity to fend for orphan children (Sefasi 2010; UNICEF 2004, in Kodero 2008). Elderly women interviewed in a rural health unit in South Africa complained about social stigma (isolation), verbal stigma (gossip), and physical stigma (isolation and separation from family members) they experienced caring for AIDS orphans, indicating the wide range of socially complex outcomes (Ogunmefun et al. 2011). A study in a rural community in Kenya revealed that 28% of orphan children were looked after by their matrilineal relatives or nonrelatives, which is contrary to accepted cultural practice and due to the huge number of orphans with which patrilineal kins could not cope (Nyambedha et al. 2003).

In recent years scholars and activists have questioned the reasons members of extended families host child orphans. For example, a Human Rights Watch investigation (2001, in Kodero 2008) revealed that foster families in Kenya were primarily interested in the benefits they could get from fostering children, even when the children were their relatives. Similar feelings were found in Botswana. Hence, it is not clear to what extent foster parents act in the best interest of orphan children or of themselves.

Kinship groups and extended families are thus increasingly being tested as alternative forms of child care. Unlike in the past, people do not always live up to the responsibility they took on to provide care for the child. Many seem enthusiastic to assume the role of caretaker, but only in expectation of financial or material benefits from institutions proposing to support orphan children or to ease social pressure from the family. It is also not uncommon, even in the presence of close kin in some instances, for the child to be pushed to be enrolled in an orphanage (Kareithi et al. 2008).

The property rights of many orphan children have been trampled on by custodians. In patriarchal families, paternal relatives generally take custody of the child. Single-female foster parents tend to be deprived of access to the resources left by the paternal relatives, who claim to have proprietary right/privilege to the resources. In the case of single paternal orphans, mothers are often pressed by the husband's relatives to give up the family's resources. Although children are legally entitled to inherit the property their parents leave behind, custodians commonly abuse the responsibility entrusted to them, embezzling the resources for personal use. The property rights of orphan children are violated even in situations where there are administrative and legal provisions to ensure the protection of such rights. Owing much to their young age and lack of awareness, the children are not able to make use of legal mechanisms to keep or reclaim the property that rightfully belongs to them (Kareithi et al. 2008).

Quality of care for orphan children in extended families: A lost cause?

From the forgoing discussion it appears that most extended host families are little prepared, capable, or willing to care for a foster child for years to come, jeopardizing the quality of their care. Kodero (2008) reported that it is often poor members of the extended family who are the custodians of orphan children, with well-off relatives tending to extend support, if any, without establishing any intimate contact with the children. Orphan children rarely find host families that meet their psychological and physical needs. UNICEF (2006) pointed out that extended families are rarely ready to meet the needs of AIDS orphans as they are likely to be facing difficult challenges themselves. This is especially true in the most affected communities, which are often economically disadvantaged and where the capacity of the family is strained by the addition of not just orphans, but also other members who are either affected or infected by HIV/AIDS. Hence, children are likely to be left with inadequate emotional and material support.

The general trend is for close relatives, particularly grandmothers, to take custody of orphans, despite their often limited interest or capacity, to fulfil societal expectations (UNICEF 2004, in Kodero 2008). Owing much to cultural norms, these relatives feel a sense of ownership in caring for the children, and they exhibit readiness to take in orphan children. The fact that foster parents are aging and tend to be single is a concern since they may be ailing and unable to generate sufficient income. They may generally not be in good stead socially, psychologically, or financially. Conversely, the fact that the many foster parents in the northern part of Rift Valley Province in Kenya are grandparents of the orphans could be positive because grandparents may provide more care and affection to children than other close relatives. Kareithi et al. (2008) emphasized the nonmaterial nature of the challenges orphans, as compared with nonorphans, face in obtaining education. The former find it difficult to get their foster parents to provide them with the support they need in their education to the extent that some had to drop out. Although school tuition was free, the children were unable to cover expenses for items such as school uniforms.

New approaches are being developed in an effort to overcome the difficulties encountered in the family setting and to address issues that have been neglected. In Zimbabwe, for example, an NGO developed a strategy based on the traditional safety net structure that assured that children in need were taken care of in their community. In this program, the community selects volunteers from among village health workers and HIV/AIDS-trained home-based caregivers to encourage local families to foster AIDS orphans, provide psychosocial and medical care to caregivers, encourage children to be HIV-tested, and follow up positive cases until they start antiretroviral (ARV) therapy (Tandi 2011). Another issue that is increasingly being addressed is the need for more support for older caregivers, who care for 40–50% of all HIV/AIDS orphans (SADC 2008). As a group, older caregivers have weak parenting skills due to the generation gap, lack information on their rights and entitlements, and tend to be poor (Laboso and Picken 2011; SADC 2008).

Recent studies and initiatives have advocated a number of child care alternatives as culturally more acceptable and cost-effective than orphanages. For example, child-headed households assisted by charities, NGOs, and governments may ensure continued social cohesiveness, minimization of psychosocial impacts on surviving siblings, retention of the family name, and maintenance of family and tenure rights (Roa 2011). Makqoko and Dreyer (2007) concluded from a study in a South African community that religious communities can effectively nurture child-headed households in an environment largely lacking the African philosophy of *ubuntu* (humanness). Another alternative, foster care by unrelated caregivers, has been found to be 5–20 times less expensive than institutional care (UNICEF 2006). A network of orphan ministries using this approach has been developed in several Central African countries (Roa 2011). These and related approaches incorporate the principles of community-based and rights-based interventions and thus deserve greater attention by researchers, donors, and administrators.

Another option is to alleviate the burden on females by increasing the commitment and number of males in care giving. This would also render home care more equitable and sustainable (Newman et al. 2011). This solution may be less feasible in the near term in view of deeply rooted male primacy and stereotyping of gendered division of work in Sub-Saharan Africa.

Institutional care

Orphanages were introduced to Africa by European missionaries and are currently supported by several African governments and many NGOs, mostly faith-based organizations and charitable groups. They are rare today in the industrialized countries, which consider them unsuitable for child care and development and largely unnecessary due to the presence of foster care, adoption services, and social security systems (McKenzie 2009).

Status and trends in institutional child care for orphans:
Denounced but growing

Institutional care in Sub-Saharan Africa has often proliferated in the aftermath of disasters such as economic crises and drought. During the 1984–1985 famine in Ethiopia, both government and nongovernment organizations launched residential orphan care programs. At that time, about 21,000 children were in 106 orphanages. Kenya, which experienced relatively few natural and human-made calamities, had a relatively small number of child care institutions (Kodero 2008) in spite of the 1.2 million HIV/AIDS orphans reported in that country in 2009 (UNAIDS 2010).

Some have criticized institutionalized orphan care for focusing solely on orphan children affected by HIV/AIDS and failing to recognize the centrality of a family-focused approach to addressing the diverse developmental needs of children. Criticisms have been leveled at reductionist approaches, claiming that they misguide interventions of varying scale because they do not take into account the far-reaching consequences of the epidemic on orphan children, their families, and communities. Interventions focusing on orphan children only and informed by such narrow approaches tend to be welfare oriented and smaller in their coverage, and they fail to mobilize relevant stakeholders, including donors, or influence national policy in health or education (Matshalaga and Powell 2002; Richter 2010).

Orphanages have received less attention in Sub-Saharan Africa than is merited by the extent and severity of AIDS impacts. This is largely due to the traditional African practice of extended families taking in orphans and the prevailing consensus that institutional care should be considered only as the last option. Orphanages are widely considered not well suited to address needs of children other than the immediate basic needs, and they are considered incapable of ensuring the psychosocial well-being of children (UNICEF 2004, in Kodero 2008).

Child development experts agree that institutional care does not promote the healthy emotional and social development of children. Problems surface particularly when children come of age and have to leave the institutions; this has been corroborated by experience from developing countries that have ardently adopted institutional care. The transition from institutional care to the community tends to strain the capabilities of former orphans, some of whom become imprisoned, are admitted to mental institutions, or end up living on the streets (UNICEF 2006). Having gone through institutional care for most of their lives, many ex-orphans lack the social skills necessary for meaningful functioning in society.

The most commonly reported impacts of institutionalization are emotional, psychosocial, developmental, and medical problems. Institutionalized children lack a sense of community and belonging, which carries a great deal of weight in defining one's self-worth in Sub-Saharan Africa (UNICEF 2006). When they grow up in institutions, children are not socialized in their cultural heritage; this impedes their reintegration into society as they cannot adapt to the norms and practices of their culture (Kodero 2008; Mukoyogo and Williams 1991, in ICAD 2002; UNICEF 2006). In addition, institutionalization makes it easier for members of the community to single out orphan children for stigma and discrimination, enabling peers to shun and tease the orphans on the grounds of their association with HIV/AIDS (Kareithi et al. 2008).

Institutional care is invariably characterized by group living with care provided by paid adults who are normally not regarded as caregivers in society. The form and quality of this care vary considerably from institution to institution. Arrangements range from large, typically impersonal, public institutions to smaller centers. The latter tend to be run by NGOs or religious organizations and 'children's villages' (UNICEF 2006). Another characteristic feature of institutional care is the lack of stable, long-term relationships between children and their caregivers (Rosas and McCall 2009, in MOWA 2009). Many communities in Malawi, for instance, are against institutional care despite the relatively superior material provisions because institutionalized children miss the sense of belonging. A sense of belonging is imperative for children to become integral members of their respective communities (Mann 2003, in UNICEF 2006). According to UNICEF, children in institutions lack adequate personal care, attention, affection, and stimulation. Child neglect, harsh and rigid discipline, maltreatment, and abuse are widespread, even in well-resourced institutions in high-income countries. There is considerable evidence that separating children from their families, community, and culture accentuates the negative elements orphans experience outside orphanages in any culture (Roa 2011).

Despite the negatives of institutional care, placement of children in institutions in Sub-Saharan Africa is growing. As families desire to alleviate the economic pressure that accompanies the addition of another child to care for, they sometimes push for orphan and vulnerable children to be enrolled in child care institutions. Some families simply find the material provisions in institutions too good to pass up as they believe they guarantee success in education and future employment. Studies in Zimbabwe and several other Sub-Saharan countries suggested that the ease of finding institutional care for orphan children can prompt many families to abdicate their responsibility toward these children (Foster et al. 1995, in UNICEF 2006; Roa 2011).

The Ministry of Women's Affairs in Ethiopia reported that an increasing number of families are eager to have orphans and vulnerable children enrolled in institutions. Sometimes children with living parents are enrolled in institutions even if their families must deny that the children's parents are alive, a coping behavior also reported from other countries (Roa 2011). Ethiopian families widely believe institutional care is beneficial for vulnerable children, offering them better life chances than they would have if they were living with their families. Many parents maintain they would be less interested in institutional care if they were assisted with the means to care for the children; they resort to institutional care only because they cannot cope alone with the responsibility of caring for children. Their perception of institutions is mixed: While they agree that institutionalization impairs children's social and life skill development, they embrace institutional care for some of its strengths, particularly material and educational provisions (MOWA 2009).

However, the lauded strength of institutional care (material provision) is questionable because most institutions lack funding (ICAD 2002; UNICEF 2006). One major limitation of orphanages is their high operational cost relative to their capacity to absorb orphans (Subbarao et al. 2001). Emphasizing the financial implications of promoting residential care, UNICEF (2004, cited in Kodero 2008) estimated that to provide adequate institutional care in Sub-Saharan Africa, 80,000 orphanages would have to be built. Another estimate (Parry 1998, in UNICEF 2006) claimed that to meet the needs of just one-tenth of the orphan population in Zimbabwe, the country would need to set up over 1,200 orphanages annually, each caring for 50 children. These requirements rule out the possibility of Sub-Saharan African countries relying on institutional care as a primary care option for orphan children. Shortage of funding greatly reduces the number of children orphanages can enroll and the quality of services they can offer, leaving many in a precarious situation (Kareithi et al. 2008). The substantial costs of infrastructure, trained staff, and appropriate regulatory mechanisms are usually not included in cost estimates for orphanages, meaning their costs are generally higher than estimates (UNICEF 2006).

Negative sentiments toward NGOs running child care institutions have been fueled by perceptions of the organizations' ulterior motives: some pursue self-aggrandizement rather than alleviating the plight of children (Kareithi et al. 2008). Such sentiments are widespread in Sub-Saharan Africa, where much is expected from NGOs in the area of social services in the absence of state-funded welfare systems. Reducing this negative publicity is one of the challenges of child care institutions.

Momentum against institutional care grew with the increasing awareness of the implications of institutional care in the lives of children. As a result, many facilities in Sub-Saharan Africa were closed. The void created by their closure is being filled by community-based alternative child care services. Between 1992 and 1997, UNICEF and Save the Children reunited 1,700 institutionalized children with their families, significantly reducing the number of children in residential care. Thirty substandard institutions were closed and the quality of care in the remaining facilities was improved. Follow-up contacts determined that care had improved for the great majority of reunited children (UNICEF 2006, p. 40).

The trend of deinstitutionalizing orphan care has decreased the interest of governments and donors in promoting institutional care services. Highly HIV-affected countries – namely South Africa, Botswana, Mozambique, Namibia, and Lesotho – are increasingly adopting family-centered interventions rather than institutional care. Large-scale programs are being evaluated in Malawi, Zambia, Kenya, Uganda, and Tanzania. Family-focused interventions have gained the support of governments and national and international development organizations (Gosh and Kalipeni 2004; Matshalaga and Powell 2002; Richter 2010). This shift is also taking place in Ethiopia, where the government's involvement in running orphanages is declining.

The paradigm shift in child care approaches highlights the negative aspects of institutional care and the belief that it should be considered only as a last resort. According to a survey by the Ethiopian Ministry of Women's

Affairs (MOWA 2009), only three government-run orphanages are operating in Ethiopia; the reduction can be attributed to government policy. The Ethiopian government's response to the plight of AIDS orphans in setting up child care institutions has been slow, as was the inadequate response of the Mengistu regime to the drought in the mid-1980s (MOWA 2009). Abebe and Aase (2007) attributed the declining involvement of the Ethiopian government in institutional child care to lack of resources for running such an expensive program.

Although government is withdrawing from institutional care, NGOs and faith-based organizations have been proliferating orphanages in Ethiopia in recent years, unperturbed by government guidance (MOWA 2009). The sharp increase in institutional care despite widespread sensitization against its impact on children's physical, emotional, and cognitive development has been described as 'paradoxical' (MOWA 2009, p. 6). Kodero (2008) predicted that institutional child care run by individuals and NGOs is likely to blossom in the future in Africa as well as globally despite the negative attitudes toward it because alternative forms of child care, such as community-based, adoption, and foster care, have not been developed adequately to accommodate the increasing number of orphan and vulnerable children. This and other arguments call for further studies exploring child care alternatives that minimize the trauma children experience from being removed from their parents.

Reasons for poor quality of care in childcare institutions

A major reason for the deficiencies of orphanages is the failure of governments to oversee, coordinate, and provide guidance to the organizations offering residential care for orphan children (Kareithi et al. 2008). The Ethiopian Ministry of Women's Affairs (MOWA 2009, p. 14) considered government supervision and oversight of orphanages inadequate and noted that the minimum care standards set out in the UN Guideline for the Appropriate Use and Conditions of Alternative Care for Children (2007) and the Ethiopian National Guidelines for Alternative Care) are seldom maintained. The ministry referenced a survey of 87 child care institutions in Ethiopia in which the quality of care was assessed using a Quality Standard Checklist based on recognized standards of institutional care described in these two guidelines. This assessment was supplemented by a qualitative study involving individual and group interviews with 388 persons. The quality of care in many institutions was low; the organizations lacked finances and professional staff and neglected child development principles. Children were exposed to discrimination, abuse, and exploitation during their stay in the institutions. Many of the institutions discouraged children from establishing meaningful relationships with their relatives, thereby undermining the possibility of reunion with extended families. At least three out of five institutions lacked proper documentation of children's profiles or a care plan for every child. When children finally leave the institution, many find it difficult to reintegrate into society for lack of life skills (MOWA 2009).

Arguments for institutional child care

Among the proponents of institutional care, Kareithi et al. (2008) claimed that the negative perception of orphanages mostly reflects administrative or policy deficiencies and negative public sentiments are unwarranted. Kareithi et al. (2008) argued that the complaints against institutional care in Kenya related more to the lack of transparency and credibility in financial matters than the poorer quality of care the children could get at the institutions compared to what they would receive from extended families. Similarly, in its national survey in Ethiopia, MOWA (2009) concluded that community members, child care staff and leadership, and some authorities tend to have a positive perception of child care in orphanages and are not aware of negative effects of institutionalization. Another factor that accounts for the relatively better quality of emotional care in orphanages in Kenya is the fact that caretakers in orphanages are much younger than those in extended families (Kodero 2008).

Despite the fact that some foster families take poor care of orphans, resentment toward institutions caring for children abounds because the presence of institutions is thought to reflect negatively on the capacity and will of relatives to care for one of their own members. However, proponents of residential care point out that property belonging to orphans in the institutions is handled legally, with the court appointing trustees as custodians of the property until the children reach legal age. Local administrations and police enforce this provision (Kareithi et al. 2008). There have been reports of members of extended families taking charge of the property the children's parents left behind and spending it for their own purpose after enrolling orphan children in institutions (Mukoyogo and Williams 1991, in ICAD 2002).

One criticism of institutional care proponents have addressed is the impersonal relationships between children and orphanage staff. Wolf and Fesseha (1998, in Kodero 2008), in their study in Eritrea, cautioned against giving heed to complaints about institutional care that are not substantiated by research and urged giving due attention to institutional care that could prove positive in the lives of orphans. Kodero's (2008) comparative assessment of the impact of selected factors on the quality of emotional care children orphaned by HIV/AIDS receive is a pioneer study. It compares children living in extended families, guardians' homes, and orphanages. The study in Kenya's Kisumu district is important in challenging the persistent extreme belief that extended families should be given priority in caring for children and institutional care considered only as a last option. Results showed that children living with extended families received poorer quality of care than children living in orphanages or with guardians. Children enrolled in orphanages enjoyed the best emotional care of the three groups.

Kodero substantiated the differences in the quality of emotional care in the various host arrangements with qualitative data he gathered about prevailing perceptions regarding orphans. The attitudes toward orphans and their needs expressed by caretakers in orphanages was positive; Kodero (2008) attributed this to the fact that many caretakers were religiously motivated and selflessly committed to their work. In a study in Ethiopia, where similar 'missionaries' were hailed as committed and selfless, the majority of the caregivers were nevertheless low-paid, disgruntled, and uninspired (MOWA 2009).

Kodero (2008) developed and used as the principal tool in his study a 13-item Quality of Caregiver–Orphan Relationship Scale to gauge the quality of emotional care across different residential options (extended family, guardian, and orphanage). The scale encompassed issues of intimacy, trust, and perceptions about food as indicators of emotional care. The instrument embraced the distinct local context as, for example, quality of emotional care can be manifested in the level of provision of food, which is in short supply.

Considering the unique nature of Kodero's findings that offer support for the continuation and strengthening of orphanages because they generally have a good record of providing quality emotional care in Kenya, studies in other settings are needed. Studies examining the reasons for the relatively good care orphanages provide and determining whether this situation would hold in other contexts and in orphanages with various caretaker motivations are urgently needed. An assessment of the accuracy and thoroughness of Kodero's scale for measuring quality of care in different communities and countries may validate this and similar tools for providing a standardized methodology for the study of emotional health in orphanages. It is also important to take note of the significance of 'food perception' in influencing the overall measurement of quality of emotional care, as children in orphanages typically have much better food and other material necessities than children in other child care arrangements.

Conclusion

Different contentions concerning who comprises orphan children in alternative forms of child care deter comparisons and contribute to the exclusion of some children in interventions. There is growing momentum in favor of community-based care for vulnerable children such as care by extended families and guardians. Barring a few studies such as the research in Kenya that identified institutional care as superior in provision of emotional care, much of the existing literature emphasizes the unfavorable impacts of institutional care on children and lack of resources. Due to donor pressure, a growing number of countries in Sub-Saharan Africa have gradually ceased providing residential care to children. However, a number of faith-based and other NGOs have established orphanages.

The literature identified two critical issues that need intervention: governmental lack of supervision and control of orphanages stemming from lack of human and financial capacity and the resulting decline in quality of care, and the incapacity of extended families to care for orphan children. Often immediate relatives assume custody of orphan children out of cultural sentiment or societal expectation with little consideration of their capacity. A significant proportion of caretakers are aged relatives with few resources and little support from other members of extended families, indicating that they need to be considered in social policies.

Overall, the literature highlights large numbers of orphan children not getting the care and support necessary for their psychosocial and physical development, regardless of the care option. There is a growing call for governments to step up their involvement in the care of HIV orphans, both in offering residential care for those with no other care option and monitoring the situation of children enrolled in orphanages, and in supporting and supervising orphanages, extended families, and guardians who are custodians of HIV orphans.

This chapter reveals that the problem of AIDS orphan care and support remains understudied, a situation that is aggravated by the failure to share information and research findings among the many institutions carrying out studies on child care alternatives (Tadele and Kifle 2007, 2010). The lack of literature is especially pronounced on the subject of community-based child care alternatives, which currently constitute the main intervention approach. The largely anecdotal information and competing terminologies and definitions of basic concepts and methodologies further complicate assessment of opportunities and constraints that must be monitored and evaluated to inform planners and managers of the merits and demerits of institutional care systems.

Development intervention has recently shifted from a needs-based approach to a rights-based approach that emphasizes entitlements over needs. Accordingly, care and assistance strategies for vulnerable children have been moving toward this latter perspective. Although many care givers increasingly understand the value of this approach, very few have taken practical steps to translate the approach into action and rarely revise their care strategies in accordance with the rights-based approach. This calls for rigorous studies on emerging child care options such as community-based child care and on how the rights-based approach may be implemented in providing optimal care to vulnerable children.

References

Abebe, T. and Aase, A. 2007. Children, AIDS and the politics of orphan care in Ethiopia: The extended family revisited. *Social Science and Medicine* 64: 2058–2069.

Akwara, P.A., Noubary, B., Ken, P.L.A. et al. 2010. Who is the vulnerable child? Using survey data to identify children at risk in the era of HIV and AIDS. *AIDS Care* 22:1066–1085.

Ayieko, M. 1997. *From Single Parents to Child-Headed Households: The Case of Children Orphaned by AIDS in Kisumu and Siaya District*. New York: HIV and Development Programme, UNDP.

Bledsoe, C. and Brandon, A. 1987. Child fostering and child mortality in sub-Saharan Africa: Some preliminary questions and answers. In van de Walle, E., Pison, G. and Sala-Diakanda, M. (eds), *Mortality and Society in Sub-Saharan Africa*, pp. 287–302. Oxford: Clarendon Press.

Case, A., Paxson, C. and Ableidinger, A. 2004. Orphans in Africa: Parental death, poverty and school enrollment. *Demography* 41:483–508.

Chuong, C. and Operario, D. 2012. Challenging household dynamics: Impact of orphanhood, parental absence, and children's living arrangements on education in South Arica. *Global Public Health* 7:42–57.

CYFO and the Italian Corporation. 1995. *Research Report on Child Abuse and Neglect In Selected Parts of Ethiopia*. Addis Ababa: Children and Youth Affairs Organization and the Italian Corporation.

de Wagt, A. and Connolly, M. 2005. Orphans and the impact of HIV/AIDS in sub-Saharan Africa. *Food, Nutrition and Agriculture* 34:24–31.

Gosh, J. and Kalipeni, E. 2004. Rising tide of AIDS orphans in Southern Africa. In Kalipeni, E., Craddock, S., Oppong, J.R. and Ghosh, J. (eds), *HIV&AIDS in Africa: Beyond Epidemiology*, pp. 305–315. Oxford: Blackwell.

ICAD (Interagency Coalition on AIDS and Development). 2002. *Best Practices for Care of AIDS Orphans*. http://www.icad-cisd.com/pdf/publications/e_orphans_web.pdf

Kareithi, J., Egesah, O. and Kong'ong'o, M. 2008. The challenges of orphan foster-age in the era of HIV/AIDS in the North Rift region, Kenya. In OSSREA (ed.), *The HIV/AIDS Challenge in Africa, an Impact and Response Assessment: The Case of Kenya*, pp. 147–189. Addis Ababa: OSSREA.

Kodero, H.M.N. 2008. Emotional care for AIDS-orphaned children in Kenya. In OSSREA (ed.), *The HIV/AIDS Challenge in Africa, an Impact and Response Assessment: The Case of Kenya*, pp. 75–145. Addis Ababa: OSSREA.

Laboso, L. and Picken, A. 2011. The gender dynamics in caregiving among older carers. Abstracts of the International Conference on AIDS and Sexually Transmitted Diseases, Addis Ababa. Abstract TUAD1104.

Makqoko, Z. and Dreyer, Y. 2007. Child-headed households because of the trauma surrounding HIV/AIDS. *HTS Theological Studies* 63:717–731.

Malinga, T. and Ntshwarang, P.L. 2011. Alternative care for children in Botswana: A reality or idealism? *Social Work and Society: The International Online-Only Journal* 9(2), www.socwork.net/sws/article/view/277

Matshalaga, N.R. and Powell, G. 2002. Mass orphanhood in the era of HIV/AIDS: Bold support for alleviation of poverty and education may avert a social disaster. *British Medical Journal* 324:185–186.

McKenzie, R.B. (ed.). 2009. *Home Away from Home: The Forgotten History of Orphanages*. New York: Encounter Books.

Messer, L.C, Pence, B.W, Whetten, K. et al. 2010. Prevalence and predictors of HIV-related stigma among institutional- and community-based caregivers of orphans and vulnerable children living in five less-wealthy countries. *BMC Public Health* 10:504.

Miller, C. 2007. *Children Affected by AIDS: A Review of the Literature on Orphaned and Vulnerable Children*. Boston: Boston University, School of Public Health.

Miller, C.M., Gruskin, S., Subramanian, S.V. et al. 2006. Orphan care on Botswana's working households: Growing responsibilities in the absence of adequate support. *American Journal of Public Health* 96:1429–1435.

Mishra, V. and Bignami-Van Assche 2008. *Orphans and Vulnerable Children in High-Prevalence Countries in Sub-Saharan Africa.* Calverton: Macro International.

MOWA. 2009. *Improving Care Options for Children in Ethiopia through Understanding Institutional Child Care and Factors Driving Institutionalization.* Addis Ababa: Ministry of Women's Affairs.

Newman, C.J., Fogarty, L., Makoae, L.N. and Reavely, E. 2011. Occupational segregation, gender essentialism and male primacy as major barriers to equity in HIV/AIDS caregiving: Findings from Lesotho. *International Journal for Equity in Health* 10:24.

Ntaganira, J., Brown, L. and Mock, N. 2011. Sexual risk behaviours among orphans heads of households in Rwanda. *Abstracts of the International Conference on AIDS and Sexually Transmitted Infections in Africa,* Addis Ababa. Abstract MOPE092.

Nyambedha, E.O., Wandibba, S. and Aagaard-Hansen, J. 2003. Changing patterns of orphan care due to the HIV epidemic in western Kenya. *Social Science and Medicine* 57:301–311.

Ogunmefun, C., Gilbert, L. and Schatz, E. 2011. Older female caregivers and HIV/AIDS-related secondary stigma in rural South Africa. *Journal of Cross Cultural Gerontology* 26:85–102.

Pharoah, R. 2005. AIDS, orphans and crime: Exploring the linkages. *South African Crime Quarterly* 13:7–14.

Richter, L. 2010. An introduction to family-centered services for children affected by HIV and AIDS. *Journal of the International AIDS Society* 13(Suppl. 2):S1.

Rivers, J., Mason, J.B., Rose, D.D. et al. 2010. The impact of orphanhood on food security in the high-HIV context of Blantyre, Malawi. *Food and Nutrition Bulletin* 31:S264–S271.

Roa, S. 2011. Community-based orphan care. *Mission Frontiers.* http://www.missionfrontiers.org/issue/article/community-based-orphan-care

SADC. 2008. *Strategic Framework and Programme of Action (2008–2015): Comprehensive Care and Support for Orphans, Children & Youth (OVCY') in the Southern African Development Community.* SADC Secretariat.

Sefasi, A.P. 2010. Impact of HIV and AIDS on the elderly: A case study of Chiladzulu district. *Malawi Medical Journal* 4:101–103.

Skinner, D., Tsheko, N., Mtero-Munyati, S. et al. 2004. *Defining Orphaned and Vulnerable Children.* Cape Town: Human Sciences Research Council.

Smart, R. 2003. *Planning for Orphans and HIV/AIDS- Affected Children: Home-based HIV/AIDS Care.* London: Oxford University Press.

Ssamula, M. 2008. Needs and coping strategies of female-headed families affected by HIV and AIDS: A case study of Masaka District, Uganda. In OSSREA (ed.), *The HIV/AIDS Challenge in Africa, an Impact and Response Assessment: The Case of Uganda,* pp. 47–100. Addis Ababa: OSSREA.

Subbarao, K., Mattimore, A. and Plangemann, K. 2001. *Social Protection of Africa's Orphans and Other Vulnerable Children: Issues and Good Practice Program Options.* Washington, DC: World Bank.

Tadele, G. and Kifle, W. 2007. Existing situation and best practices in the area of information management related to children living in vulnerable circumstances in Ethiopia. Paper prepared for the Italian Cooperation Program in Support of Children and Adolescents in Vulnerable Circumstances, Addis Ababa.

Tadele, G. and Kifle, W. 2010. Assessment of the information management practices of organizations working with children living under difficult circumstances in Ethiopia. In Yntiso, G. (ed.), *Inter-generational Challenges in Ethiopia: Understanding Family, Children and the Elderly. Proceedings of the Sixth Annual Conference of the Ethiopian Society of Sociologists, Social Workers and Anthropologists*, pp. 95–110. Addis Ababa: United Printers.

Tandi, M.D. 2011. Grandmother of kindness: A social and health safety net for children orphaned by HIV in Zimbabwe. *Abstracts of the International Conference on AIDS and Sexually Transmitted Diseases*, Addis Ababa. Abstract TUAD1105.

UNAIDS. 2008. *Report on the Global AIDS Epidemic.* Geneva: UNAIDS.

UNAIDS. 2010. *Report on the Global AIDS Epidemic.* New York: UNAIDS.

UNICEF. 2006. *Caring for Children Affected by HIV and AIDS.* Florence, Italy: Innocenti Research Center. http://www.hsrc.ac.za/Document-2455.phtml

World Vision. 2008. *2009 New Project Opportunity, Fighting Child Labor in East Africa: Helping AIDS-impacted Children Stay in School in Four Countries.* http://www.volusion.com/assets/images/company/worldvisionvolusionpdf1.pdf

Yamano, T., Shimamura, Y. and Sserunkuuma, D. 2005. Living arrangements and schooling of orphaned children and adolescents in Uganda. *Economic Development and Cultural Change* 54:833–856.

Young Lives. 2009. *The Impact of Parental Death on Child Outcomes: Evidence from Ethiopia.* Policy Brief. http://www.younglives.org.uk/pdf/publication-section-pdfs/policy-briefs/YL_PB7_EthiopiaOrphans.pdf

Books, papers, and other resources for further reading

Audemard, C. and Viknikin, K. 2006. *Orphans and Vulnerable Children in Sub-Saharan Africa.* Baltimore: Johns Hopkins University Press.

Foster, G., Levine, C. and Williamson, J. (eds). 2005. *A Generation at Risk: The Global Impact of HIV/AIDS on Orphans and Vulnerable Children.* Cambridge, MA: Cambridge University Press.

Grannis, S.W. 2011. *Hope Amidst Dispair: HIV/AIDS-Affected Children in Sub-Saharan Africa.* London: Pluto Press.

Joslin, D. (ed.). 2002. *Invisible Caregivers: Older Adults Raising Children in the Wake of HIV/AIDS.* New York: Columbia University Press.

10

Mainstreaming HIV Interventions into Education Systems

Anne A. Khasakhala

Introduction

The HIV epidemic continues to threaten the achievement of national developmental agendas and, by extension, the Millennium Development Goals, including the goals for education. The United Nation's 2011 Political Declaration on HIV and AIDS set the ambitious target of halving by 2015 the percentages of young people below 15 years who had sexual intercourse (UNAIDS 2011). This and related goals are to be achieved largely by expanding access to children aged less than 15 years to information and education for the improvement of life skills. This strategy was based on the premise that education is a 'window of hope' and a social 'vaccine' against HIV since it equips individuals with knowledge necessary for survival (Hargreaves and Boler 2006; World Bank 2002). According to UNICEF (2002), the education sector shoulders the task of finding lasting solutions that mitigate the impacts of the HIV pandemic.

The impacts of the pandemic on the education sector are varied and significant, ranging from HIV infections and AIDS disease among teachers and students to effects on the quality of local educational services. In Swaziland, KwaZulu-Natal, and the Central African Republic, for example, school enrolment fell by 10–36% largely due to AIDS at the beginning of the millennium (Badcock-Walters 2001; UNAIDS 2002, p. 50). HIV and AIDS represent a direct threat to achieving the goal of 'Education for All' as the epidemic affects the supply of and demand for primary and secondary schooling, especially in high-HIV-prevalence countries. Moreover, education remains one of the most effective interventions against the epidemic (Global Campaign for Education 2004). Education is effective in part because it provides access to health information and care to poor and disadvantaged children who would otherwise have few opportunities (WHO 2008, p. 2). The crucial role of the education sector in national responses is further indicated by the fact that about 60% of the public sector workforce is in the education sector in many countries (Bundy et al. 2010, p. xii).

The relationship between AIDS and the education sector is circular. That is, as the epidemic worsens in the general population, it also worsens in the education sector, and the high incidence of HIV transmission in the education sector is likely to maintain current incidence rates in the general population (AVERT 2011). Similarly, while HIV/AIDS threatens the achievement of education goals set by the international community, global commitments to interventions that reduce HIV vulnerabilities among children and youth cannot be met without the contribution of the education sector (UNAIDS 2008).

Progress to date in mainstreaming HIV/AIDS in education in Sub-Saharan Africa has been uneven. A major incentive to accelerate mainstreaming programs is the premise that mainstreaming is the main route toward ensuring comprehensive realization and implementation of country plans for preventing HIV infection and mitigating the impacts of HIV/AIDS on the education sector (Bundy et al. 2010). Although major achievements have been made in recent years in the education sector in protecting individuals and communities from HIV/AIDS (UNESCO 2010), numerous challenges persist in regard to the planning, coordination, and implementation of programs (Visser-Valfrey and Pronk 2007). The objective of this chapter is to review literature on mainstreaming HIV/AIDS interventions within the educational infrastructure in Sub-Saharan Africa.

Definition of mainstreaming HIV/AIDS in education systems

UNAIDS, World Bank, and UNDP (2005) defined mainstreaming as a process that enables development actors to address the causes and effects of HIV and AIDS as they relate to their mandates in an effective and sustainable manner, both through their usual work (what they do) and through their workplace (where they do their work). This process involves both external mainstreaming (interventions aimed at HIV prevention and mitigation of HIV/AIDS impacts on the education sector) and internal mainstreaming (interventions responding to HIV/AIDS impacts on teachers and educational staff). At a more general level, mainstreaming HIV/AIDS is a process of changing policy in a systemic manner toward achieving broad social goals of controlling the spread of the epidemic and mitigating its effects. In the context of the education sector, mainstreaming is conceptualized as a deliberate and strategic change in education policy to address the effects of HIV in the education sector and achieving the sector's set goals, plans, and actions nationwide. Thus mainstreaming requires that attention be given to the impacts and feasible responses to HIV/AIDS in education systems processes, including education sector infrastructure, curriculum integration, teacher training, HIV prevention, and monitoring and evaluation of outcomes (Bundy et al. 2010, p. 16; Rugalema and Khanye 2002).

Rationale for mainstreaming

Mainstreaming HIV/AIDS in education aims at integrating HIV/AIDS prevention and mitigation efforts in education policies, programs, and projects. This approach can ensure that addressing HIV and AIDS is not an add-on or an isolated activity but an integral part of education sector policy, strategies, curricula, actions, and monitoring and evaluation efforts. It also means that HIV/AIDS should not be seen as a separate issue, but as part of overall educational plans and priorities, including those related to life skills, social skills, health, and nutrition. Mainstreaming should be a joint effort involving teachers' organizations and other key stakeholders, including those in the health sector and national AIDS programs (UNAIDS 2008).

Rugalema and Khanye (2002) developed a model for mainstreaming HIV/AIDS in the education sector that influenced early research and interventions. Their framework elucidates major links in the bi-directional relationship between HIV/AIDS and education that require that educational planning in the context of HIV/AIDS takes into consideration two aspects in particular: the impact of the disease on educational systems and the role of education in reducing the spread of the disease and mitigating its impacts (Commonwealth Secretariat 2006; Kelly 2008). Because much has been written on HIV/AIDS impacts, this chapter focuses mainly on prevention and mitigation, both promising intervention strategies that are inadequately understood.

Mainstreaming should take place in both curriculum-based and extracurricular programs. Rugalema and Khanye's (2002) conceptual framework has four fundamental conditions that must be met for successful mainstreaming of HIV/AIDS in education:

1. The strategies should be innovative, well designed, and implemented to maintain the quality of education despite the effects of the epidemic on the system.
2. Policies and programs should be developed that target teachers because HIV/AIDS is an important workplace issue.
3. Education managers and support staff working with schools should also be targeted. HIV/AIDS must be seen not only as a problem 'out there' but also as a problem 'within'.
4. A robust management information system on HIV/AIDS should be designed and maintained.

Recent progress in mainstreaming

A 2004 survey of progress with mainstreaming HIV/AIDS in education in 14 Commonwealth countries in Sub-Saharan Africa found that only four countries had a specific HIV and AIDS policy and only five countries had a workplace policy in place (Commonwealth Secretariat 2006, p. 15). Slow and inadequate responses of stakeholders in the region to the epidemic, related mainly to the failure of the educational sector to address HIV/AIDS systematically and associated underutilization of available resources, prompted the UNAIDS Inter-Agency Task Team (IATT) on Education to establish in 2002 the working group known as the Accelerate Initiative Working Group. This initiative addresses these and other challenges and supports countries in accelerating and improving responses to the crisis. The five objectives of the initiative are as follows:

1. Promote leadership and demand for the response to HIV/AIDS in the education sector.
2. Harmonize support among partners to assist countries in better and more cost-effective ways.
3. Promote coordination between partners and national AIDS authorities for funding purposes.
4. Share HIV/AIDS information relevant to the education sector and strengthen the technical content of that information.
5. Implement the sectoral response to HIV/AIDS (Bundy et al. 2010).

The Girls' Education Initiative of the United Nations was launched in 2000 as a partnership of organizations seeking to narrow the gender gap in education and ensure that, by 2015, all children complete primary education. United Nations Girls' Education Initiative (UNGEI) is providing the gender context for the Accelerate Initiative by promoting the mainstreaming of gender into the education sector's HIV/AIDS responses and strategies (Bundy et al. 2010).

By 2007, 37 countries representing 85% of school-aged children in Sub-Saharan Africa and 76 agencies, NGOs, and development partners participated in the Accelerate Initiative; 75% of the participating African governments used both education and AIDS funds to support their school health programs (Bundy et al. 2010, p. 16). In regard to the first objective described above, 26 of the 37 governments participated in subregional workshops. Of these, 26 ministries of education proceeded to develop and implement actions. The outcome of efforts to achieve Objective 2 was also encouraging: a total of 76 organizations collaborated throughout the 2002–2007 period, holding 24 workshops supported by UNAIDS-affiliated agencies, bilateral donors, and civil society organizations. All 37 participating ministries of education achieved Objective 3 by communicating with their respective national AIDS authorities, with 26 of them subsequently obtaining national funding. Wide distribution of key documents on HIV/AIDS and education, together with the establishment of subregional networks of HIV/AIDS focal points, met Objective 4. By the end of 2007, 76% of 34 countries had an education-specific HIV/AIDS strategy; 32 countries had focal points at their ministries of education; 30 countries were training teachers to protect themselves; and all countries provided some prevention for primary or secondary students, 31 countries providing this information to pre-puberty students (Bundy et al. 2010, p. 37). These achievements bode well for the provision of HIV prevention services and social support for affected educators and learners and protecting the sector's capacity to provide quality education (UNAIDS 2007; UNESCO 2005). UNAIDS (2008) developed a toolkit for mainstreaming HIV and AIDS in the education sector for education staff at managerial and operational levels with the objective of providing orientation, identifying specific outcomes, and monitoring progress.

Education policies on HIV and AIDS

Most Sub-Saharan countries reported significant progress in developing national responses to HIV/AIDS, including implementing national policies to guide national responses toward HIV/AIDS prevention and control. The existence of sector-wide approaches, such as the formulation and implementation of explicit education HIV/AIDS strategic plans, noted above, is an indicator of commitment to fight the HIV epidemic within institutions (Nzioka and Ramos 2008).

After a slow start, universities and other higher education institutions also have begun to introduce HIV prevention strategies. The University of Botswana provided an early example of effective prevention and support for students as well as teaching and support staff. The school consistently targeted high-risk behaviors, including excessive drinking and sexual intimidation of female students in hostels. Clinics and student counseling services (including confidential HIV testing) have also been strengthened (Bennell 2004). The UN Family Planning Association in Ethiopia developed an HIV prevention program that provides voluntary counseling and testing (VCT) services and HIV/AIDS information to students and staff of Addis Ababa and Bahir Dar universities and strengthened networking and partnership with university and Ministry of Health-based partners (UNFPA 2007).

In Kenya, the Ministry of Education implemented a range of school-based HIV education and behavior change interventions through Primary School Action for Better Health (PSABH) in 1999. In September 2004, the government of Kenya, with the assistance of UNESCO, launched several additional school-based education sector initiatives on HIV and AIDS. The Ministry of Education has an AIDS Control Unit, which provides proactive leadership and ensures that HIV/AIDS prevention and control priorities become integrated into mainstream ministry functions (Nzioka et al. 2007).

HIV/AIDS and education sector infrastructure

Different international organizations and individual countries have implemented initiatives in the education sector in the forms of different strategies and programs, although not all of these have been systematically documented. At the national level, some countries have taken steps to address the impact of HIV and AIDS on the education sector and, as described above, adapt systems to respond to the epidemic.

During the past decade, ministries of education in Sub-Saharan African countries have seriously assessed actual and potential impacts of the epidemic in the education sector and have actively pursued the development of infrastructure. Apart from the establishment of ministerial AIDS control units, the creation of high-powered and well-resourced national AIDS commissions was a major achievement. For the first time, countries exhibited the political and bureaucratic will to make a comprehensive multisectoral approach a reality. The emergence of sector-wide approaches with budget support meant that the main donors became centrally involved in both policy design and implementation. They were therefore in a much better position to ensure that HIV/AIDS issues were addressed throughout the education sector. Ring-fenced donor funding for AIDS and education programs was readily forthcoming though hampered by nonaccountability of a number of governments (Bennell 2004).

HIV and AIDS education programs in schools

Recognition of the impact of HIV/AIDS on the education sector has led to the development of school-based programs. Such programs are essential in reaching a great majority of children and young people, and they also tend to benefit the wider community. Although evidence on the impact of these programs is anecdotal, the evidence suggests that the programs are able to influence attitudes and beliefs at an early stage of life (Jukes et al. 2008). School programs also have the benefit of equipping staff with teaching and learning tools (Mathews et al. 2006). As teachers tend to be role models for the Sub-Saharan African communities, schools may be the only places where adolescents seek information on reproductive health.

There is evidence that school-based programs in Sub-Saharan Africa have been innovative, introducing new teaching methods into the curriculum, such as life skills education (LSE). LSE is a methodology that develops the ability of children and young people to reason and helps them develop agency and social competence in order to act. It may help children and young people to better deal with the challenges of HIV and AIDS, including issues of gender, violence, and human rights (Hoffman 2006). In a review of literature on interventions targeting the sexual behavior of youths, Hubley (2000) found that children and adolescents are more likely to abstain or delay first sex after exposure to life skill programs. The beneficial effect of classroom teaching on teenage child bearing, a useful indicator of the incidence of unprotected sex, is less obvious. Whereas child bearing rates of 15- to 17-year-old girls attending teacher training schools in Cameroon declined over the course of a six-year study (Arcand and Wouabe 2010), no changes were found among female students in Kenya (Dupas et al. 2009).

Successful implementation of HIV/AIDS programs varies geographically and depends to a large extent on the availability of adequate resources and trained teachers. While analyzing the impact of HIV and AIDS life skills programs on secondary school students in KwaZulu-Natal, South Africa, James et al. (2006) found a significant increase in student knowledge about HIV/AIDS, but the programs had no effect on safe sex practices or on measures of psychosocial determinants of these practices. The study showed that implementation of the program for teachers was selective or partial in some schools. LSE is not value free, and its success depends on striking acceptable balances among the duty of the school to impart the knowledge and skills, the capacity of the learner, and parental authority (Ngwenya 2003). Unclear strategies, poor design and evaluation of effectiveness and sustainability, and scaling up are additional challenges that must be addressed in any LSE program (Hoffman 2006).

Curriculum integration

Past efforts at mainstreaming HIV/AIDS in the education sector focused mainly on learners in primary and secondary schools (Rugalema and Khanye 2002). Tertiary institutions are just beginning to be brought on board. A number of courses, both voluntary and compulsory, have been introduced in various institutions at different levels, even though these do not constitute 'mainstreaming' HIV/AIDS throughout the curricula (Otaala 2003). In Kenya, for example, the majority of public universities have introduced a compulsory course on HIV/AIDS. However, the course is very general and academic in nature, failing to impart life skills to learners. The University of Namibia has introduced a compulsory module for all first-year students. The module, entitled 'Social Issues', deals with gender, ethics, and HIV/AIDS. Various departments have also made efforts to incorporate aspects of HIV/AIDS education in their curricula. At other universities, HIV/AIDS interventions have been incorporated into the formal curricula and extracurricular activities such as sports and creative arts. In Kenya and Uganda, HIV/AIDS interventions are now part of professional studies at teacher training colleges (Nzioka and Ramos 2008). The effectiveness of curriculum-based education programs in reducing risky sexual behaviors is well documented (Kirby et al. 2005).

One weakness in school-based health intervention programs in Sub-Saharan Africa is the paucity of evaluation studies. Variations in the content, duration, and intensity of interventions, together with differences in evaluation design and instruments, further impede objective comparisons across countries or even subregions (Kaaya et al. 2002). Nevertheless, several studies have demonstrated positive effects of school-based programs on knowledge, attitudes, and communication about sexuality and sexual health (Kelley 2006). These findings emanate mostly from case studies (see Rugalema and Khanye 2002; Sherman and Bassett 1999), including one revealing that children enjoy peer-led HIV and AIDS sessions because they not only provide opportunities for discussion, but also encourage appropriate and successful socialization in the school environment (Rugalema and Khanye 2002).

Condom distribution in schools

Pragmatic governments accept that greater condom use among young people has to be at the heart of any effective HIV prevention strategy (Johnson 2000). Given the strong religious convictions of many leaders, this is not a palatable policy for some. However, as the epidemic remains severe, there are few alternatives; abstinence and pleas to be faithful have proven to be unpopular with youth. Beginning in 2007, condoms and information on sexuality and reproduction as well as access to HIV testing were made available to secondary school students free of charge in a few high-prevalence countries. NGOs took the lead in implementing this policy. In South Africa, these services were made available through the Children's Act to children aged 12 and older (Han and Bennish 2009) but this provision was strongly opposed by teachers' unions in Zimbabwe and Zambia (Condom distribution 2012; We will not 2012). Condom distribution in schools created a storm of protest also from many churches and generated resistance from school administrators throughout Sub-Saharan Africa, but governments steadfastly upheld the practice, which proved to be successful overall (Nzioka et al. 2007; Risley and Bundy 2007).

Programs targeting teachers

To be effective, programs aimed at teachers need to address both aspects of the role of the educational system in preventing and mitigating the effects of HIV/AIDS in Sub-Saharan African countries: the impact of the disease on teachers and students, and the role of education in reducing the spread of the disease and mitigating its impacts.

Teacher training

Teachers provide direct implementation of school-based programs and must therefore be trained properly to reduce HIV risk in schools and promote health-seeking behaviors. A study of South African school-based programs affirmed that teacher training improves the implementation of HIV/AIDS education by raising awareness among pupils and teachers about the problem of HIV/AIDS and the importance of proper responses (Mathews et al. 2006). In Kenya, the Primary School Action for Better Health (PSABH) program, which trained head teachers, senior classroom teachers, and parents/community representatives on HIV/AIDS and sex and sexuality, was successful in reducing HIV risk and transmission levels (Maticka-Tyndale et al. 2007). According to Maticka-Tyndale et al. (2007), around 11,000 out of 19,000 Kenyan schools had implemented PSABH by June 2006. Evaluations of the program revealed positive results – condom use increased among boys and girls were more likely to decrease or delay sexual activity. In Nigeria, a promising prevention strategy was designed and implemented in secondary schools and a national NGO assisted 12 community organizations in equipping teachers in 24 secondary schools with skills to teach gender equality so they could serve as peer educators, but the outcomes of these strategies remain to be evaluated (Oladeji et al. 2011). Nevertheless, throughout much of Sub-Saharan Africa, teacher training is carried out in a piecemeal manner and takes place outside of working hours; teachers are burdened with increasing workloads due to absenteeism and sick leave related to their own health and the deaths of colleagues and relatives, impeding programs (Commonwealth Secretariat 2006, Section 7; PlusNews 2008).

Several challenges beyond the widespread programming, infrastructure, and resource constraints confront teacher education programs. Beyers and Hay (2011) questioned the ability of teachers to meet the educational needs of HIV-positive students in the absence of support from education support services and resource centers. Wiese (2011), addressing issues surrounding the changes from an authoritarian to a democratic form of education in South Africa, identified the need for greater competence of teachers in dealing with the sensitivities and controversies of HIV/AIDS education in the changing political context.

This observation has implications for other teacher training programs in Sub-Saharan Africa operating in similar political contexts.

Teachers infected or affected by HIV

Because teachers are central pillars in the education system, their survival and well-being are essential for the sustainability of the system. Teachers in Sub-Saharan Africa face huge challenges, including an increasing workload due to absenteeism, sick leaves, deaths of colleagues, the responsibility for the care of sick relatives, and the need to provide assistance to infected and affected pupils (Education International 2006). HIV/AIDS has led to an increase in teacher mortality and absenteeism, severely reducing both teaching time and quality. One of the most extensive studies of teacher attrition in southern Africa, carried out in all 41 education districts in KwaZulu-Natal, found that while relatively few teachers died in 1999 due to AIDS, nearly 5% of all teachers were estimated to die annually by 2010 (Badcock-Walters 2001). According to UNESCO (2005), the permanent or temporary absenteeism of one teacher can have strong repercussions on as many as 100 students.

Despite the impact of HIV/AIDS on teachers, most education ministries have not paid adequate attention to school-based HIV and AIDS programs.

Although practically all countries have policies regarding programs that support infected and affected educators, they do not have action plans or resources with which to implement them. In many countries, programs designed to give support and care to educators have started only recently or do not exist.

Some interventions have demonstrated effectiveness. The provision of antiretrovirals (ARVs) to teachers as part of government health programs in Botswana and Namibia since the late 1990s led to almost immediate declines in AIDS-related deaths, declines that were sustained (Bennell 2004). From 2004 onward, teachers and other education support personnel in other high-prevalence countries have been able to access ARVs either as part of improved government medical services or in national antiretroviral therapy (ART) rollouts. Earlier concerns about patient compliance proved to be largely unfounded, and the new generation of ARVs has been easier to take with few serious side effects. In some cases, affected teachers were transferred to schools located close to clinics (Bennell 2004; Haile Gabriel 2008).

New regulations concerning sick leaves and medical leaves ensured that ill teachers could take long-term sick leave and be quickly replaced by temporary teachers (Bennell 2004). National gender and education strategies have been introduced in all countries, although the exact policies and interventions vary widely. They include national sensitization programs; the establishment of girls-only schools and classes; bursaries/stipends for girls, particularly for girls in secondary and tertiary education; and girls-only education voucher schemes that have enabled poor households to choose the schools they prefer for their daughters (Bennell 2004). Mozambique effectively implemented a workplace program aimed at teachers and nonteaching staff that provides assistance with health problems, including HIV/AIDS. The training and deployment of more than 3,000 social workers in all districts of the country has resulted in a solidly mainstreamed workplace program integrated into existing Ministry of Education structures and mechanisms that has led to improved collection of data on the well-being of staff (Machwira et al. 2011).

Challenges in the education sector

One of the key challenges in addressing HIV/AIDS continues to be the level of denial about the disease (Nzioka et al. 2007). In many countries and contexts, HIV/AIDS has traditionally not been thought of as a substantial educational problem. Instead, it is considered a health issue in Sub-Saharan Africa (Haile Gabriel 2008; Nzioka et al. 2007). Therefore, governments and their development partners tend to give insufficient attention to education and other nonhealth sectors in developing HIV/AIDS policy, plans, and funding mechanisms. In 2004, for example, 60% of funding to the education sector for HIV did not pass through national AIDS coordinating mechanisms (Visser-Valfrey and Pronk 2007). Moreover, many educational organizations and ministries of education are unaware of the various sources of HIV funding available to them as part of multisectoral responses to the epidemic.

Although the political will to tackle HIV/AIDS has grown enormously over recent years, a wide gap remains between the global agenda and actual implementation of that agenda. On a positive note, HIV/AIDS plans that are focused and adapted to reach those most at risk of HIV infection are starting to be implemented worldwide (UNAIDS and WHO 2006). However, such plans have often not been implemented at the school level because they were developed in isolation from other policy and budgetary processes (Boler et al. 2003).

The AIDS epidemic has disabled the education sector's core functions in many eastern and southern African countries. However, with a few exceptions, governments, and ministries of education in particular have failed to take the decisive steps necessary to protect schools from the ravages of the epidemic. In some countries, the conflicting findings and recommendations of donor-funded HIV/AIDS impact assessments have increasingly confused and sometimes frightened politicians and senior civil servants. Experts insist that in the face of the AIDS threat, schools must take on a whole new set of responsibilities. Given that this 'transformation' agenda is just not feasible, doing little or nothing has become the preferred option (Castro et al. 2007).

Massive decentralization efforts in some countries of Sub-Saharan Africa have shifted implementation responsibilities to the district level, with the result that the head offices of ministries of education have become even more detached from front-line school-level delivery issues. Public sector reform has resulted in large-scale retrenchments, with neither sizeable improvements in incentives nor the technical and management competencies of senior and middle-level education managers at both national and district levels. Thus, the overall capacity of ministries of education to design and implement education policies has declined still further. Most teachers' unions have failed to mobilize around the threat to their memberships posed by the epidemic, and in several countries they have been fractured, although a few interventions have taken place in Kenya and South Africa. The main exception is South Africa, where the largest teachers' union has been instrumental in pushing through the implementation of a comprehensive HIV/AIDS workplace program (World Bank 2002).

Ministries of education in Sub-Saharan Africa were unable in the past to introduce LSE as a time-tabled subject with professionally trained teachers; in 2002 they begun to train teachers in the life skills approach and by 2007, most countries taught HIV using the life skills approach (Bundy et al. 2010, pp. 45–46). One reason for the change is that countries have managed to wrest control of schools from faith-based organizations, many of which had been vehemently opposed to sexual and reproductive health education in schools. Only 'moral education' was acceptable, but moral education does not tackle underlying social and cultural beliefs that fuel high-risk behavior. Although parental resistance to sex education in schools also remains strong in many countries, parents are increasingly perceiving some aspects of these programs useful. In Dar es Salaam, for example, while parents were aware of the cultural restriction prohibiting them from talking to their children about sexuality and reproductive behavior and they opposed the use of condoms as a step to promiscuity, most of them approved of these programs (Mbonile and Kayombo 2008). Similarly, in Port Harcourt, Nigeria, nearly all parents of pregnant girls rarely discussed sexual matters with their adolescent daughters and considered contraceptives unacceptable and harmful but wanted a school-based sex education program to prevent unwanted pregnancy (Briggs 1998).

The reluctance to discuss both sex and HIV/AIDS within schools and communities greatly devalues and reduces the effectiveness of school-based programs (Boler et al. 2003). The fact remains that teachers have been afraid to address issues such as HIV/AIDS and sex education due to cultural, religious, and socialization factors, as reported from Botswana (Mhlauli 2011). Furthermore, many teachers are unsure whether broaching such subjects is their responsibility or the purview of the parent. Moreover, many education experts feel that the HIV/AIDS curriculum, which adopts the scientific approach, serves to 'dehumanize' HIV, making it difficult for students to connect with HIV as a real human issue that could affect them (Boler et al. 2003).

Some of the silence that clouds HIV and AIDS within the education sectors in Sub-Saharan Africa has been attributed to the lack of information on the occurrence of AIDS-related illnesses (Katohoire and Kirumira 2008). This situation has not been helped by the strong moral backlash in many communities severely affected by the epidemic. The power of the churches, both established and evangelical, has increased with the deepening economic crisis (Rose et al. 2004).

But it is governments that must take charge because they play a leading role in HIV/AIDS education as they set policy and facilitate the implementation of policy. However, one of the reasons Africa is over-represented in the statistics for infection and death related to HIV/AIDS is that many African countries do not have the resources or the infrastructures to carry out effective prevention programs (Gachuhi 1999). Without sufficient funding, health care budgets are grossly inadequate to provide basic health care, let alone implement effective prevention programs. Furthermore, governments are expected to disburse the modest funds they have across all sectors of society, impeding responses to HIV/AIDS in the education setting in many African countries.

Conclusion

This chapter reveals that a number of eastern and southern African countries have implemented HIV/AIDS strategies and programs in their education sectors, although most of them have not been systematically documented and evaluated. Integrating HIV/AIDS education in the education curriculum at all levels of learning (from primary school to tertiary institutions) has proven to be an effective approach in maximizing coverage and benefits to targeted populations. Some success in mitigating the impact of HIV/AIDS has been achieved by including HIV/AIDS information in the curriculum, providing ARVs to teachers as part of government health services, distributing condoms in schools, and empowering teachers and students by creating an environment in which life skills and personal choice can be effectively taught. Increasing participation of governments in several initiatives to implement and expand school health programs is particularly promising. One challenge in moving forward is to assess the extent to which these actions bring about beneficial results for teachers, learners, and the broader education sector.

The challenges that impede the effective implementation of HIV/AIDS intervention strategies in the education sector in Sub-Saharan Africa could result in millions of additional infections among young people. The inability of ministries of education in some countries to design and implement education policies may be overcome if government, donors, and civil society work together more systematically and transparently to create policy inertia on HIV/AIDS in education. At the school level, the powerful role educators play in forming societal values and attitudes and thus the unique platform they have can be used to combat stigma, fear, and apathy, and break moral taboos through open discussion of sex and the risks of HIV and other sexually transmitted pathogens.

References

Arcand, J.L. and Wouabe, E.D. 2010. Teacher training and HIV/AIDS prevention in West Africa: Regression discontinuity design evidence from the Cameroon. *Health Economics* 19:36–54.

AVERT. 2011. *Impact of HIV/AIDS in Africa.* www.avert.org/aids-impact-africa.htm

Badcock-Walters, P. 2001. *The Socioeconomic Impact of HIV/AIDS on Education in Kwa-Zulu Natal.* Durban: KZNDEC Provincial Education Development Unit.

Bennell, P. 2004. AIDS in Africa: Three scenarios for the education sector. Report prepared for the UNAIDS project AIDS in Africa: Scenarios for the Future. Geneva: UNAIDS.

Beyers, C. and Hay, J. 2011. Supporting HIV-positive learners in inclusive classes in South Africa: Is it the responsibility of teachers? *Journal of Social Science* 26:99–104.

Boler, T., Adoss, R. Ibrahim, A. and Shaw, M. 2003. *The Sound of Silence: Difficulties in Communicating on HIV/AIDS in Schools.* London: ActionAid.

Briggs, L.A. 1998. Parents' viewpoint on reproductive health and contraceptive practice among sexually active adolescents in Port Harcourt local government area of Rivers State, Nigeria. *Journal of Advanced Nursing* 27:261–266.

Bundy, D., Patrikios, A., Mannathoko, C. et al. 2010. *Accelerating the Education Sector Response to HIV: Five Years of Experience from Sub-Saharan Africa.* Washington, DC: World Bank.

Castro, V., Duthilleul, Y. and Caillods, F. 2007. *Teachers' Absence in an HIV AIDS Context: Evidence from Nine Schools in Kavango and Kaprivi, Namibia.* Paris: UNESCO International Institute for Education Training.

Commonwealth Secretariat. 2006. *Education Sector Responses to HIV and AIDS: Learning from Good Practices in Africa.* London: Commonwealth Secretariat.

Condom distribution (Condom distribution in Zambia schools not the best option). 2012. June 22. ZNUT. http://www.mwebantu.com/2012/06/22/condom-distribution-in-zambian-schools-not-best-option-znut-efz/

Dupas, P., Duflo, E., Kremer, M. and Sineis, S. 2009. *Teacher Training for HIV Prevention through Primary Schools (Kenya).* Berkeley: University of Berkeley, Center for Effective Global Action.

Education International. 2006. Training for life: Teacher training on HIV/AIDS. Draft report. Brussels: Education International.

Gachuhi, D. 1999. The impact of HIV/AIDS on education systems in the Eastern and Southern Africa region, and the response of education systems to HIV/AIDS: Life skills programmes. Paper presented at the All Sub-Saharan Africa Conference on Education for All, Johannesburg, 6–10 December.

Global Campaign for Education. 2004. Learning to survive: How education for all would save millions of young people from HIV/AIDS. www.Campaignforeducation. org

Haile Gabriel, A. 2008. The challenges and opportunities of mainstreaming HIV and AIDS intervention in Ethiopia's higher education system: What roles for tertiary education? In OSSREA (ed.), *The HIV/AIDS Challenge in Africa, an Impact and Response Assessment: The Case of Ethiopia,* pp. 1–69. Addis Ababa: OSSREA.

Han, J. and Bennish, M.L. 2009. Condom access in South African schools: Law, policy and practice. *PLoS Medicine* 6(6):e1000006. doi:10.1371/journal.pmed.1000006

Hargreaves, J. and T. Boler, T. 2006. *Girl Power: The Impact of Girls' Education on HIV and Sexual Behaviour.* Johannesburg: Action Aid International.

Hoffman, A.M. 2006. HIV prevention: Is life skills education making a difference? Paper presented at the Regional Workshop on Good Practices in Education Sector Responses to HIV and AIDS in Africa. IIEP Workshop on the Impact of HIV/AIDS on Education. Paris, International Institute for Educational Planning, UNESCO, 27–29 September.

Hubley, J. 2000. *Interventions Targeted at Youth Aimed at Influencing Sexual Behaviour and AIDS/STD.* Leeds: Leeds Health Education Database.

James, S., Reddy, P., Ruiter, R.A.C. et al. 2006. The impact of HIV and AIDS life skills programs on secondary school students in KwaZulu- Natal, South Africa. *AIDS Education and Prevention* 18:281–294.

Johnson, S. 2000. The impact of AIDS on the education sector in South Africa. Paper presented at the Workshop on the Impact of HIV/AIDS on Education, International Institute for Educational Planning, Paris, 12–15 September.

Jukes, M., Simmons, S. and Bundy, D. 2008. Education and vulnerability: The role of schools in protecting young women and girls from HIV in southern Africa. *AIDS* 22:S41–S56.

Kaaya, S.F., Mukoma, W., Fisher, A.J. and Klepp, K. 2002. School based sexual health interventions in Sub-Saharan Africa: A review. *Social Dynamics* 28:64–88.

Katohoire, A. and Kirumira, E. 2008. *The Impact of HIV and AIDS on Higher Educational Institution in Uganda.* Paris: UNESCO, International Institute for Education Training.

Kelley, M.J. 2006. Education and AIDS: Are we too optimistic? Paper presented at the Regional Workshop on Good Practices in Education Sector Responses to HIV and AIDS in Africa, Johannesburg, 12–14 September.

Kelly, M.J. 2008. *Education for an Africa without AIDS.* Nairobi: Paulines Publications.

Kirby, D., Laris, B.A. and Rolleri, L. 2005. *Impact of Sex and HIV Education Programs on Sexual Behaviours of Youth in Developing and Developed Countries.* Durham, NC: Family Health International.

Machwira, P., Roberto, E., Rodrigues, Z. and Willems, Z. 2011. Strengthening education sector GIV and AIDS workplace programmes in Mozambique. *Abstracts of the 16th International Conference on AIDS and STIs in Africa*, Addis Ababa, Abstract MOPE276.

Mathews, C., Boon, H., Flisher, J. and H. Schaalma. 2006. Factors associated with teachers' implementation of HIV/AIDS education in secondary schools in Cape Town, South Africa. *AIDS Care* 18:388–397.

Maticka-Tyndale, E, Wildish, J. and M. Gichuru. 2007. Quasi-experimental evaluation of a national primary school HIV intervention in Kenya. *Evaluation and Program Planning* 30:172–186.

Mbonile, L. and Kayombo, E.J. 2008. Assessing acceptabilityof parents/guardians of adolescents towards introduction of sex and reproductive health education in schools at Kinondoni Municipal in Dar es Salaam City. *East African Journal of Public Health* 5:28–31.

Mhlauli, M.B. 2011. Teaching controversial issues in primary schools in Botswana: Reality or illusion? *British Journal of Art and Social Sciences* 2:143–156.

Ngwenya, C. 2003. AIDS in schools: A human rights perspective on parameters for sexuality education. *Acta Academia* 35:184–204.

Nzioka, C., Karongo, A. and Njiru, R. 2007. *HIV/AIDS in Kenyan Teachers Colleges: Mitigating the Impact.* Paris: UNESCO International Institute for Education Planning.

Nzioka, C. and Ramos, L. 2008. *Training Teachers in the Context of HIV and AIDS: Experiences from Ethiopia, Kenya, Uganda and Zambia.* Paris: UNESCO International Institute for Education Planning.

Oladeji, A., Taiwo, A., Mojisola, F. et al. 2011. It is time to mainstream human rights issues and gender equality information into HIV preventive interventions among in-school young people. *Abstracts of the 16th International Conference on AIDS and STIs in Africa*, Addis Ababa, Abstract TUAD0805.

Otaala, B. 2003. Institutional policies for managing HIV/AIDS in Africa. An overview paper prepared for the Regional Training Conference on Improving Tertiary Education in Sub-Saharan Africa: Things That Work! Accra, 23–25 September.

PlusNews. 2008. South Africa: Sex education – the ugly stepchild in teacher training. *Global HIV/AIDS News and Analysis* Newsletter, 22 May.

Risley, C. and Bundy, D. 2007. *Estimating the Impact of HIV and AIDS on the Supply of Basic Education.* London: Partnership for Child Development, Imperial College.

Rose, K., Maito, M., Dolata, S. and Ikeda, M. 2004. *Data Archive for the SACMEQ 1 and 2 Projects.* Paris: IIEP-UNESCO.

Rugalema, G. and Khanye, V. 2002. Mainstreaming HIV/AIDS in the education systems in sub-Saharan Africa: Some preliminary insights. In Coombe, C. (ed.), *The*

HIV Challenge to Education: A Collection of Essays, pp. 81–103. Paris: UNESCO, International Institute for Educational Planning.

Sherman, J.B. and Bassett, M.T. 1999. Adolescents and AIDS prevention: A school-based approach in Zimbabwe. *Applied Psychology* 48:109–124.

UNAIDS. 2002. *Report on the Global AIDS Epidemic.* Geneva: UNAIDS.

UNAIDS. 2007. *Accelerating Education's Response to HIV and AIDS.* Geneva: UNAIDS.

UNAIDS. 2008. *Toolkit for Mainstreaming HIV and AIDS in the Education Sector: Guidelines for Development Cooperation Agencies.* UNAIDS, Inter-Agency Task Team on Education. http://unesdoc.unesco.org/images/0015/001566/156673E.pdf

UNAIDS. 2011. *Global AIDS Response Progress Reporting 2012: Guidelines Construction of Core Indicators for Monitoring the 2011 Political Declaration on HIV/AIDS.* Geneva: UNAIDS.

UNAIDS and WHO. 2006. *2006 AIDS Epidemic Update.* Geneva: UNAIDS.

UNDP. 2005. *Mainstreaming HIV/AIDS in Sectors and Programs: An Implementation Guide for National Responses.* Geneva: UNAIDS.

UNESCO. 2005. *UNESCO's Response to HIV and AIDS.* Paris: UNESCO HIV/AIDS Coordination Unit.

UNESCO. 2010. *Report of the Workshop on Mainstreaming HIV and AIDS in the Education Sector.* Paris: UNESCO.

UNFPA (United Nations Family Planning Association Ethiopia). 2007. *Preventing HIV/AIDS.* http://countryoffice.unfpa.org/ethiopia/2008/12/30/278/preventing_hivaids/

UNICEF. 2002. *HIV/AIDS Education: A Strategic Approach.* New York: UNICEF.

Visser-Valfrey, M. and Pronk, H. 2007. *Mainstreaming HIV&AIDS and Sexual Reproductive Health & Rights into Education: Challenges and Reality.* Report of the UNAIDS IATT on Education Symposium, 6 November, 2006. Amsterdam.

We will not (We will not allow condoms in schools: ZIMTA). 2012. Radio Vop Zimbabwe, 14 April. http://www.radiovop.com/index.php/national-news/8713-we-will-not-allow-condoms-in-schools-zimta.html

WHO. 2008. *Promoting Adolescent Sexual and Reproductive Health through Schools in Low-Income Countries: A Information Brief.* Geneva: WHO.

Wiese, E.F. 2011. Teacher sensitive issues: Teacher training, education for democracy and HIV/AIDS in South Africa. PhD dissertation, University of Birmingham, School of Education.

World Bank. 2002. *Education and HIV/AIDS: A Window of Hope.* Washington, DC: World Bank.

Books, papers, websites, and other resources for further reading

Website for Education Internationals' HIV/AIDS Links: http://www.ei-ie.org/educ/aids/eelinks.htm

Maticka-Tyndale, E., Tiemoko, R. and Makinwa-Adebusoye, M. (eds.) 2007. *Human Sexuality in Africa: Beyond Reproductuion.* Auckland Park: Action Health Incorporated, see Chapters 2–4.

11
Monitoring and Evaluation of HIV/AIDS Prevention Programs

Anne A. Khasakhala and Helmut Kloos

Introduction

Monitoring and evaluation of HIV occurrence and responses allow countries to track the epidemic and their prevention and control efforts. Scientists use standardized indicators to assess progress and challenges over time and make cross-national comparisons. Governments and international donors in Sub-Saharan Africa are giving increasing attention to the need to develop effective monitoring and evaluation (M&E) programs to provide reliable data in a timely fashion that can guide and help to improve programs. Spending on the various national programs and initiatives in different Sub-SaharanAfrican countries, ranging from $12.0 million in Madagascar to $2.09 billion in South Africa in 2009, is largely determined by the stage and intensity of the epidemic, health policy, national resources, and donor support (UNAIDS 2010a). These massive inputs and the colossal and urgent needs at hand make systematic monitoring and evaluation of control and prevention of HIV infection and AIDS patient care programs critical to maximizing their cost effectiveness, particularly in resource-poor countries (World Bank 2006). HIV prevention programs in particular may benefit from improved M&E systems because spending commitment and funding for prevention has failed to keep up with spending on AIDS treatment (Carty and Nieburg 2010; Henderson et al. 2009). In addition, current emphasis in HIV prevention on combined biomedical, behavioral, and structural approaches (see Chapter 8) requires accurate, appropriate, timely, and evidence-based information that M&E systems can provide.

The aim of M&E programs and activities is to track changes in target indicators and relate them to interventions. Monitoring is the routine tracking of information about programs and projects and their intended outputs, outcomes, and impacts; it is aimed at measuring progress toward achieving program and project objectives. In the prevention and control of HIV/AIDS, monitoring most often involves reporting program/project activities, noting changes in trends in the epidemic and major determinants, tracking costs and expenditures, and examining their functioning. Monitoring is an internal activity and is usually carried out during project implementation, preferably regularly, at monthly, quarterly, or other intervals, for optimum results. Thus monitoring can track the overall implementation of projects at different levels, focusing not only on inputs and processes, but also on project outputs (Adamchak et al. 2000; Global AIDS Program 2003).

Evaluation, on the other hand, is based on research and analysis of the conceptualization and design of programs, the monitoring of program interventions, and the assessment of program utility. It focuses on why results are or are not being achieved and on unintended consequences or issues of interpretation, relevance, effectiveness, efficiency, impact, or sustainability. Evaluation is usually rigorous and based on quantitative and qualitative analysis of information about program activities, characteristics, and outcomes to determine the merit of a specific program (Adamchak et al. 2000; Global AIDS Program 2003).

Monitoring and evaluation are closely related, mutually supportive, and interdependent. Monitoring can provide quantitative and qualitative data using selected indicators, data that can serve as inputs to evaluation exercises. Evaluation also supports monitoring, serving as a source of lessons that can be applied in the development of conceptual or methodological innovations for use in refining the monitoring function, for example, by devising appropriate indicators for future projects. Process evaluation, which focuses on program implementation, is included in this discussion to provide information on implementation and operational functioning of programs and projects. In process evaluation, data are collected and detailed analysis is conducted on the delivery of interventions, differences between the target population and the population served, and access to the intervention. This chapter examines the status of M&E of HIV/AIDS programs in Sub-Saharan Africa with an emphasis on prevention programs especially among young people, and it describes efforts to support capacity building in M&E in Sub-Saharan Africa.

Declarations and principles

Three political declarations made at the United Nations level have promoted a policy environment conducive to the development of monitoring and evaluation systems. Building on the 2001 UN General Assembly Special Session on HIV/AIDS Declaration of Commitment on HIV/AIDS (UNGASS) and the 2006 Political Declaration on HIV/AIDS, the 2011 Political Declaration on HIV/AIDS generated new commitments among member states and adopted ambitious new targets for 2015 (UNAIDS 2011a). The UN member states unanimously adopted seven targets: (1) reducing HIV transmission in the general population and among sex workers, men having sex with men (MSM), and people who inject drugs by 50%; (2) reducing tuberculosis deaths of people living with HIV/AIDS (PLWHA) by 50%; (3) providing access to antiretroviral therapy (ART) for 15 million PLWHA; (4) reducing mother-to-child transmission by 90%; (5) lowering AIDS-related maternal deaths by 50%; (6) increasing funding to $22–24 billion annually; and (7) ensuring that critical enablers and synergies are generated in various development sectors to address structural issues. The new targets also included increasing access to HIV services for people at high risk of infection (MSM, users of illicit drugs, and sex workers) and empowering females through the elimination of gender inequality, gendered abuse, and violence.

The United Nations issued guidelines in 2011 to all member countries on the use of the 25 core indicators and 5 other Millennium Development Goals (MDG) indicators for improving the quality and consistency of data collected and presented in the annual United Nations General Assembly Special Session (UNGASS) reports. Countries were encouraged to select and include additional indicators in their national M&E plans depending on the type(s) of epidemic they faced and prevailing exposure risk patterns. Although most of the core indicators applied to all countries, the countries were encouraged to disaggregate data by age and sex to allow for more detailed analyses of trends than what was possible with the data used in many country reports in the past (UNAIDS 2011a). The development of standardized indicators, the issuance of guidelines for monitoring key programmatic areas since 1993, and the availability of more than 400 HIV-related indicators through the Indicator Registry established in 2007 have considerably strengthened M&E efforts (UNAIDS 2008a).

The International Conference on AIDS and STIs in Africa (ICASA), held in 2003 in Nairobi, brought together officials from the national coordinating bodies and relevant ministries of African nations, major bilateral and multilateral funding agencies, nongovernment organizations (NGOs), and the private sector for a consultative meeting to review principles for national-level coordination of the HIV/AIDS response. The officials agreed to use the 'Three Ones' principles to guide their HIV/AIDS M&E systems. That is, they agreed that each country would put in place the following three elements in their response to HIV/AIDS: an HIV/AIDS action framework that would provide the basis for coordinating the work of all partners, a national AIDS coordinating authority with a broad-based multisector mandate, and a country-level monitoring and evaluation system (UNAIDS 2005).

Based on these principles, most countries in the Sub-Saharan region developed strategic management frameworks, providing a common understanding of the expected results, outputs, impacts, performance measures, and reporting mechanisms to be followed by all key stakeholders involved in the AIDS response. The Three Ones principles have served as a model in many countries for increasing aid effectiveness (UNAIDS 2010b).

Considerable progress has been made toward achieving the objectives set forth by the Three Ones principles. Between 2005 and 2007 alone, the number of Sub-Saharan African countries with the basic elements of a functioning M&E system in place increased from 8 to 15, including 10 countries in eastern and southern Africa (UNAIDS 2008b, p. 22). These elements (a national monitoring and evaluation plan that includes budgetary requirements and is secured by funding, a functional national monitoring and evaluation unit and/or monitoring and evaluation working group, and a central national HIV database) have greatly strengthened M&E systems and improved methods of tracking the accuracy and reliability of national prevalence, incidence, and mortality data. In 2010, 43 Sub-Saharan countries reported on at least some of the 25 core UNGASS indicators (UNAIDS 2011b), although the capacity of M&E systems and the quality, distribution, and use of the data need to be further improved, as described below. We discuss below some of the implications and remaining challenges of using core indicators for young people in the region.

Monitoring the status of HIV/AIDS and determinants: A focus on young people

Eighteen of the 25 core UNGASS indicators are relevant to young people and four relate exclusively to young people. We summarize here some data on young people in the 2010 UNGASS country progress reports because achievement of the MDG to halt and reverse the spread of HIV/AIDS prevalence among 15 to 24-year-olds depends to a large degree on meeting the needs of people in this age group and respecting and protecting their human rights. Young people accounted for 41% of all new adult HIV infections and young women for 64% of the infections among young people in 2010. The huge transmission potential of this group, accentuated by high-risk populations within the group (young people injecting drugs, MSM, and sex workers) and by difficulties this segment of the population faces in accessing health services, as described in previous chapters, demands an understanding of corresponding M&E activities aimed specifically at young people (UNAIDS 2011b). One country – Lesotho – has made young people a priority in its national HIV/AIDS strategic plan (UNAIDS 2011b).

The 42 Sub-Saharan countries submitting UNGASS reports in 2010 reported on progress toward most of the 25 core indicators, but coverage of different indicators varied considerably. Table 11.1 shows the reporting for eight key indicators. Whereas progress on some indicators such as budgets (Indicator No. 1) and HIV prevalence (Indicator No. 22) was reported by practically all countries, progress on some behavioral and structural indicators for high-risk groups was reported by far fewer countries.

Results for Indicators 13 and 15 were reported by more countries than results for the other behavioral indicators, but reported values varied considerably by gender. The mean value for Indicator 13 (percentage of 15- to 24-year-olds with knowledge of HIV prevention and transmission) was

Table 11.1   Number of Sub-Saharan countries reporting on eight core indicators in their 2010 UNGASS country progress reports

Indicator (by UNGASS indicator no.)	No. of countries[a]
No. 22: HIV prevalence	40,40
No. 1: Total domestic and international AIDS spending (in US$) for youth, orphans, and vulnerable children	42(18)
No. 13: Percentage of young women and men who both correctly identify ways of preventing the sexual transmission of HIV and who reject major misconceptions about HIV transmission	36,35(4)
No. 15: Percentage of young women and men who have had sexual intercourse before the age of 15[b] in the last 12 months	36,35
No. 17: Percentage of young women and men[c] who had more than one sexual partner in the last 12 months and report the use of a condom during their last intercourse	25,30(3)
No. 7: Percentage of young women and men[c] who received an HIV test in the last 12 months and who know the results	31,31(4)
No. 10: Percentage of orphans and other vulnerable children whose households received free basic external support for caring for the child	33(1)
No. 9: Percentage of adults in MARPS reached with HIV prevention programs[d]	13(12)

[a]Where data are available, number of females followed by males; number of countries with incomplete data or submitting last report before 2005 in parentheses.
[b]Includes DHS data.
[c]Males and females aged 15–19.
[d]Includes sex workers, MSM, and people who inject drugs, all below 25 years.
Sources: Various 2010 UNGASS Country Reports (UNAIDS 2010b).

higher for males (38.1%) than females (33.8%), and the mean value for Indicator 15 (percentage of youth who had sexual intercourse before age 15 and during the 12 months preceding the survey) was higher for females (16.2%) than males (14.6%). This pattern indicates that males had more knowledge of HIV prevention and transmission than females and females had earlier sexual initiation, as described in other chapters of this volume. The gender differential for Indicator 15 may be higher than these values suggest due to possible underreporting in societies where virginity before marriage is highly valued, an issue requiring further study.

Relatively few countries reported progress on Indicator 17 (the percentage of 15- to 19-year-olds who had more than one sexual partner in the last

12 months and used a condom during their last intercourse), especially for women, a pattern also found for 20- to 24-year-old women in Sub-Saharan countries and in most other regions. Significantly more males aged 15–19 (47.9%) than females (31.9%) used condoms, with values for males ranging from 3.4% in Madagascar to 93.7% in Nigeria and for females from 3.9% in Madagascar to 85.2% in Botswana. Similarly, according to Indicator 16 (not shown in Table 11.1), mean percentage reduction in 14- to 25-year-olds having had sex with multiple partners in the past year in the period between 1997 and 2010 was greater among males (47.9%) than females (31.9%) in 15 Sub-Saharan countries, with no reductions reported for females in Kenya and Uganda during that period and an increase of 3% in Tanzania (UNAIDS 2011b). More countries in Sub-Saharan Africa reported progress on Indicator No. 7 (utilization of HIV testing during the 12 months prior to the survey and knowing the test results) than in any other region. Nevertheless, use of VCT services by youth remained low in Sub-Saharan Africa overall; fewer than 20% of young people in 10 countries with large numbers of young people at high risk of infection (Botswana, Côte d'Ivoire, Ghana, Malawi, Mozambique, South Africa, Swaziland, Tanzania, Zambia, and Zimbabwe) were tested in 2010 (UNAIDS 2011b).

Only 13 Sub-Saharan countries reported progress on Indicator 9 (percentage of most-at-risk populations [MARPs], reached with HIV prevention programs), fewer than any other region (Table 11.1). Only Nigeria reported on sex workers, MSM, and people who inject drugs. This low reporting appears to be due to a combination of low access to health services of these three groups, especially MSM and people who inject drugs, relatively low use of injectable drugs in the region, stigma attached to MSM, and the denial of human rights to these groups in many countries, as discussed in Chapters 2, 4, and 8.

Government and civil society in about one-third of the Sub-Saharan countries have laws, regulations, and policies that constitute obstacles for HIV/AIDS programs for young people (UNAIDS 2011b). Progress on structural Indicator No. 10, measuring the percentage of orphans and other vulnerable children (OVC) whose households received free external support, was reported by 33 countries and reveals a very wide range of support levels, from 1% in Sierra Leone to 75% in South Africa. In nine countries, mostly poor counties, fewer than 10% of the affected households received aid for orphans and OVC (Table 11.1), corroborating the reports in Chapters 6 and 9 of family members experiencing extreme hardship as they attempt to provide care and support to orphans and other vulnerable children.

Age-specific gendered treatment data are needed to better evaluate the effect of interventions on the dynamics of infection. Whereas the number of children newly infected with HIV is estimated to have declined 15% between 2001 and 2010 as a result of ART preventing mother-to-child transmission

(MTCT) (UNAIDS 2010a), the impact of interventions on HIV infection in the 15–24 age group is not known because the current UNGASS indicator that measures the effect of ART refers only to children and adults (UNAIDS 2011b). In Tanzania, one of the few countries disaggregating HIV infection data for age groups at four-year intervals rather than the ten-year intervals reported by most countries, the ratio of infected females/males was highest in the 20–24 age group and declined consistently until the 35–39 age group (United Republic of Tanzania 2010, p. 11). This is a strong indication of the increasing HIV risk to women age 20–35 compared to men and presents a case for stepped-up efforts to reduce HIV transmission in girls. Prevention of HIV in youth, including the most-at-risk youth populations, is more challenging than prevention of MTCT due to numerous transmission pathways and the many barriers affecting interventions in different socioeconomic, cultural, and political settings, requiring context-specific approaches and information (UNAIDS and WHO 2011).

A glaring discrepancy persists between the high HIV transmission potential of highly vulnerable groups and their neglect in prevention programs. For example, although sex workers, MSM, and people who inject drugs accounted for an estimated 30% of all new infections in Burkina Faso, 28% in Côte d'Ivoire, and 43% in Ghana, only 1.7%, 0.4%, and 0.2% of prevention expenditure in these countries, respectively, were devoted to programs targeting these groups (UNAIDS and World Bank 2010). Similarly, in Kenya only 0.35% and in Mozambique 0.25% of all AIDS spending was allocated for HIV prevention among people who injected drugs, even though they constituted one-quarter and one-third of all new infections (Colvin et al. 2009; NACC 2009).

The relative neglect of these vulnerable groups is also indicated by the failure of a number of countries to endorse the Declaration of Commitment on HIV/AIDS and to report on core indicators pertaining to high-risk populations in the 2010 UNGASS country reports. Only 20 of the region's 42 reporting countries reported on the use of condoms by sex workers, three countries reported on MSM, and two countries on people who inject drugs (UNAIDS 2011b). Incomplete reporting for these groups extends across the developing world and indicates not only priorities in resource-poor countries, but also persisting failure to follow through on commitments to protect human rights (Persson et al. 2011). In South Africa, for example, lack of resources and inadequate policies are impediments to meeting the needs of children and other high-risk populations. Although South Africa's M&E system operates in an environment of political will and commitment to addressing women's issues, the country has not made a policy initiative to address the concentrated epidemics within sex workers and other MARPs (MSM and migrant miners) and is unable to meet the needs of its large youth population at risk of infection partly due to a lack of social workers (Republic of South Africa 2010, pp. 32–33).

Improved country-level monitoring and evaluation and combination prevention strategies that have been developed as part of second-generation surveillance systems are facilitating evidence-informed responses to the epidemic even though some countries are still trying to put in place routine data collection systems, identify additional resources, and upgrade strategies and activities for HIV surveillance for specific populations. Since HIV/AIDS was first recognized, approaches and methodologies for monitoring and responding to the epidemic have continually improved (UNAIDS 2008a). During the last few years, new information technologies such as the use of electronic medical records, Web-based systems, and mobile phone networks have improved timely reporting and accuracy of data and strengthened health systems in most Sub-Saharan countries (Ekouevi et al. 2011). As a result, it has become easier to estimate HIV prevalence and incidence to determine the extent of program coverage, to characterize and evaluate national responses, and to gauge the levels of available and required funding for HIV programs in poorer countries (UNAIDS 2008a).

Temporal and spatial changes in the epidemic necessitate M&E systems that can track the dynamics and impacts of the epidemic in different socioeconomic, cultural, and political settings (UNAIDS and WHO 2011). Evolving combination prevention tools described in Chapter 8 may facilitate the implementation of M&E programs tailored to the uniqueness of HIV epidemics and subepidemics in different countries and population groups.

Agencies supporting M&E capacity building

International efforts have been made to harmonize and align support for M&E systems, outlined in the Three Ones principles (UNAIDS 2005). A number of countries in Africa have adopted the principles, but the extent to which development partners and international and local NGOs have embraced them is not known. The precarious HIV/AIDS funding environment, duplication of efforts among the various programs, and widespread lack of coordination point to the need for global leaders to apply the Three Ones principles in HIV/AIDS funding because the coordination of national responses enshrined in the principles can increase the coordination of funding and programs. Spicer et al. (2010) suggested that better coordination at the global level may not only result in more efficient use of available resources, but may also prevent duplicate spending; increase the possibility of initiating new programs, including more effective prevention programs; and promote transparency and coordination between global health initiatives and local programs, further discussed below.

International efforts to harmonize and align support for M&E systems, entrenched in the Three Ones principles, have gathered momentum. The Global Monitoring and Evaluation Team (GAMET) was set up by UNAIDS in 2001 to improve the quality of HIV/AIDS M&E and build national capacity to achieve the third 'One' principle (one country-led and country-owned M&E system) by working closely with 31 partner countries in Sub-Saharan Africa and international partners (World Bank 2009). A 2009 report by GAMET concluded that major progress had been made in the rapid growth in resources for HIV/AIDS, progress accompanied by increased recognition of the importance of and investment in M&E systems. In many countries, resources are no longer a major constraint to the development of functioning M&E systems. In 2009, GAMET provided support to national HIV/AIDS authorities in 32 Sub-Saharan countries, focusing primarily on improving the quality of HIV/AIDS monitoring and evaluation and building national capacity (World Bank 2009).

Apart from GAMET, the United States Agency for International Development (USAID) continues to support efforts toward M&E of HIV/AIDS prevention programs at the local, regional, and national levels. The efforts have been directed mainly toward the support of the development of standardized indicators in consultation with other national governments, multilateral donors, technical experts, and nongovernmental organizations that enable program managers to monitor similar results over time and among countries. The system includes two basic categories of data – HIV seroprevalence data and survey data from human behavioral surveys (USAID 2009).

There is also broad consensus about the importance of harmonizing the elements of an effective M&E system and the need to effectively coordinate financing and technical assistance. In most countries, M&E teams and development partners have developed road maps to ensure that all partners on the ground work together to support implementation of a national M&E system. Nigeria, for example, developed a road map for enhancing monitoring and evaluation of HIV/AIDS (NACA 2008). In the absence of a clear road map, HIV/AIDS programs supported by large international agencies such as the Global Fund may create vertical and parallel service delivery structures that undermine health systems and lead to inefficiencies, as reported from Ghana (Atun et al. 2011).

Status of monitoring and evaluation of HIV/AIDS programs in five Sub-Saharan African countries

About half of the 32 Sub-Saharan countries supported by GAMET had developed M&E frameworks and operational plans by 2007, but fewer than one-third had M&E systems in place that were regularly reporting on key performance indicators (World Bank 2009). For the five countries reviewed in this section (Uganda, Kenya, Ethiopia, Tanzania, and Nigeria), essential documentation has been developed, including M&E indicator guides, country operational manuals, illustrative country plans and budgets, toolkits, and road maps for effective partner coordination and implementation of M&E

systems. It is important to note, however, that monitoring and evaluation systems are being strengthened largely with external funds because countries are only beginning to follow the standard guideline specifying that up to 10% of program funds be directed to strengthening such systems. Most Sub-Saharan countries have established AIDS coordinating agencies (UNAIDS 2008b) but are at different stages, as illustrated by the case studies from five countries presented below.

Uganda

An M&E subcommittee composed of various key stakeholders from government, nongovernment, and development partners was established in Uganda in 2005 to guide the national M&E functions. The subcommittee has since played a key role in guiding the development of the performance measurement and management plan and the operational handbook for the National Strategic Plan 2007/08–2011/12, which addresses the concerns raised in the 2005 evaluation of the M&E framework for the previous National Strategic Framework 2001–2006 (Government of Uganda 2010, p. 58). The new M&E plan is linked to the national integrated M&E system of the National Development Plan, which recognizes HIV/AIDS as a cross-cutting development issue in Uganda. The Uganda AIDS Council (UAC) is strengthening its M&E unit with more skilled staff and in-house training and is also strengthening its linkages with HIV and AIDS stakeholders through a partnership arrangement in order to champion information sharing and feedback systems at both national and decentralized levels. By 2009, 58 indicators at the national level had been identified for monitoring the national response and 47 indicators for monitoring service delivery output from districts, 10 of which had completed district-level plans (Government of Uganda 2010, p. 59).

In spite of these and other achievements, technical assistance and capacity building at all levels of the M&E system need to be further strengthened; for example, the UAC does not regularly receive information from line ministries and other stakeholders, preventing updating of the database regarding key indicators, and few sectors besides health have developed HIV/AIDS strategic plans. Due to these problems, delays in programs implementation, and human resource constraints, the M&E system has not been adequately operationalized (Government of Uganda 2010, pp. 58–63).

Kenya

In Kenya, the National AIDS Control Council (NACC) developed a national HIV/AIDS M&E framework in 2005. The framework, guided by the Three Ones principles, specifies 55 national indicators, data collection methods, reporting schedules, and organizations responsible for reporting. The framework provides an environment for inclusion of new ideas on monitoring and evaluation and improvement of indicators in line with efforts by experts and organizations working on monitoring and evaluation of HIV/AIDS (NACC 2008, 2010). The M&E system was put in place with an operational manual to facilitate data collection on 55 national HIV indicators, reporting, data analysis, and decision making (NACC 2010). The M&E system is integrated into the multisectoral HIV/AIDS strategic plan Kenya developed in 2000. The strategic plan for 2009/10–2012/13 emphasizes four main strategies, including the provision of cost-effective prevention, treatment, care, and support services informed by an engendered rights-based approach (NACC 2010).

In addition to outlining the achievements in reporting and data analysis, the UNGASS 2010 report by the NACC (2010) also identified a number of weaknesses in the country's M&E: low compliance in submitting reports to the NACC, attributed to some partners and implementers sending their reports instead to donors who support them; weaknesses in the M&E subsystems that hindered data compilation and reporting processes; the need for harmonization of the data management information system at the national level with the growing number of indicators; and the need for detailed analysis. A more serious deficiency of reporting in Kenya (and most other Sub-Saharan countries) was the failure to report on behavioral indicators for MARPs as a result of criminalization of commercial sex workers, MSM, and people who inject drugs, even though these groups constitute a major driver of the epidemic (NACC 2010, pp. 44, 67).

Ethiopia

In Ethiopia, the Federal HIV/AIDS Prevention and Control Office (FHAPCO) developed a comprehensive and sustainable M&E system covering the period 2009–2013, but monitoring activities date from 1989. The framework has been generally successful at harmonizing the collection of data at impact and outcome levels. Health sector reporting has been aligned by ongoing updates to the health management information system. Other achievements between 2005/6 and 2008/09 include improvements in human resources for M&E; availability of training and IT support to implementing institutes; allocation of a budget for M&E; initiation of population-based HIV surveillance because antenatal client-based surveillance underestimated HIV prevalence for HIV/TB, sexually transmitted infections (STIs), MARPs, and other entities; further progress by Federal HIV/AIDS Prevention and Control Office (Ethiopia) (FHAPCO) toward establishing a central national warehouse that makes available health facility and community-level HIV-related data, allowing for easy sharing of data among the databases of the different levels; sharing of data and reports between key government organizations and major donors in an effort to decide on a single national measure for each indicator; and development of a reporting format and an integrated supportive supervisory checklist to gather and compile regional-level inputs (FDRE 2008, 2010).

By 2010, 25 core indicators had been included in the M&E system but the knowledge/behavioral indicators for the general population had not been updated since 2005. However, information on the sizes, high-risk behavior and HIV prevalence of MARPS was inadequate due to low levels of social mobilization and low coverage of school-based interventions. Despite rapid expansion of behavioral change communication programs in and out of school, increasing awareness of HIV/AIDS was not accompanied by reduction in risk behavior. Another worrisome trend is the increase in condom use by sex workers with paying customers that reached 99.4% in 2008. This trend, coupled with a decline in condom use with nonpaying customers (66.0%) (FDRE 2010, pp. 9, 16, 39, 62), indicates the impact of the element of trust between steady sexual partners.

Other remaining challenges in implementing the M&E system include difficulties of the system to fully collect all relevant information, including care and support activities both planned and implemented; incompatibility or nonmeasurability of some indicators; lack of baseline for various indicators and inadequate organization of information, largely due to lack of personnel skilled in information management; and poor communication infrastructure at the regional level. A major problem has been the failure to report on specific indicators at the lower level, particularly at *kebele* service points that are manned by health personnel. In order to overcome the problems that arose because health workers were not responsible for reporting nonhealth indicators, the Ministry of Health has started the process of establishing a community management information system. This system will gather nonclinical data from all implementing partners at different levels (FDRE 2010).

Tanzania

In Tanzania, the M&E system, based on the Three Ones principles, comprises a set of documents, tools, and processes that define all aspects of monitoring and evaluating the HIV response in the country. The national M&E framework was developed and launched in 2004 and the M&E operational plan was developed in 2005. The findings of a situational analysis conducted by World Bank/GAMET in collaboration with UNAIDS and the Tanzania Commission for AIDS (TACAIDS) were used to revise the M&E operations plan and develop the Tanzania Output Monitoring System for HIV/AIDS (TOMSHA) and the costed national HIV M&E road map (TACAIDS 2008).

The main data sources for the M&E system are HIV surveillance, behavioral surveillance, population-based surveillance, surveys on quality of health-related HIV services, a condom quality and condom availability survey, a workplace survey, and smaller surveys. For process monitoring, the data sources used include TOMSHA Ministry of Health and Social Welfare medical HIV services monitoring data, Ministry of Education and Vocational Training program monitoring data, and Public Expenditure Review and TACAIDS financial system data (TACAIDS 2008). The M&E system was strengthened between 2004/05 and 2008/09 by analyzing the data regularly for the preparation of reports for the various indicators; carrying out two HIV indicator surveys; harmonizing the indicators for reporting, data collection, and data flow among partners; revising the systems for data collections and analysis to facilitate data use at the points of collection to promote evidence-based planning; and making available at all levels guidelines and protocols for data collection, analysis, and quality improvement (Republic of Tanzania 2010, p. 29; TACAIDS 2008).

A number of managerial and technical weaknesses need to be overcome to further improve Tanzania's M&E system. These include limited capacity at subnational levels in data collection, management, analysis, and reporting, a problem that also affects most other countries in eastern and southern Africa (WHO 2010). Furthermore, the improvement of HIV prevention programs will also require data for specific population groups including MARPS, workplace interventions, and a number of behavioral indicators for youth (Republic of Tanzania 2010, p. 29).

Nigeria

Nigeria's National Agency for the Control of AIDS (NACA) established an M&E unit appropriately staffed and supported by M&E working groups with membership from key stakeholders. Specific responses have been coordinated and scaled up at the national, state, and local government levels toward achieving the targets specified in the 2001 Declaration of Commitment on HIV/AIDS in the areas of universal access to comprehensive prevention, treatment, care, and support programs (NACA 2008, 2010).

These efforts called for a robust and standardized monitoring and evaluation framework. Consequently, the Nigerian National Response Information Management System (NNRIMS) was officially launched in April 2004. By 2006, the majority of state AIDS coordinating agencies had been formed and inaugurated, programming at the state level had been initiated based on state strategic plan (SSP) documents (developed in line with the national strategic framework), and reporting based on NNRIMS protocols had commenced. By 2010, personnel in all 36 states, in the Federal Capital Territory, and at service delivery points had been trained in the use of the harmonized M&E tools (NACA 2010). A well-defined organizational structure had been put in place by 2009, including an HIV M&E unit in the Ministry of Health and supporting M&E systems in 28 federal ministries, departments, and agencies and among public/private sector stakeholders and donors, and 29 states had installed an electronic database for M&E (NACA 2010). These achievements were possible because the political and policy environments were favorable (Odutolu et al. 2006).

Further improvements in the M&E system are being planned in the areas of structure, manpower development, and program monitoring. The improvements include defining the responsibilities and roles of the Ministry of Health, line ministries, and NGOs; strengthening leadership in line ministries and NGOs; strengthening the capacity of and ensuring funding for M&E systems at the state level; promoting research; improving the evaluation of prevention, treatment, care, and support programs; harmonizing multiple data systems for prompt decision making; strengthening human capacity at all levels; linking state and sectoral M&E plans to the national plan; addressing issues of underreporting and late reporting; and improving filing and record systems in some facilities (NACA 2010).

These brief assessments of five national M&E systems reveal that considerable progress has been made by governments since the turn of the millennium in developing systems that can contribute to the HIV/AIDS response. They also show that political will is instrumental in generating a favorable policy environment and the technical, manpower, and managerial capacities necessary to operationalize harmonized, fully functional, and efficient M&E systems, as shown in Nigeria. The urgency is growing to successfully meet the numerous challenges in reaching the objectives set forth in the Three Ones principles and using M&E as a tool for providing timely, reliable, and comprehensive information for multisectoral HIV/AIDS interventions. The need is increasing for correct, evidence-based decisions in an environment of funding uncertainties and increasingly complex and expensive HIV prevention programs.

Other challenges relate to the linkages of different but relevant databases in a single health information management system. Lack of systems for tracking resources for HIV/AIDS impedes M&E activities, given the massive donor resources that are being channeled into M&E activities. Similarly stifling for decision making is the lack of data due to inadequate capacity in data analysis and interpretation. The decentralization of health services has added to the problem of collecting data, a problem that is exacerbated by the failure of many private and NGO-run health facilities to report information. The continuing use of multiple information and reporting systems associated with specific vertical programs and funding in many Sub-Saharan countries contributes to work overload and lack of timely and accurate data (WHO 2010).

Agencies supporting M&E capacity building: A focus on PEPFAR

The President's Emergency Plan for AIDS Relief (PEPFAR), the largest component of the U.S. Global Health Initiative, is one of a number of government agencies and NGOs that have been at the forefront of supporting programs for building capacity in HIV/AIDS monitoring and evaluation around the world. Between 2004 and 2008, PEPFAR contributed $15 billion to prevention, treatment, and care programs in 15 'focus countries', 12 of them in

Africa (Botswana, Côte d'Ivoire, Ethiopia, Kenya, Mozambique, Namibia, Nigeria, Rwanda, South Africa, Tanzania, Uganda, and Zambia). These countries are among the countries most severely impacted by the HIV pandemic and least able to adequately respond on their own (Sessions 2008).

PEPFAR uses a two-pronged approach to facilitate capacity building for M&E in a number of countries: strengthening country monitoring systems to track program service delivery and supporting evaluation studies toward effective, evidence-based programming (PEPFAR 2010). The PEPFAR program has been instrumental in significantly increasing HIV and tuberculosis testing and reducing HIV-related mortality (Benadavid and Bhattacharya 2010; Gunneberg et al. 2011). It is considered by many the most successful of President George W. Bush's foreign policy initiatives (Brown 2008).

In spite of its achievements, the PEPFAR program has fallen short of its potential contribution. Criticism has been leveled at PEPFAR because of its emphasis on the abstinence and 'be faithful' (A and B) components of the ABC approach that discourages and ignores condom promotion and related health education. Although the program claims to target high-risk groups, commercial sex workers are underserved because of the requirement that grantees explicitly oppose prostitution, and youth were not given condoms out of fear that condom distribution might increase premarital sex. Similarly, anti-gay organizations conducted prevention activities using messages stigmatizing MSM, and this drove MSM further from access to prevention services. A panel of experts considered the implementation of the AB directives, which were not inclusive and involved little policy discussion at the country level and thus did not consider country-level needs and conditions, to pose obstacles to the development of effective, evidence-based programs. This situation impeded country-based programming, particularly integration of prevention, treatment, and care programs, including family planning and sexual and reproductive health services (Cohen 2005; Evertz 2010; GAO 2008).

The most frequently cited country example of PEPFAR's shortcomings is Uganda, which had pursued a highly effective AIDS prevention program since 1990 using an ABC approach that stressed the use of condoms and reduction in the number of sexual partners. Two years after adopting the PEPFAR program in 2001, the number of new HIV infections nearly doubled in Uganda and the social bias embedded in the program and its implementation by conservative, faith-based organizations helped spawn an anticondom and antigay climate that resulted in a state-sponsored homophobic environment that led to imprisonments and deaths (Epstein 2005; Evertz 2010).

The reauthorization of PEPFAR in 2008, although eliminating some restrictions on funding, failed to eliminate all impediments to the development of evidence-based and equitable programs; it kept the funding restriction against organizations refusing to explicitly state their opposition to prostitution and it maintained the preference for abstinence-only programs by denying support to the integration of family planning and HIV services. This piecemeal approach perpetuated the funding problems of many programs targeting commercial sex workers and made many commercial sex workers, MSM, and youth hesitant to seek health services out of fear of being penalized (Evertz 2010). PEPFAR also prohibited PEPFAR-funded organizations from distributing condoms in South African schools or providing information on condoms to students 14 years old and younger. These regulations disregarded the South African government's policy of letting individual schools decide whether to distribute condoms to students (Han and Bennish 2006).

In 2011, PEPFAR appeared to proceed toward a more human rights and nondiscriminatory approach when it issued a guidance note encouraging program administrators to develop interventions that consider the needs of MSM and called for implementers to offer nondiscriminatory programs and for government leaders in host countries to revise existing legislation (Council for Global Equality 2011). This discussion and results of global health initiatives illustrate the need for greater country oversight in the monitoring and evaluation of activities and behaviors at all levels of HIV/AIDS programs. In Ghana, for example, where the Global Fund contributed nearly 85% of the national AIDS control program budget, structures parallel to national systems emerged that led to inefficiencies that could be overcome only with strong government leadership (Atun et al. 2011). Various organizations working in the field of global health, including the Commission on Smart Global Health Policy at the Center for Strategic and International Studies, emphasize the need for increased accountability and transparency that would foster more objective evaluation of country programs. These objectives may be achieved by adhering to publicly stated outcome targets, implementing acceptable measurement frameworks within partnership agreements with host governments, and utilizing results generated by PEPFAR programs, among others (Evertz 2010).

Conclusion

During the last decade, most Sub-Saharan countries have developed M&E systems, especially in the areas of building human and institutional capacity and resource allocation; the coordination, implementation, and strengthening of M&E activities, especially at the local level; and questions regarding quality and use of information.

Despite the achievements, Sub-Saharan countries are still faced with a myriad of challenges. Some of these challenges are related to the adherence to the Three Ones principles. Although nearly all countries have adopted these three principles, many programs obtaining their funding from NGOs often fail to comply with central government regulation and guidelines. We hope this problem will be overcome with information and education.

Countries also face a number of challenges related to lack of M&E capacity at lower levels to provide timely reporting, causing delays in decision making. Other challenges include inadequate manpower for M&E activities and training requirements as well as lack of clear indicators, tools, and guidelines.

One of the greatest challenges in M&E is the difficulty in bringing all stakeholders on board to support M&E endeavors. In many organizations M&E is still viewed as the exclusive domain of the M&E unit. There is a need to engage all stakeholders to embrace M&E in order to overcome some of the challenges stated above. Another issue that cannot be ignored is the failure of a number of Sub-Saharan African countries to allocate program funds to strengthening these systems due to continuing dependency on international donors. Dependency on external funding has increased in recent years in Sub-Saharan Africa and there is a need for further studies examining the policies and practices of international donors to ensure that responses are grounded in science and guided by humanitarian principles, not religious ideology or political maneuvering, and are realistically aimed at achieving universal access and meeting the MDGs.

The sustainability of M&E of HIV/AIDS programs at the local, regional, and national levels is a high priority of most Sub-Saharan countries. The need to continually monitor and evaluate the HIV/AIDS epidemics and the impact of interventions in the various countries obtains further urgency in view of the growing patient population and the expansion and increasing complexity of prevention, control, and care and support programs. The effectiveness and sustainability of M&E systems in tracking the implementation of projects, monitoring program interventions, and assessing the utility of programs also requires transparency and accountability in the utilization of financial and material resources.

Because M&E programs are at the center of sound governance, they are necessary for the achievement of evidence-based policy making, budget decisions, management, and accountability in Sub-Saharan Africa's HIV/AIDS prevention programs. If properly carried out, M&E activities can generate a range of benefits, including contributions to project planning and policy development, enhancing governance at all levels, providing project managers with necessary information, and ensuring that the lessons learned from previous projects are incorporated into the design and implementation of new projects.

References

Adamchak, S., Bond, K. and MacLaren, L. 2000. *Monitoring and Evaluating Adolescent Reproductive Health Programs*. Washington, DC: Focus on Young Children.

Atun, R., Pothapregada, S.K., Kwansah, J. et al. 2011. Critical interactions between the Global Fund-supported HIV programs and the health system in Ghana. *Journal of Acquired Immune Deficiency Syndromes* 57(Suppl. 2):S72–S76.

Benadavid, E. and Bhattacharya, J. 2010. PEPFAR in Africa: An evaluation of outcomes. *Annals of Internal Medicine* 19:685–695.

Brown, D. 2008. AIDS funding binds longevity of millions to U.S. *Washington Post,* July 26.

Carty, L. and Nieburg, P. 2010. *Prevention of New HIV Infections: Priorities for U.S. Action.* Washington, DC: Center for Strategic and International Studies.

Cohen, A.S. 2005. U.S. global AIDS policy and sexually active youth: A high-risk strategy. *The Guttmacher Report on Public Policy* 8(3):1–4.

Colvin, M., Gorgens-Albino, M. and Kassed, S. 2009. *Analysis of HIV Prevention Response and Modes of HIV Transmission: The UNAIDS GAMET Supported Synthesis Process.* Sunninghill, South Africa: UNAIDS Regional Support Team for Eastern and Southern Africa.

Council for Global Equality. 2011. U.S. President's Emergency Plan for AIDS Relief (PEPFAR) releases MSM technical note. Washington, DC: May 19. http://globalequality.wordpress.com/tag/pepfar/

Ekouevi, D.K., Karcher, S. and Coffie, P.A. 2011. Strengthening health systems through HIV monitoring and evaluation in Sub-Saharan Africa. *Current Opinions in HIV and AIDS* 6:245–250.

Epstein, H. 2005. *The Invisible Cure: Africa, the West and the Fight against AIDS.* London: Penguin Books.

Evertz, S.C. 2010. How ideology trumped science: Why PEPFAR has failed to meet its potential. Council for Global Equality. www.americanprogress.org and www.globalequality.org

FDRE (Federal Democratic Republic of Ethiopia). 2008. *Report on Progress towards Implementation of the UN Declaration of Commitment on HIV/AIDS.* Addis Ababa: Federal HIV/AIDS Prevention and Control Office.

FDRE (Federal Democratic Republic of Ethiopia). 2010. *Report on Progress towards Implementation of the UN Declaration of Commitment on HIV/AIDS.* Addis Ababa: Federal HIV/AIDS Prevention and Control Office.

GAO (U.S. Government Accountability Office). 2008. *Global HIV/AIDS: A More Country-based Approach Could Improve Allocation of PEPFAR Funding.* Report to Congressional Requesters. www.gao.gov/new.items/d08480.pdf

Global AIDS Program. 2003. *Monitoring and Evaluation Capacity Building Program Improvement: Field Guide.* Atlanta: Centers for Disease Control and Prevention.

Government of Uganda. 2010. *UNGASS Country Progress Report Uganda, January 2008-December 2009.* http://data.unaids.org/pub/Report/2010/Uganda_2010_country_progress_report_en.pdf

Gunneberg, C., Sculler, D., Reid, A. et al. 2011. Comparison of progress in provision of HIV testing and ART for TB patients: African region, the rest of the world and PEPFAR supported countries. Rome: Abstracts of the 6th International Conference on HIV Pathogenesis, Treatment and Prevention. Abstract TUPE485.

Han, J. and Bennish, M.L. 2006. Condom access in South African schools: Law, policy and practice. *PLoS Medicine* 6(1):e1000006. doi: 10.1371/journal.pmed.1000006

Henderson, K., Worth, H., Aggleton, P. and Kippax, S. 2009. Enhancing HIV prevention requires addressing the complex relationship between prevention and treatment. *Global Public Health* 4:117–130.

NACA. 2008. *Roadmap towards Repositioning the HIV/AIDS Monitoring and Evaluating System in Nigeria.* Abuja: National Agency for the Control of AIDS.

NACA. 2010. *2010 UNGASS Progress Report Nigeria.* Abuja: National Agency for the Control of AIDS.

NACC. 2008. *UNGASS 2008 Country Report for Kenya*. Nairobi: National AIDS Control Council.

NACC. 2009. *Kenya HIV Prevention Response and Modes of Transmission Analysis*. Nairobi: National AIDS Control Council.

NACC. 2010. *UNGASS 2010 Country Report-Kenya*. Nairobi: National AIDS Control Council.

Odutolu, O., Jerome, O., Mafeni, P.O. and Oluwole, A.F. 2006. Monitoring and evaluation of HIV/AIDS in Nigeria, in Adeji, O., Kanki, P.J. and Otutolu, O. (eds.), *AIDS in Nigeria: A Nation on the Threshold*, pp. 537–558. Cambridge, MA: Harvard University Press.

PEPFAR (U.S. President's Emergency Plan for AIDS Relief). 2010. *Monitoring and Evaluation*. Washington, DC: USAID.

Persson, A., Ellard, J., Newman, C. et al. 2011. Human rights and universal access for men who have sex with men and people who inject drugs: A qualitative analysis of the 2010 UNGASS narrative country progress reports. *Social Science and Medicine* 73:467–474.

Republic of South Africa. 2010. *Country Progress Report on the Declaration of Commitment on HIV/AIDS, 2010 Report*. Report was submitted to UNAIDS, Geneva.

Sessions, M. 2008. *Overview of the President's Emergency Plan for AIDS Relief (PEPFAR)*. Center for Global Development. http://www.egdev.org/section/initiatives/_archive/hivmonitor/funding/pepfar_overview

Spicer, N., Aleshkina, J., Biesma, R. et al. 2010. National and subnational HIV/AIDS coordination: Are global health initiatives closing the gap between intent and practice? *Global Health* 6:3.

TACAIDS (Tanzania Commission for AIDS). 2008. *UNGASS Country Progress Report: Tanzania Mainland: Reporting Period January 2006-December 2007*. http://data.unaids.org/pub/Report/2008/tanzania_2008_country_progress_report_en.pdf

UNAIDS. 2005. *The 'Three Ones' in Action: Where We Are and Where We Go From Here*. Geneva: UNAIDS.

UNAIDS. 2008a. *Guidance and Specifications for Additional Recommended Indicators*. Geneva: UNAIDS.

UNAIDS. 2008b. *Report on the Global AIDS Epidemic*. Geneva: UNAIDS.

UNAIDS. 2010a. *World AIDS Day Report*. Geneva: UANIDS.

UNAIDS. 2010b. *UNGASS Country Reports 2010*. http://www.unaids.org/en/dataanalysis/monitoringcountryprogress/

UNAIDS. 2011a. *Global AIDS Response Progress Reporting 2012: Guidelines, Construction of Core Indicators for Monitoring the 2011 Political Declaration on HIV/AIDS*. Geneva: UNAIDS.

UNAIDS 2011b. *Securing the Future Today: Synthesis of Strategic Information on HIV and Young People*. Geneva: UNAIDS.

UNAIDS and WHO. 2011. *Guidelines on Surveillance among Populations Most at Risk for HIV*. Geneva: UNAIDS.

UNAIDS and World Bank. 2010. *New HIV Infections by Mode of Transmission in West Africa: A Multi-Country Analysis*. Dakar: UNAIDS Regional Support Team for West and Central Africa.

United Republic of Tanzania. 2010. *UNGASS Reporting for 2010 (Tanzania Mainland and Zanzibar)*. http://www.unaids.org/en/dataanalysis/monitoringcountryprogress/2010progressreportssubmittedbycountries/tanzania_2010_country_progress_report_en.pdf

USAID. 2009. *Strategic Information for HIV/AIDS.* http://www.usaid.gov/our_work/global_health/aids/TechAreas/multisectoral/strategic.html

WHO. 2010. *Joint WHO-UNICEF-UNAIDS-PEPFAR Capacity-Building Workshop: Strengthening Reporting and Monitoring in the Health Sector for the African Region.* Johannesburg, 27–30 September.

World Bank. 2006. *Global HIV/AIDS Program: HIV/AIDS M&E – Getting Results: New Approaches to the 'Third One' in a Changing M&E Landscape.* Washington, DC: World Bank.

World Bank. 2009. *Global Monitoring and Evaluation Team (GAMET).* http://web.worldbank.org

Books, papers, websites, and other resources for further reading

McCoy, K.L., Ngari, P.N. and Krumpe, E.E. 2005. *Building Monitoring, Evaluation and Reporting Systems for HIV/AIDS Programs.* Washington, DC: Pact.

Website for the AIDS and Clinical Trials Group. www.actgnetwork.org/login.aspx?ReturnUrl=%2findex.aspx

Website for the *Journal of HIV/AIDS Surveillance and Monitoring.* http://www.ieph.org/ojs/index.php/jHASE/issue/view/4

Website of the GAMET HIV Monitoring & Evaluation Resources Library. http://gametlibrary.worldbank.org/pages/15_M_Eplan_English.asp?getContent=Tutorials&All=1

Website of the Global Health Sciences Department of the University of California, San Francisco. http://globalhealthsciences.ucsf.edu/prevention-public-health-group/publications-reports

Website of Global HIV M&E Information. http://www.globalhivmeinfo.org/PagesHomePage.aspx

12
Ethical Issues in HIV/AIDS Biomedical Research

Anne A. Khasakhala and Helmut Kloos

Introduction

The aim of biomedical research is to improve the health of individuals through more effective medical diagnostics, clinical care, and therapeutics as well as through public health practices oriented to the community. The pharmaceutical industry and government sponsors are increasingly moving clinical research to developing countries. Between 2002 and 2008, the number of U.S. Food and Drug Administration–regulated investigators carrying out biomedical research outside the USA increased by 15% annually while the number of U.S.-based researchers declined by 5.5% (Getz 2007).

One indicator of an increased focus on Africa for biomedical research is the number of African countries in which HIV vaccine trials are being conducted. Whereas researchers had conducted an HIV vaccine clinical trial in only one country (Uganda) prior to 2000 (Mugerwa et al. 2002), they have since conducted HIV vaccine, microbicide, and/or preexposure prophylaxis trials in eight eastern and southern African countries (South Africa, Botswana, Zimbabwe, Malawi, Tanzania, Kenya, Rwanda, and Uganda) (AVAC 2011). The pace of biomedical research is particularly fast in southern Africa, where research ethics capacity is reportedly in danger of falling behind the pace of research activities (Moodley and Rennie 2011).

Three key factors drive Western pharmaceutical firms to outsource clinical research to developing countries: (1) substantial cost savings due to low labor cost in developing countries; (2) shorter timelines for clinical testing and thus cost savings in countries with large pools of potential research participants and lower research costs that permit rapid recruitment; and (3) the weak and low-cost regulatory environment in developing countries (Glickman et al. 2009), including low risk of litigation (Moodley and Myer 2007). Ideally, ethical legal frameworks should ensure not only that scientific goals are reached but also that the health and human rights of research participants are protected (Andana et al. 2011).

A number of factors affect the conditions under which clinical trials are conducted, such as differences in cultures; standards of care that vary by sponsors and participants in studies; and differences manifested in political, legal, and social contexts. A number of ethical issues have emerged in the course of HIV/AIDS and other disease-specific biomedical interventions in Africa. They are generally viewed from the perspective of the adequacy and equitability of the research guidelines, standards, and protocols used and the competency and integrity of the ethics committees in the countries where the research is being conducted (Moodley 2002). This chapter examines these and other pertinent issues related to ethical biomedical research, such as research collaboration, the role of bioethical research committees in Sub-Saharan Africa, and research funding. The central argument of this chapter is that despite the existence of national and international guidelines, standards, and protocols that govern biomedical research undertakings in Sub-Saharan African countries, many gaps and challenges relating to ethical issues still need to be addressed to ensure just, transparent, and optimal research processes.

Ethical principles relevant to biomedical research

The three principles on which codes of biomedical research ethics are based are autonomy, beneficence, and justice (Ijsselmuiden and Faden 1992). Autonomy refers to an individual's personal liberty of thought and action and is justified by respect for persons with the right to determine their own destiny. Autonomy gives research participants the freedom to deliberate and perform acts of their choosing and allows for special measures to protect the interests of those whose autonomy is diminished. Beneficence denotes the moral obligation to minimize possible harms and to actively maximize potential benefits. It involves explicit consideration of benefits commensurable to risk and includes stringent obligations not to injure intentionally (sometimes expressed as the separate principle of nonmaleficence). Justice refers to treating each person fairly and properly and translates into an ethical obligation to ensure that the burdens and benefits of research are fairly and equitably distributed. These guidelines, which cover a wide range of activities in research involving human participation, formed the basis for the national guidelines adopted by many countries (WHO 2000).

Although human experimentation in health research has been in existence for centuries (Caballero 2002), organized efforts to protect human subjects participating in experiments date only from 1947, when the Nuremberg Code banned forced experiments on humans. The central feature of the Nuremberg Code was the protection of the integrity of the person participating in research. This ban subsequently led to the Helsinki Declaration of 1964. The declaration, which has been revised seven times, sets out the principles to be observed in research on human participants and has become the cornerstone of research related to health care. The declaration has been criticized for not fully protecting local populations; it requires only that researchers need be 'aware of' other ethical and legal requirements. Procedures for enforcement and penalties for breach of the declaration are absent, and the declaration, like all international ethical codes, does not have the force of law (Macklin 2009; World Medical Association 2000).

The application of these and other principles to Sub-Saharan Africa has often been incomplete and occasionally contentious. In particular, autonomy in the choice to participate in a study, provided through a clear understanding of the study protocol and indicated by the signature of informed consent, has been criticized as emanating from an Anglo-American perspective that may not be shared by cultures that place greater importance on community. The situation in Africa, plagued by poverty, cumbersome sociocultural traditions, and high illiteracy, has introduced vulnerability and coercion into the debate (Jegede 2008; Meda 2003). Meda observed that autonomy of choice might not exist in the context of poverty when potential participants are faced with the privileges offered them by the study, such as a standard of care significantly better than the rest of the population receives.

Ethical issues

The process of obtaining informed consent

The process of obtaining informed consent is a core feature of any research undertaking that involves human subjects. A number of studies have examined ethical, legal, and social implications of this process. According to the international ethical guidelines, the informed consent process requires that ethical standards governing human subject research be no less stringent in developing nations than in developed nations (CIOMS/WHO 2002). However, this is not always possible, given the lower levels of literacy; language barriers; and limited understanding of medical concepts, procedures, and disease causation in most developing countries. Additional factors, including monetary inducement (a form of coercion) and lack of understanding of research projects, often preclude well-informed, culturally relevant voluntary consent.

Consent forms need to be prepared and administered in an understandable and culturally acceptable manner, a requirement often inadequately considered by researchers. Mystakidou et al. (2009) offered suggestions on how to overcome the many ethical and practical challenges in obtaining informed consent. They noted that enrolling women, including pregnant, perinatal, and breast-feeding women and adolescent girls, in HIV/AIDS clinical trials is particularly problematic because of gender issues and stigma, discussed in various chapters in this volume. A community-based challenge is to ensure the anonymity of research participants, which may be compromised by close social networks and lack of privacy space that often enable neighbors and others to intrude during interviews, potentially biasing responses and jeopardizing participation in research (Shaibu 2007).

Moodley (2002) noted that using the process of obtaining informed consent as applied in the West assumes that participants in South Africa and other developing countries can be isolated from kinship and community ties. In Africa, however, decision-making has traditionally been the prerogative of communities. For that reason, Mystakidou et al. (2009) suggested that counselors and community leaders might be more effective than others in communicating as middle men with target populations. Other challenges relate to the ways researchers and ethics review committees interpret and apply informed consent (Jegede 2009).

Annas and Grodin (1998) suggested that obtaining informed consent in Africa is difficult and problematic not only because of cultural barriers, but also because research subjects tend to confuse research with treatment in an environment of scarce health care. Thus they tend to accept any offer of 'medical assistance' made by research projects. Annas and Grodin considered it therefore unethical to obtain consent from impoverished populations in the absence of a realistic plan to deliver the outcome products of the research to the population. Many other researchers have concluded that truly voluntary informed consent is rarely obtained in clinical research in Africa and other parts of the developing world (Campbell 2010).

The inability of research participants in Africa and other developing regions to give valid informed consent may render them highly susceptible to exploitation (Rothman 2003). The principles of obtaining informed consent have been challenged in Zambia, where voluntary informed consent was compromised in two cases. In a case involving herbal remedy trials, payments and unrealistic promises were made to predominantly poor study participants. In the second case, inadequate information was provided to community members and research participants in a microbicide trial that resulted in negative publicity, complaints about women participating in the trial becoming infected with HIV, and allegations that the trials were unethical (Andana et al. 2011). Problems such as these illustrate the need for appropriate administration of informed consent requests.

Although international ethics guidelines address the issue of post-trial access to any benefits resulting from research, this issue continues to defy clear solutions in resource-constrained countries (Merritt and Grady 2006). A related concern is how voluntary participation can be ensured in settings where community leaders exert pressure on communities to enroll in clinical trials.

In order to make obtaining informed consent context-specific and thus culturally and socially more acceptable in Africa, Ijsselmuiden and Faden (1992) recommend that procedures for obtaining voluntary informed consent in developing countries be tailored to local customs and culture.

In the USA and many other industrialized countries, for example, regulatory procedures require written consent and focus on the informed consent document itself rather than on the process of obtaining the informed consent (NBAC 2001). The Ethics, Law and Human Rights Collaborating Centre of the WHO/UNAIDS African AIDS Vaccine Program (in Mamotte et al. 2010) issued a report recommending that improvements be made in the formulation and administration of consent forms in order to reduce misunderstandings between researchers and study participants. The center expressed a need to share simple and effective consent templates and procedures across disease areas and to focus on the process of obtaining consent rather than on the forms alone. The report further recommended that comprehensive tests be administered to participants prior to and during participation in clinical trials to ensure that they understand the concepts (Mamotte et al. 2010).

Although signed forms make it easy to audit informed consent (one useful dividend of this process), there are other ways to ensure that informed consent has been obtained. An ethically sound alternative to written consent is oral consent that has been witnessed and verified (Taiwo and Kass 2009). In many countries, it is important that researchers obtain permission from local leaders to seek individual informed consent and to discuss other aspects of the research, such as any benefits to the community and anonymity of informants. Although it may be difficult to identify the members of the community who should be consulted and to determine the level of authority they should have in permitting researchers to approach potential participants, such consultations can be helpful in improving both the informed consent process and the overall research design. Mystakidou et al. (2009) suggested that counseling prior to consenting is crucial for some population subgroups such as adolescents and should be coupled with consent from parents and legal guardians. Consultations with community leaders and other local decision-making structures are required in many African countries as a first step in the consent process; consultations may be followed by community, familial and individual consent. Chokshi et al. (2007) emphasized that all social units involved must grant consent to validate it.

Research collaboration in HIV/AIDS

Collaboration among individuals, institutions, and countries has been increasing steadily for decades, covering different disciplines, development categories, institutions, geographical regions, and countries. Katz and Martin (1997) believed that all are propelled by the notion that collaboration in research is good and should be encouraged. It is a well-accepted axiom in scientific research that collaboration has become an inevitable and essential research component in every field, given its numerous benefits that include enabling researchers to share knowledge, skills, and resources. In the case of African countries, researchers within the continent publish the majority of their research as a result of international collaboration (Narvaez-Berthelemot et al. 2000). Conducting research through collaboration tends to reduce costs and the need for biomedical infrastructure in host countries. Many African countries have taken note of these benefits and, as a result, some have launched initiatives aimed at encouraging and strengthening collaboration among researchers and institutions. Current trends indicate that securing research grants is to a large extent dependent on whether the intended research is to be carried out through collaboration.

Nevertheless, collaboration in HIV/AIDS research in Africa has not been without friction. Both successes and strains have characterized most projects undertaken by researchers in Africa, especially in conjunction with foreign colleagues (Cohen 2000). Cohen noted that tensions have been especially high with regard to equity, including access to financial resources and facilities, participation, transfer of technology, self-reliance, training opportunities, credit, and the use of laboratory facilities by African researchers for personal transactions. Even greater controversy stems from the conflict generated between domestic and international researchers surrounding appropriate ethical research in different countries, especially when conducting HIV clinical trials on humans.

For example, a dispute arose in 2001 between the Department of Microbiology at the University of Nairobi, Kenya, and the Human Immunology Unit of Oxford University concerning research on vaccine development for HIV/AIDS (Patel 2006). The research began with study findings revealing that some HIV-infected Kenyan sex workers from Majengo, an informal settlement in Nairobi, had an immune response that protected them from developing the disease. Researchers from the two countries extracted genetic material from the sex workers and explored whether the material might form the basis for an effective vaccine. The researchers from Oxford patented the process the study teams had developed but did not acknowledge the contributions of the scientists from the University of Nairobi. The study was halted and trials of the vaccine postponed until researchers from the two countries agreed to a new memorandum of understanding (Patel 2006).

As this case illustrates, it is imperative that collaborative research protocols state clearly the contribution of each individual to the project. One problem that plagues most researchers from the developing world is inadequate documentation of the process of the collaborative research and of their individual contributions. In the above-mentioned case, when the Kenyan researchers were asked to state their contribution to the research process they were unable to do so; hence the controversy (Patel 2006).

Vaccine research

As with drug trials, ethical challenges have arisen in vaccine trials in Africa, where HIV-vaccine trials were completed or were underway in 17 countries by 2008 (AVAC 2008). The challenges are compounded when trials involve more than one vaccine; HIV, tuberculosis (TB), and malaria vaccine trials, for instance, present their own unique ethical challenges, requiring careful planning and close collaboration with study communities (Mamotte et al. 2010). Smit et al. (2005) emphasized the need for social and behavioral ethics in HIV vaccine trials, particularly in issues such as assessing individuals' and communities' willingness to participate in vaccine research, participant retention and default patterns, and the study of participants' sexual risk behavior. HIV-vaccine trials are unique in that discrimination and stigma are often directed at participants, who may be perceived to be at high risk of HIV. In malaria vaccine research, the ethics of testing transmission-blocking vaccines that do not protect study subjects from infection or disease but prevent infecting others needs to be taken into consideration. In TB research, the use of placebos may be considered to be unethical when there is a BCG tuberculosis vaccine that could be given to the control group (see Mamotte et al. 2010), although placebos are considered unethical also in HIV trials (Annas and Grodin 1998).

A review of ethical/legal frameworks for biomedical research in Cameroon, Malawi, Nigeria, Rwanda, and Zambia, all countries where HIV-vaccine trials are taking place, found that while these frameworks were able to support vaccine research and protect the rights of research participants, the complexity of the issues at hand was often beyond the capacity of national health research committees and local research ethics committees (Andana et al. 2011). For example, informed consent and post-trial access were variably addressed in these frameworks, with only Malawi and Rwanda addressing the needs and rights of vulnerable groups such as children, pregnant women, elderly persons, and orphans in their guidelines; this situation prevailed also in other countries. These comparative studies hold many lessons for other African countries in capacity building and implementation of ethical/legal frameworks (Andana et al. 2011).

Each trial requires a review of research protocols and follow-up monitoring to ensure their scientific merit and compliance with ethical standards. This is a complex process particularly in the case of HIV-vaccine trials in view of their collaborative nature with the involvement of researchers from Africa and industrialized nations. Monitoring of research after approval is crucial for the optimization of the research process, particularly the protection of the rights and welfare of study participants (Nyika et al. 2009).

Discourse of care and treatment during vaccine clinical trials often centers on standards of care and treatment to be provided when a participant becomes infected (Mamotte et al. 2010). This issue is especially relevant to trials related to AIDS, which, unlike malaria and TB, remains incurable. Mamotte et al. (2010) examined standards of care in multistudy centers in Sub-Saharan countries and found them to be of higher quality than those provided by national health care systems; this means that the standards are not sustainable after the projects are terminated. This finding argues for the integration of multistudy centers with national healthcare systems to provide uniform care and treatment to participants who may become infected instead of offering them preferential treatment only during the duration of the trials.

Genetic and genomic research

The rapidly expanding field of genetic and genomic science, which promises to provide novel insights into the role of human genetic variation in health, presents numerous challenges outside the health 'box' that need to be met to optimize interaction between researchers and study populations. Particularly urgent are the development of new approaches that ensure that participants are adequately informed about the dynamics and complexities of the scientific and ethical issues arising during genomic trials (Rotini and Marshall 2010). For example, existing guidelines for participation in research have largely failed to ensure that researchers explain unfamiliar concepts such as DNA and genetic database. The large number of factors in the epidemiology of HIV and other common infections, together with the heterogeneous distribution of certain genetic effects in different communities and regions, often calls for the collection of large numbers of samples and phenotypic information in a wide variety of cultures and socioeconomic groups, rendering the acquisition of informed consent particularly challenging (Chokshi et al. 2007). A genetic study of podoconiosis, another stigmatized disease, has implications for HIV/AIDS research. Participants hesitated to give their consent, fearing aggravation of stigmatization, and demanded that genetic studies be approved at the household level prior to commencement of surveys (Tekola et al. 2009).

HIV prevention research

Another widely debated ethical issue in HIV prevention research in Sub-Saharan Africa and other developing regions revolves around the provision of long-term antiretroviral therapy (ART) to research subjects who contract HIV during clinical trials. It is inevitable that some participants will become infected during HIV trials because they continue their high-risk behaviors during the research. Host communities are vulnerable to infection due to poverty, illiteracy, and the stigma associated with HIV/AIDS. The ethical complexities of conducting HIV vaccine trials in developing countries include ensuring meaningful community participation; fair selection of volunteers; sound, culturally sensitive consent processes; monitoring of ongoing social harms; obligations of sponsors to ensure HIV treatment to volunteers who become HIV infected during trials in resource-poor contexts; and ensuring fair access to post-trial benefits, capacity development, and effective products (Milford et al. 2006).

Participants who become infected with HIV may begin to require ART four to five years after initial HIV infection, possibly many years after the end of Phases I and II vaccine trials (carried out with relatively small numbers of healthy participants at low HIV risk to assess safety issues and immune responses). There is some scientific interest in providing HIV vaccine to trial participants, particularly in Phase III therapeutic vaccine trials (which typically enrol thousands of volunteers at high risk of HIV infection to assess the efficacy of an HIV vaccine in preventing HIV infection or progression to AIDS-related diseases); the scientific interest is due to the fact that the main objective of these trials is to measure vaccine efficacy in disease amelioration (Fitzgerald et al. 2003). Continuous administration of ART after termination of trials is important because most people in developing countries do not have health insurance.

There is evidence that despite the usually observed aggregate decrease in risk behavior during clinical trials, some individual risk behavior does increase (Bartholow et al. 2005). The ethical concern is the extent to which treatment and care are not directly related to the research design – and not usually available in the host community or country. Slack et al. (2004) recommended that sponsors and investigators be responsible for the treatment of all infections acquired during the course of HIV vaccine trials. However, it is not always possible to identify participants who meet the requirements for the clinical trials.

In the absence of binding international regulations and standards for vaccine research, WHO (2011) is providing guidance, coordination, and support to developing countries to ensure that vaccine trials adhere to widely accepted medical practices. In addition, UNAIDS (2007) has issued guidelines stating that sponsors have the responsibility to ensure access to internationally optimal care and treatment regimens, including antiretroviral therapy for those who become infected during HIV prevention trials. As part of the long-standing debate over what standards of care ought to be set in vaccine trials, the issue of whether researchers have an obligation to provide medical care for trial participants who become infected with HIV as a result of their behavior (and not the vaccine) during the course of the trial has not been settled (Tarantola et al. 2007). Some researchers have opposed the provision of care, arguing that care and treatment would impose a huge cost and logistic burden on sponsors and thus threaten the future of vaccine trials (Teck-Chuan et al. 2008). For example, the government of Cameroon suspended ongoing placebo-controlled trials of the drug tenofovir to prevent HIV infection in sex workers when the government could not reach an agreement with the sponsors and investigators on the level of treatment and care that should be provided to those who develop HIV antibodies during the trials (Mills et al. 2005). Some sponsors are not able to use research funds for such treatments. For example, a U.S. Congressional statute states that research funds from the National Institutes of Health cannot be used to pay for treatment that is not a specific focus of the research (Fitzgerald et al. 2003). Volunteers may become clinically eligible for treatment only several years after a trial is over but there may be challenges in administering the treatment because trial sites are usually closed and trial staff has left the country soon after the trial has ended; in addition, certain trial sites are not equipped as treatment delivery sites. Furthermore, not all researchers are clinicians, and those who are may lack the competence to treat HIV infections.

An especially challenging issue is that of ensuring vulnerable individuals are treated fairly, both during and after a trial. Although ethical issues that might arise during a study may have been extensively discussed, the particular circumstances surrounding research sponsored and conducted by investigators from economically developed countries and performed in economically underdeveloped countries have focused increased attention on poststudy issues. This concern is sometimes described as an issue of post-trial obligations surrounding the question of what obligations trial sponsors and researchers have, if any, to participants at the end of a study. Shaffer et al. (2006) investigated the concerns and priorities of key stakeholders in a developing country regarding the ethical obligations of researchers and perceptions of equity, or 'what is fair', for study participants in an HIV/AIDS clinical drug trial. They concluded that potential clinical trial participants, clinician researchers, and administrators are of the opinion that discontinuing therapy following an HIV/AIDS clinical trial would be unfair. Notwithstanding continuing arguments for and against sponsor responsibility for post-trial treatment, it is becoming increasingly accepted that researchers have a long-term obligation to treat HIV/AIDS clinical trial participants (Shaffer et al. 2006).

Ethical issues arise at the conclusion of all clinical trials. According to the Declaration of Helsinki Principle 30, every patient participating in a study should be assured of access to the best-proven prophylactic, diagnostic, and therapeutic methods identified by the study when the study terminates (World Medical Association 2000). Other international documents either have similar post-trial provisions or call for the best efforts of sponsors and researchers to secure benefits for the participants in the trial and, in some cases, for other persons who might be candidates for the successful intervention (World Medical Association 2000). Having a plan for the routine provision of a successful new intervention to participants after a trial is a way to ensure that the study is responsive to the health needs of the host country. The ethical obligation to provide the intervention to nonstudy members in the community who might benefit from it is much less clear, but a plan to do so would help reduce the risk of exploitation.

Preexposure prophylactic trials

Preexposure prophylactic (PrEP) trials in developing countries have generated much controversy, particularly with regard to care for trial participants and provision of prevention tools. This is because the prevailing weak socioeconomic conditions, limited health care access, and little experience and understanding of research almost inevitably lead to potential exploitation of study participants by corporations from industrialized nations carrying out clinical trials in developing countries (Benatar 2000; Resnik 2004). New or improved drugs resulting from research in research-friendly African countries can reach the market in developed countries relatively quickly but may not ever be sold in Africa because they are unaffordable (Anangwe 2005). Further, the demand for the great majority of these drugs in the host countries is lower than in the affluent countries for which they are being developed, and health services for their delivery are absent in the host countries (Glickman et al. 2009). Consequently, research participants and communities in African countries bear the major share of the burden of research without receiving a fair share of the benefits.

It is widely thought that individuals and communities in developing countries assume the risks of research, but most of the benefits may accrue to people in developed countries (Benatar 2000). The situation is further compounded by poverty, limited health care services, illiteracy, cultural and linguistic differences, and limited understanding of the nature of scientific research in the developing countries. These factors increase the possibility of exploitation (Emanuel et al. 2000). Furthermore, the regulatory infrastructures and independent oversight processes that might minimize the risk of exploitation tend to be less well-established, less supported financially, and less effective in developing countries. For efficacy trials of any biomedical HIV prevention product, the populations with the highest incidence of HIV are those most likely to be considered for participation and those most likely to benefit from an effective intervention. However, for a variety of reasons, these populations may be relatively vulnerable to exploitation and harm in the context of biomedical HIV prevention trials (UNAIDS 2007).

Bioethics research committees

The low capacity of research ethics committees (RECs) in developing countries to review research proposals is a frequently cited problem. RECs are required to interpret international ethics guidelines in specific socioeconomic and cultural conditions and often operate in complex environments characterized by power inequalities among governments, donors, researchers, and/or communities. Several factors often compromise their independence in decision making, including interests of governments and other institutions, money, prestige, customs, and lack of adequate knowledge. In places where challenging authority and debating complex issues are difficult, RECs may lack transparency, and conflicts of interest frequently impede fair negotiations in developing countries (Moodley and Myer 2007; Rugemalila 2001).

Although RECs in Sub-Saharan Africa are still inadequate in numbers and quality, the conclusion by Rwabihana et al. (2010) that the region lacks trained and independent personnel who can serve on RECs fails to consider the realities on the ground. The numerous socioeconomic and political factors discussed in this chapter and the employment of many researchers by large pharmaceutical firms are more likely impediments. Thus issues such as bias and favoritism may be effectively addressed only after these problems are solved.

Another problem that seems to bedevil the research ethical committees in Africa is lack of continuity of expertise due to high turnover of staff. Emanuel et al. (2004) observed the extremity of these challenges in developing countries' contexts relative to the developed countries. HIV vaccine trials – which are often international collaborations between resource-poor nations and organizations from more resourced countries – may be especially challenging to RECs in developing countries. RECs and researchers working in Africa have the responsibility of safeguarding patients' rights in the same way they would in industrialized nations. However, they have not always done so; rather, researchers from the North tend to side-step local ethical committees in the developing world when they know it would be difficult to obtain clearance for their studies from the committees. They are able to circumvent local ethical committees in part because of the prevailing corruption in most African countries. In some cases, they are aided by the fact that the polity overshadows the academy; many academicians heading scientific institutions do so under the pressure of powerful politicians and may not have the expertise to review technical proposals.

Political influence on RECs is strong in African countries, where most medical research institutes are public entities whose heads are politically appointed and maneuvered. They lack the independence and guidelines to objectively review research initiated and funded by the developed world and carried out in developing countries (Nyika et al. 2009). An example is a 2004 case involving illegal and unethical export of blood samples from a Kenyan children's home without proper approval. The researcher at the orphanage who had been working officially on the study claimed that scientists from Oxford University came to Kenya and illegally took blood samples of patients from the facility. The National Council for Science and Technology investigated the charge and determined that a research proposal had been appropriately prepared by the university but the protocol in the proposal had not indicated that blood samples were to be exported to the UK. The oversight was reported and an application was made in 2001 for which the ethical clearance was given in 2002. In the meantime, samples had been exported. The Oxford scientists insisted that they had not meant to do anything unethical; they had been given verbal approval to take the samples and assumed the oral permission was adequate (Patel 2006).

Some Western researchers and pharmaceutical firms have taken advantage of the lack of local legislation and have ignored rudimentary local guidelines, suggesting paternalism and double standards (Nyika et al. 2009). For instance, Pfizer was accused of unethical behavior during trials of the drug trovafloxacin mesylate (Trovan) in Nigeria. It was alleged that several children were denied effective alternative treatment so that clinical data could be obtained to support approval by the regulatory agency. Later Pfizer claimed that the trial did not seek to gather clinical data, but to help sick children in a poor region of Nigeria (Pfizer 2009).

In response to the complexities of conducting research in African countries, numerous initiatives have been set up aiming at increasing capacity for ethical review of health research (Nyika et al. 2009). These initiatives involve a number of nonprofit African organizations in capacity-building programs. For example, the South African Research Ethics Training Initiative, which is based at the Universities of KwaZulu-Natal and Pretoria, provides training in ethics to African researchers and REC members through short-term fellowships and long-term educational programs. Despite these initiatives, little empirical research has been conducted in Sub-Saharan countries to determine REC capacity to review and approve clinical trial protocols, including protocols for HIV vaccine trials (Sumathipala et al. 2004).

Research to date reveals the need to develop appropriate local ethical guidelines and policy to train REC members and to increase RECs' independence, diversity of membership, and monitoring of approved protocols. A study in Uganda showed that research on HIV vaccines faces many barriers – social, political, legal, ethical, and behavioral. The barriers include public misconceptions and media misinformation, a lengthy review process, and inadequate national regulatory mechanisms (Hyder et al. 2004). In Kenya, reviewers frequently reported that they often do not have the training to understand complex immunological concepts.

Funding of biomedical research and patent issues

Research in developing countries is often financed by well-resourced developed countries and conducted in vulnerable host communities with diverse cultural backgrounds (Anangwe 2005; Milford et al. 2006). Multinational research is frequently conducted according to the regulatory frameworks of wealthier sponsor countries, which may be inappropriate for host country conditions and raises ethical concerns about potential exploitation of host communities and participants, insensitivity to community ethos, the scope of sponsor-investigator obligations, and the appropriate communication of research results to participants (Kilama 2003; Milford et al. 2006).

Clinical research in developing countries is conducted primarily to respond to local health needs, but it can also be exploratory research conducted to test the feasibility or effectiveness of interventions or to respond to national regulatory requirements, which may require clinical trial experience in different ethnic groups or in a number of different health care settings. Clinical trials in developing countries are typically complex and costly, and the lack of infrastructure and complex ethical and regulatory requirements makes conducting clinical research in developing countries a formidable challenge (Anangwe 2005; Milford et al. 2006). Researchers must consider the local context in which research will take place and obtain and follow guidelines from local experts, committees, and institutions as necessary. These steps must be taken as part of an interactive learning experience if the research is to be implemented successfully.

The many resources required in biomedical research, including human and financial resources, equipment, drugs, and vaccines, make this research area a preserve of pharmaceutical multinationals, which are driven by profit motives. The developed countries have traditionally dominated North–South collaboration in biomedical research and pharmaceutical trade, nearly all in a one-way direction (Anangwe 2005). The rapid increase in South–South collaboration in biotechnology is decreasing the dependence of African countries on the North and boosting competitiveness and growth of the pharmaceutical sector in developing countries. South African firms have more South–South collaborations than any other developing country after Brazil, including China and India, and nearly as many South–South as North–South collaborations. Collaborations within Africa exist between South Africa and all southern African countries except Zambia and Angola and with Kenya, Uganda, Nigeria, Ghana, Sudan, and Egypt. The growing number of bilateral, multilateral, and regional agreements among African and non-African countries is promoting the development of HIV diagnostic kits, drugs, and vaccines and, equally important, is addressing shared health problems (Thorsteinsdóttir et al. 2010).

Resnik (1998) considered the international distribution of biomedical research resources to be highly inequitable and unjust for two reasons. First, multinational pharmaceutical and biotechnology companies do not regard research and development (R&D) investments in health problems of developing nations to be economically profitable. Second, government biomedical research agencies in developed countries face little political pressure to allocate funds for the problems of developing nations. R&D on new drugs, vaccines, and other biological materials is very expensive, and part of the cost of bringing a new product to the market is generally considered R&D and part is considered a capital expenditure (Mahmoud et al. 2006). Nevertheless, developers of a new product must follow the stipulations of the International Conference on Harmonization of Good Clinical Practices and adhere to acceptable international scientific and ethical standards (Kilama 2009).

Developing a new product and bringing it to market is not only costly; it also takes a relatively long time, usually 10–12 years (Resnik 2004). The patent a company obtains usually lasts 20 years, during which time the patent holder has exclusive rights to make, use, or commercialize its invention, with some exceptions mentioned below. Once a patent expires, the company still has exclusive rights over the trademarked name of its invention, but other companies can manufacture, use, or commercialize the invention under a non-trademarked (generic) name. As a result, drug companies prioritize their R&D activities depending on the factors that affect the profitability of a new product, such as the size of the potential market, consumer demand, the scope of intellectual property protection, the expected time from the laboratory to the market, and liability costs. Few companies capitalizing R&D are interested in spending money on drugs and vaccines for diseases that afflict the developing world, where consumer demand for them is weak and intellectual property protection is uncertain (Resnik 2001), although they may decide to allocate funds to projects for the developing world as a social responsibility (Resnik 2004).

Politics has been cited as the main barrier to increasing government funding for R&D on health problems in the developing world (Resnik 2004). First, R&D on problems that have their main impact on the developing world does not have as much popular support in the North as R&D on problems that have their main impact on the developed world. Second, even research that has popular appeal will not obtain government support if no advocacy group lobbies the government for money.

Patent issues, although highly technical and legal in nature, have made their way into the ethical debate with respect to their place in prior agreements and as obstacles to access to treatment and to the development of new treatment in developing countries. The Trade Related Aspects of Intellectual Property Rights (TRIPS) agreement set by the World Trade Organization (WTO 2005) in 1995 provide a legal framework that promotes the profit motives of the pharmaceutical industry. It guarantees pharmaceutical companies patent protection of a product for a period of 20 years, giving them the legal power to prevent African countries from importing cheaper generics. However, the TRIPS Agreement provides low-income countries with flexibilities in implementing laws and regulations that allow them to overcome impediments in pricing, tariffs, and trade agreements in increasing access to affordable and quality antiretrovirals (ARVs) and diagnostics. The Doha Declaration on the TRIPS Agreement and Public Health elaborated on the flexibilities of the TRIPS Agreement that can promote access to ART for all (UNAIDS 2011). These provisions include compulsory licenses, mechanisms authorizing governments or third parties to use a patent-protected drug without the consent of the patent holder; parallel imports, the simultaneous importing and local purchase of the same products for price advantages; and exemptions for least developed countries that exempt these countries from mandatory compliance with the TRIPS Agreement for extended periods (UNAIDS 2011). Differential pricing for ARVs between high-, middle-, and low-income countries, a strategy compatible with the TRIPS Agreement that has ensured that the lowest prices were charged in low-income countries, has apparently been used by more countries than the other four incentives (Yadav 2010).

Although more than 60 low- and middle-income countries have obtained generic ARVs in large quantities since the Doha Declaration (Hoen et al. 2011), relatively few Sub-Saharan countries have amended their laws to incorporate flexibilities optimally since the Doha Declaration (Beall and Kuhn 2012; WIPO 2010). Moreover, challenges to further increases in the ARV rollout may be expected if new drugs are more widely patented in Sub-Saharan Africa, if policy provisions impede the importation or local production of ARVs, and if funding lags behind needs (Hoen et al. 2011). UNAIDS (2011, p. 9) and WTO (2011) urged low- and medium-income countries to identify their priority needs to the TRIPS Council for implementing the TRIPS Agreement and high-income countries and international organizations to provide support to least developed countries to address the needs effectively.

Drug prices are still among the major obstacles to ARV treatment access in poor countries even though prices have continued to decrease, between 40% and 60% between 2008 and early 2010 (UNAIDS 2011). Second-line combination treatments with protease inhibitors cost up to four times as much as the first-line drug cocktails, which averaged $150–$200 per adult person per year in 2010 (PlusNews 2010) and the Global Fund (2010) estimated that by 2020, 50% of the cost of ART worldwide will be used to treat 24% of all AIDS patients on second-line treatment regimens (PlusNews 2010). The cost of first-line generic combinations needs also to be reduced further to close the monetary gap between overall needs and available funding.

Conclusion

This review of pertinent ethical issues in biomedical research with a focus on HIV/AIDS in Sub-Saharan Africa reveals that the continent's socioeconomic and regulatory context increasingly attracts biomedical research projects by international corporations and research institutions. Despite the adoption of universal declarations and national regulations that protect human subjects participating in research, effective protection of human subjects continues to be generally inadequate across countries, and the increasingly multinational nature of research activities by international corporations has underscored these disparities. We conclude that in view of the weakness of existing international ethical guidelines, biomedical research in Sub-Saharan Africa may benefit from national regulations that provide guidance on the role of local research ethics committees, informed consent procedures, standards of care, and compensation for injuries caused by sponsored research. The ethical concerns raised by the use of placebo control trials emanate from the fact that these trials are used to establish standard treatment protocols. However, given the controversy surrounding the Helsinki Declaration revisions, the debate over the best-proven and best available treatments remains at the core of clinical trial design in African countries, where, for the most part, the best-proven treatment is not available to the population in need of it.

High poverty levels and perceived desperation of people in Sub-Saharan Africa have convinced some Western medical corporations that this region is the cheapest destination for testing their biomedical products and ideas. This has given rise to potentially risky trials with little regard for safety and ethical issues, a situation attributable partly to the absence of clear policies in African countries to guide biomedical trials.

African companies that have the capacity to produce generic products may benefit from incentives to produce ARV drugs and vaccines, even though this may lead to competition over the control of underserved markets. This conflict of interest may be ameliorated by requiring that Western multinationals that want to enter these markets negotiate partnership agreements aimed at reducing the gap caused by high-level technology and market penetration. These processes and a number of international agreements and guidelines, particularly the TRIPS Agreement, promise to result in further reductions in drug prices and thus further increases in the availability and accessibility of ARVs and, hopefully, of vaccines in the future. South–South collaboration in biotechnology development represents another promising route to the development of Sub-Saharan Africa's biotechnology.

References

Andana, P., Awah, P., Ndebele, P. et al. 2011. The ethical and legal regulation of HIV-vaccine research in Africa: Lessons from Cameroon, Malawi, Nigeria, Rwanda and Zambia. *American Journal of AIDS Research* 10:451–463.

Annas, G.J and Grodin, M.A. 1998. Human rights and maternal-fetal HIV transmission prevention trials in Africa. *American Journal of Public Health* 88:560–563.

AVAC (AIDS Vaccine Advocacy Coalition). 2008. *The Search Must Continue* (AVAC Report 2008). New York: AVAC.

AVAC. 2011. A quarterly update on HIV prevention research. *Px Wire* 4(1):1–4.

Bartholow, B.N., Buchbinder, S., Celum, C. et al. 2005. HIV sexual risk behavior over 36 months of follow-up in world's first HIV vaccine efficacy trial. *Journal of AIDS* 39:90–101.

Beall, R. and Kuhn, R. 2012. Trends in compulsory licensing of pharmaceuticals since the Doha Declaration: A database analysis. *PLoS Medicine* 9:e1001154, epub 2012 Jan 10.

Benatar, S. R. 2000. Avoiding exploitation in clinical research. *Cambridge Quarterly on Health Ethic* 9:562–565.

Caballero, B. 2002. Ethical issues for collaborative research in developing countries. *American Journal of Clinical Nutrition* 76:717–720.

Campbell, B. 2010. Informed consent in developing countries: Myth or reality. http://www.dartmouth.edu/~ ethics/docs.Campbell_informed consent.pdf

Chokshi, D.A., Thera, M.A., Parker, M. et al. 2007. Valid consent for genomic epidemiology in developing countries. *PLoS Medicine* 4(4):e95. doi: 10.1371/journal.pmed.0040095.

CIOMS/WHO 2002. *International Guidelines for Biomedical Research Involving Human Subjects*. Geneva: Council for International Organizations of Medical Sciences (CIOMS) in collaboration with the World Health Organization.

Cohen, J. 2000. Balancing the collaboration equation. *Science* 288(5474):2155–2158.

Emanuel, E.J., Wendler, D. and Grady, C. 2000. What makes clinical research ethical? *Journal of the American Medical Association* 283:2701–2711.

Emanuel, E.J., Wood, A. and Fleischman, A. 2004. Oversight of human participants research: Identifying problems to evaluate reform proposals. *Annals of Internal Medicine* 141:282–291.

Fitzgerald, D., Pape, J.W., Wasserheit J. et al. 2003. Provision of treatment in HIV-1 vaccine trials in developing countries. *Lancet* 362:993–994.

Getz, K.A. 2007, Sept. 1. Global clinical trials activity in the details. *Applied Clinical Trials*. http://www.appliedclinicaltrialsonline.com/appliedclinicaltrials/article/articleDetails. jsp?id=453243

Glickman, S.W., McHutchison, J.G., Peterson, E.D. 2009. Ethical and scientific implications of the globalization of clinical research. *New England Journal of Medicine* 360:816–823.

Global Fund. 2010. *Resource Scenarios for 2011–2013 and the Long-term Cost and Health Impact of Global Fund Programs*. The Global Fund 3rd Voluntary Replenishment 2011–2013, First Meeting, The Hague, Netherlands, 24–25 March.

Hoen, E., Berger, J., Calmy, A. and Moon, S. 2011. Driving a decade of change: HIV/AIDS, patents and access to medicines for all. *Journal of the International AIDS Society* 14:15.

Hyder, A.A., Wali, S.A., Khan, A.N. et al. 2004. Ethical review of health research: A perspective from developing country researchers. *Journal of Medical Ethics* 30: 68–72.

Ijsselmuiden, C.B. and Faden, R.R. 1992. Research and informed consent in Africa: Another look. *New England Journal of Medicine* 326:830–834.

Jegede, A.S. 2008. Understanding informed consent for participation in international health research. *Developing World Bioethics* 9:81–87.

Jegede, S. 2009. African ethics, health care research and community and individual participation. *Journal of Asian and African Studies* 44:239–253.

Katz, J.S. and Martin, B.R. 1997. What is research collaboration? *Research Policy* 26:1–18.

Kilama, W. 2003. Malaria vaccine research and testing in Africa. *Acta Tropica* 88(2):153–159.

Kilama, W. 2009. From research to control: Translating research findings into health policies, operational guidelines and health products. *Acta Tropica* 112(Suppl. 1): S91–S101.

Macklin, R. 2009. The declaration of Helsinki: Another revision. *Indian Journal of Medical Ethics* 6:2–4.

Mahmoud, A., Danzon, P.M., Barton, J.M. et al. 2006. Product development priorities. In Jamison, D.T., Breman, J.G. and Measham, A.R. (eds.), *Disease Control Priorities in Developing Countries*, Chapter 6. Washington, DC: World Bank.

Mamotte, N., Wassenaar, D., Koehn, J. and Essak, Z. 2010. Convergent ethical issues in HIV/AIDS, tuberculosis and malaria vaccine trials in Africa: Report from the WHO/UNAIDS African AIDS vaccine programme's ethics, law and human rights collaborating centre consultation 10–11 February 2009, Durban, South Africa. *BMC Medical Ethics* 11:3. doi: 10.11/1472-8939-4-3

Meda, N. 2003. HIV/AIDS clinical research in Africa: Ethical aspects. In Sukovski, K. (ed.), *The Ethical Aspects of Biomedical Research in Developing Countries: Proceedings of the Round Table Debate*, pp. 33–42. Luxembourg: Office for Official Publications of the European Communities.

Merritt, M. and Grady, C. 2006. Reciprocity and post-trial access for participants in antiretroviral therapy trial. *AIDS* 20:1791–1794.

Milford, C., Wassenaar, D. and Slack, C. 2006. Resources and needs of research ethics committees in Africa: Preparations for HIV vaccine trials. *IRB: Ethics and Human Research* 28:1–9.

Mills, E.J., Rachlis, B., Wu, P. et al. 2005. Media reporting of tenofovir trials in Cambodia and Cameroon. *BMC International Health and Human Rights* 5(6). doi:10.1186/1472-698x-5-6

Moodley, K. 2002. HIV vaccine trial participation in South Africa: An ethical assessment. *Journal of Medical Philosophy* 27:197–215.

Moodley, K. and Myer, L. 2007. Health research ethics committees in South Africa 12 years into democracy. *BMC Medical Ethics* 8:1.

Moodley, K. and Rennie, S. 2011. Advancing research ethics training in Southern Africa (ARESA). *South African Journal of Bioethics and Law* 4:1004–1005.

Mugerwa, R.D., Kaleebu P., Mugyenyi, P. et al. 2002. First trial of the HIV-1 vaccine in Africa: Ugandan experience. *British Medical Journal* 324:226–229.

Mystakidou, K., Panagiotou, I., Katsaragakis, S. et al. 2009. Ethical and practical challenges in implementing informed consent in HIV/AIDS clinical trials in developing or resource-limited countries. *Journal of Social Aspects of HIV/AIDS* 6(2):46–57.

Narvaez-Berthelemot, N., Russell, J.M., Arvanitis, R. et al. 2000. Science in Africa: An overview of mainstream scientific output. Paper presented at 8th International Conference on Scientometrics and Informetrics, Sydney, 16–20 July.

NBAC (National Bioethics Advisory Commission). 2001. *Ethical and Policy Issues in Research Involving Human Participants*. Bethesda, MD: NBAC.

Nyika, A., Kilama, W., Chilengi, R. and Tangwa, P. 2009. Composition, training needs and independence of ethics review committees across Africa: Are the gate-keepers rising to the emerging challenges? *Journal of Medical Ethics* 35:189–193.

Patel, V. 2006. *Clinical Trials in Kenya*. Amsterdam: Stichting Onderzoeg Multinationale Ondernemigen (SOMO). http://www.somo.nl/html/paginas/pdf/Kenya_clinical_trials_2006_EN.pdf

Pfizer (Pfizer sued over alleged drug experiment on Nigerian children: District Court Jurisdiction Under Alien Tort Statute at Issue). 2009. *Judicial View*. http://jv.onebeep.com/Court-Cases/Torts/Pfizer-Sued-Over-Alleged-Drug-Experiment-on-Nigerian-children/44/5865

PlusNews. 2010. Second-line drugs often cost up to four times more than first line drugs. 2010. *Plus News Newsletter*, Office of the Coordination of Humanitarian Affairs, United Nations.

Resnik, D.B. 1998. The ethics of HIV research in developing nations. *Bioethics* 12:286–306.

Resnik, D.B. 2001. Developing drugs for the developing world: An economic, legal, moral and political dilemma. *Bioethics* 1:11–32.

Resnik, D.B. 2004. The distribution of biomedical research resources and international justice. *Developing World Bioethics* 4:42–57.

Rothman, D.J. 2003. Clinical trials in 'developing' countries: Is there a special 'Third World' ethic? *Zeitschrift für Ärztliche Fortbildung und Qualitätssicherung* 97:695–702.

Rotini, C.N. and Marshall, P.A. 2010. Tailoring the process of informed consent in genetic and genomic research. *Genome Medicine* 2:20.

Rugemalila, J.B. 2001. Health research ethics for African countries. *Acta Tropica* 78:S99–S103.

Rwabihana, J.-P., Girre, C. and Duguet, A.-M. 2010. Ethics committees for biomedical research in some African emerging countries. *Journal of Medical Ethics* 36: 243–249.

Shaffer, D.N., Yebei, V.N., Ballidawa, J.B. et al. 2006. Equitable treatment for HIV/AIDS clinical trial participants: A focus group study of patients, clinician researchers, and administrators in western Kenya: Research ethics. *Journal of Medical Ethics* 32:55–60.

Shaibu, S. 2007. Ethical and cultural considerations in informed consent in Botswana. *Nursing Ethics* 14:503–509.

Slack, C., Stobie, M., Milford, C. et al. 2004. Provision of HIV treatment in HIV preventive vaccine trials: A developing country perspective. *Social Science and Medicine* 60:1197–1208.

Smit, J., Middelkopp, K. and Myer, L. 2005. Socio-behavioural challenges to phase III vaccine trials in Sub-Saharan Africa. *African Health Sciences* 5:198–206.

Sumathipala, A., Siribaddana, S. and Patel, V. 2004. Under-representation of developing countries in the research literature: Ethical issues arising from a survey of five leading medical journals. *BMC Medical Ethics* 5:5–10.

Taiwo, O.O. and Kass, N. 2009. Post-consent in oral health subjects' understanding of informed consent in oral health in Nigeria. *BMC Medical Ethics* 1:10.

Tarantola, D., Macklin, R., Reed, Z.H. et al. 2007. Ethical considerations related to the provision of care and treatment in vaccine trials. Paper read at the 4th IAS Conference on Pathogenesis, Treatment and Prevention, Sidney, Abstract No. MOAC304.

Teck-Chuan, V., Cinn, J., and Campbell, A.V. 2008. Multinational research. In Crowley, E.M. (ed.), *From Birth to Death and Bench to Clinic: Briefing Book for Journalists, Policymakers, and Campaigns*, pp. 107–110. Garrison, NY: The Hastings Center.

Tekola, F., Bull, S., Farsides, B. et al. 2009. Impact of social stigma on the process of obtaining informed consent for enetic resaerch on popoconiosis: A qualitative study. *BMC Medical Ethics* 10:13. doi:10.1186/1472-6939-10-13.

Thorsteinsdóttir, H., Melon, C.C., Ray, M. et al. 2010. South-South entrepreneurial collaboration in health biotech. *Nature Biotechnology* 5:407–416.

UNAIDS. 2007. *Ethical Considerations in Biomedical HIV Prevention Trials*. Geneva, Switzerland: UNAIDS.

UNAIDS. 2011. *Using TRIPS Flexibilities to Improve Access to HIV Treatment*. Geneva: UNAIDS.

WHO. 2000. *Operational Guidelines for Ethics Committees that Review Biomedical Research*. WHO Report TDR/PDR/Ethics/2000.1. Geneva: WHO.

WHO. 2011. Vaccine Research and Development. http://www.who.int/vaccine_research/en/

WIPO (World Intellectual Property Organization). 2010. *Patent Related Flexibilities in the Multilateral Legal Framework and Their Legislative Implementation at the National and Regional Levels*. Geneva: WIPO.

World Medical Association. 2000. *Declaration of Helsinki: Ethical Principles for Medical Research Involving Human Subjects*. Edinburgh: World Medical Association.

WTO (World Trade Organization). 2005. *Amendments to the TRIPS Agreement: General Council Decision of 6 December 2005*. http://www.wto.org/english/tratop_e/trips_e/wt1641_e.htm

WTO (World Trade Organization). 2011. Least developed countries' priority needs in intellectual property. http://www.wto. org/English/tratop_e/ldc_e.htm

252 *Impacts and Responses to HIV/AIDS*

Yadav, P. 2010. *Differential Pricing for Pharmaceuticals: Review of the Literature, New Findings and Ideas for Action.* Report prepared for the U.K. Department of International Development. Zaragoza: Zaragoza Logistics Center.

Books, papers, websites, and other resources for further reading

Braude, H.D. 2009. Colonialism, Biko and AIDS: Reflections on the principle of beneficence in South African medical ethics. *Social Science and Medicine* 68:2053–2060.

Website of the science and technology regional collaboration network IBSA network: http://www.ibsa-trilateral.org

Website of the science and technology regional collaboration network New Partnership for Africa's Development: http://www.nepad.org

13
Conclusion

Damen Haile Mariam and Helmut Kloos

This volume demonstrates that the social sciences can contribute significantly to a better understanding of the complexities of the HIV/AIDS epidemic and to developing effective and appropriate prevention, care, and support programs in Sub-Saharan Africa during this time of stepped-up responses. Disciplinary blindness and biased research pursuing biomedical objectives, procrastination by some governments and the international community in responding to the epidemic in a timely fashion, and the vested interests of aid organizations contributed to discrepancies between national research agendas and the realities of HIV risk, impacts, and vulnerabilities and the needs of the African people. The lesson that is still being learned in some quarters is that most HIV prevention programs in Africa have failed mainly because biomedical researchers and administrations failed to adequately address the social, cultural, economic, and political context of HIV/AIDS and human sexuality. Where collaboration between the social and biomedical sciences was achieved, research results were not always considered in policies and interventions. For example, the global governance of HIV/AIDS still fails to take into account local perceptions, experiences, and responses to the disease, as noted by Getnet Tadele in the Introduction. These shortcomings are also apparent in the design and implementation of some programs at the local level in Sub-Saharan Africa, reflecting deeprooted traditions, perceptions, and practices that cannot be changed without adequate understanding of socioeconomic and cultural constraints affecting the participation of HIV-infected and affected people and communities.

In addressing the multifaceted themes of sexuality and inequalities in social and sexual relations, Chapters 2–4 draw attention to significantly higher female than male HIV vulnerability in the social and economic contexts of different Sub-Saharan African countries. Cultural perceptions of masculinity and femininity are identified in Chapters 2, 3, and 4 as some of the major impediments to reducing high-risk sexual behavior, sexual inequities, and violence against women. This information can broaden understanding of these and related driving forces of the HIV epidemic, which were until recently neglected by researchers and policy makers. The empowerment of women, the transformation of gender relations, and decreasing female and male vulnerability to HIV infection will require sexually more conciliatory and equitable positions of religious, cultural, and social norms of masculinity and femininity. A number of useful frameworks developed by various declarations and conventions emphasize sexual and reproductive rights, together with other social, economic, and political rights that must inform HIV/AIDS policy and programs to render interventions more effective (Tallis 2002, pp. 16–20, 50). With the ongoing up-scaling of HIV services, additional aspects of the masculinity factor need to be examined, such as the relationship between the use of HIV testing and treatment services and local understandings of manhood, a major barrier to the utilization of services by males. In an effort to provide a balanced assessment of these and other intransigent obstacles to HIV prevention, Getnet Tadele and Woldekidan Amde point out that multiple-partner sex, stigma, denial, and blame casting are not more prevalent in Sub-Saharan Africa than in industrialized countries in the North and that some of the behaviors labelled in the literature as 'traditionally African' are of recent origin. These findings help to dispel the notion that Africans are inherently more prone to transmit HIV and may guide prevention and control programs in assessing vulnerabilities and opportunities for community participation.

Chapters 2–5, on gender, youth, and socioeconomic issues in HIV risk, describe some of the variable relationships between poverty and HIV vulnerabilities. They point out that while poverty contributes to women's vulnerabilities and exacerbates HIV impacts at all levels of society, it may also interact with education, sexual networks, and high-risk behavior in ways that may put relatively affluent males at high risk of infection. The extensive national Demographic and Health Survey (DHS) data showing a direct relationship between HIV rates and socioeconomic status and recent findings that extramarital sex by men declined with increased poverty (Skovdal et al. 2011) underscore the complexities of the role of socioeconomic status on infection. While this information supports the view by de Walque and Kline (2010) that the relationships between education, poverty, and HIV status may be amenable to change through policies and programs, the role of poverty in HIV transmission needs to be studied more thoroughly in different contexts (Muchini et al. 2010).

The discussion of the interrelationship between food insecurity, poverty, and HIV/AIDS vulnerability by Ayalew Gebre and colleagues helps to shape the contour of HIV vulnerability at the individual, household, and community levels, particularly in eastern and southern Africa, which include some of the most rural economies and some of the most food insecure and poor countries in Sub-Saharan Africa. HIV/AIDS is now well known to have reduced farm production and damaged livelihoods by shrinking and weakening labor forces, reducing land areas cultivated, and effecting changes in agricultural practices. Poverty alleviation and food security programs must consider the two emerging issues of increasing feminization of poverty and currently sharp increases in the cost of food in Sub-Saharan Africa. The increasingly recognized links between nutrition and HIV infection outcomes and between food security and HIV vulnerability, particularly among women and children, are further evidence of the need to ensure food security as an enabling and empowering strategy in HIV prevention efforts.

The examination of vulnerability to the impact of HIV/AIDS at the individual, household, workplace, and community levels by Ayalew Gebre and colleagues in Chapter 6 brings together information on HIV/AIDS impacts, risk, and adaptive or coping behavior that can inform policy makers and program managers. The authors' examination of social and cultural dimensions contributes to a better understanding of the impacts of HIV at the household level beyond the economic analyses of most studies. In particular, the differential impacts on women and girls caring for ill family members, to the point that many students drop out of school and engage in transactional sex and grandmothers go begging, further illustrate the heavy HIV burden females bear. A considerable amount of information is presented on the impacts of the disease on social relations and economic wellbeing beyond infected individuals and households that supports the view that HIV/AIDS contributes to increasing poverty and inequality in the wider community, also noted by Haaker (2010), although causal pathways and synergisms still need to be identified in different socioeconomic and cultural settings. For instance, Chapter 6 presents understudied relationships between natural resources and HIV/AIDS in people's quest for food, including the accelerated exploitation of natural resources by AIDS-affected communities and, vice versa, increasing HIV vulnerability among fishermen caused by altered fishing practices necessitated by water pollution in Lake Victoria, practices that affected sexual behavior. The impacts of these and other understudied and complex relationships between HIV/AIDS, ecosystems, and societal well-being must be better understood to improve and up-scale preventive, treatment, care, support, and impact mitigation services and create a socioeconomic and psycho-social environment that empowers affected individuals, groups, and institutions and overcomes persisting stigma.

Continuing the discussion of workplace-related impacts and responses, Chapter 7 describes the high HIV vulnerability of migrant laborers in the socioeconomic context of southern African mines and commercial farms, where some of the highest infection rates anywhere have been recorded. Gender inequality, labor exploitation, the creation of high-risk living conditions by corporations, and generally weak and unenforced labor policies have contributed to the high HIV transmission levels and limited access to health services among migrant laborers, particularly females. The role of these workers in the spread of HIV at the workplace, within national boundaries, and in their home areas in other countries is far from understood, as is the impact of HIV/AIDS programs recently implemented by mines and farms. Further research may shed new light on these issues and the legacy of HIV/AIDS in southern Africa (see, for example, Barnett and Whiteside 2008) as companies make more information available.

The information in Chapters 2, 6, and 8 on traditional and contemporary social and political organizations and leaders, previously neglected in HIV/AIDS discourse but increasingly considered to have the potential to be key players in HIV/AIDS interventions, points to a large potential human resource for community-initiated and community-owned interventions. The generally greater success of Africans themselves than international organizations in running AIDS projects has been attributed to feelings of solidarity, compassion, and mutual aid that prompt collective action in communities (Epstein 2007, p. xiv). Faith-based organizations, burial associations, traditional healers, traditional community leaders, community conversations and dialogues, and youth organizations have contributed significantly to prevention, care, and support programs. More studies will be required to determine how to streamline their contributions in multisectoral HIV/AIDS programs and how traditional institutions of governance can be aligned harmoniously with the modern state. Further research may identify suitable partners and coalitions for the development of a broader support base in comprehensive HIV/AIDS programs, especially in underserved rural areas and among hard-to-reach populations.

The remarkable progress made in rapidly up-scaling antiretroviral treatment programs, implementing combined prevention programs, and creating awareness; recent advances in the care and support of AIDS patients; as well as initiatives in school health, orphan care, and monitoring and evaluation of programs in Sub-Saharan Africa indicate that the HIV/AIDS epidemic can be controlled and its impacts mitigated if the necessary resources are allocated in a timely, equitable, and sustainable manner. Our guardedly optimistic outlook contrasts with the more pessimistic view prevailing a decade ago (see, for example, Kalipeni et al. 2004), prior to the massive antiretroviral therapy (ART) rollout. Achievements to date clearly reveal the crucial role of humanitarian vision, political will, and innovative policies and programs that emphasize equity and collaboration among stakeholders at all levels of society, from the community to the national levels. Governments and international partners are gradually extending multisectoral HIV/AIDS programs to most-at-risk groups, including men having sex with men (MSM), sex workers, injection drug users, and adolescents, in recognition of their significance in HIV transmission, although progress in this area is often elusive due to deeply entrenched sociocultural inequities, stigma, and discrimination. These various efforts and the strengthening of health services through task shifting in line with decentralization and primary health care strategies and new HIV prevention strategies, particularly those aiming at structural changes and prevention of mother-to-child transmission of HIV, hold promise for further reducing HIV transmission.

In spite of the significant achievements made to date, ART cannot be considered a 'magic bullet', and its success will, to a considerable degree, depend on overcoming a number of persisting socioeconomic, cultural, infrastructure, political, and funding problems. Levelling off and even declining funding for HIV/AIDS programs, due largely to donor fatigue and the world economic crisis, threaten the progress made so far by interrupting ART. Interrupting ART would invariably increase the risk of virological failures in resource-poor areas (Pisani 2010) and also the number of eligible infected people failing to obtain ART. It may be possible for declining funding to be offset by increasing cost-effectiveness and efficiency of interventions and realizing greater ownership of the HIV/AIDS response by African countries. There is an emerging trend in several African countries to increasingly contribute to interventions in the form of joint ventures, technology transfers, and direct investments toward the development of antiretrovirals (ARVs) and other medical products. This trend bodes well for further mobilization of domestic resources, capacity building, and sustainability of HIV/AIDS interventions. More than half a dozen major African agreements and initiatives are promising, including the 2011 African Consensus and Position on Development Effectiveness; the African Union Health Strategy 2007–2015; ongoing collaboration among the United Nations Economic Commission for Africa, the African Union, the African Development Bank, and the Harmonization of Health in Africa; the 2007 Pharmaceutical Manufacturing Plan for Africa; and the 2006 Abuja Call for Accelerated Action towards Universal Access to HIV and AIDS, Tuberculosis, and Malaria Services in Africa. These provide the framework for alleviating Africa's dependency crisis and increasing African ownership of development investments, two goals that have eluded traditional development cooperation approaches (UNAIDS 2012).

Several other emerging issues related to the up-scaling of treatment programs need urgent attention. For example, different investigators have reported both positive and negative effects of ART on stigma in different contexts (Maughan-Brown 2010; Wilhelm-Solomon 2010), and the impact of treatment on the sexual behavior of infected persons is still unclear (Shafer et al. 2011; Venkatesh et al. 2010). The ballooning orphan and surviving people living with HIV and AIDS (PLWHA) populations require that alternative care services, particularly community-based care and chronic care and support services, be upgraded in ways that improve their quality and sustainability. The weakening of the traditional African care system of the extended family, now overstretched largely because of poverty and the widespread familial AIDS burden, makes it prudent to consider alternative AIDS patient and orphan care and support systems, as suggested by Getnet Tadele and Woldekidan Amde in Chapter 9.

Although many traditional HIV/AIDS prevention programs have failed in Sub-Saharan Africa, strategies designed to encourage safer sexual behavior were highly successful, particularly in Uganda and Senegal (Green 2003; UNAIDS 1999). These positive outcomes are corroborated by more recent information in various chapters, particularly in the chapter on mainstreaming HIV interventions into educational systems by Anne Khasakhala. Her review evaluates how education policies and the school environment in Sub-Saharan Africa affect the vulnerability of people in the education system to HIV infection and progress made by some recent initiatives Both issues need to be better understood for the development of appropriate policies and effective prevention, treatment, and care programs and efforts to ameliorate the impact of the epidemic. The fact that mainstreaming efforts have increased coverage and benefits to targeted populations, including HIV/AIDS information in the curriculum and distribution of ARVs and condoms in schools, suggests that reductions of the high HIV transmission rates among students, teachers, and support staff are possible.

It is increasingly recognized that monitoring and evaluation will become more important as a management tool with the ever-increasing demands for programs that track the dynamics and impacts of the HIV/AIDS epidemic, assess the effectiveness of the increasing number and complexity of interventions, and up-scale promising programs. Because HIV/AIDS in Sub-Saharan Africa is, as in other regions, a politically charged issue, monitoring and evaluation can be powerful in convincing policy makers, donors, and the general population to support programs (UNAIDS 2000). But the data presented must be scientifically valid rather than merely politically correct, an issue raised, among others, by critics of national HIV estimates that had to be adjusted downward (Chin 2007). The impending funding crisis facing HIV/AIDS programs will increase the need for monitoring and evaluation programs that can maximize their cost-effectiveness. Anne Khasakhala's and Helmut Kloos's review of the literature on monitoring and evaluation programs, including recent national UNGASS reports, reveals that, notwithstanding the considerable achievements in capacity building and implementation, many gaps remain in the timely collection, completeness, quality, and use of data for evidence-based decision making. Their examination of monitoring and evaluation (M&E) reporting by Sub-Saharan countries shows continuing underreporting of behavioral and socioeconomic indicators for children and other high-risk groups as a serious impediment to planning and implementing equitable and comprehensive HIV/AIDS programs.

The chapters by Getnet Tadele, Ayalew Gebre, and colleagues on the major intervention strategies provide ample evidence that while the biomedical approach has done much in preventing the spread of the HIV/AIDS epidemic, it cannot improve the health of populations in isolation. The authors' main argument is that interventions should not only target individuals for treatment and behavioral change, but also promote health-enhancing social, economic, and cultural environments, an approach largely neglected in the past. Several recent research projects in different African countries indicate that endogenous behavior change, while still inadequate and uneven among countries and communities, has been achieved through structural interventions (Glick 2010). While these findings underscore the importance of contextualizing HIV/AIDS studies in different locales and socioeconomic groups, there is a need to link reported behavior changes with epidemiological data to validate results of HIV risk studies, a task social scientists often failed to carry out in an environment of frail biomedical/social science relations.

The final chapter of this volume addresses human rights and social justice issues surrounding the development of antiretroviral drugs and vaccines in Sub-Saharan Africa that have come to the fore in recent years as part of the massive ART roll-out and intensified efforts to develop a vaccine for use in humans. The combination of corporate greed, regulatory weakness, and undereducated participating populations provides a fertile ground for exploitive and culturally insensitive biomedical research that may not be in the best interest of host countries and target populations. Upgrading biomedical research and strengthening local research committees, adhering to established guidelines and informed research procedures and standards of care, and establishing partnerships between multinational pharmaceutical corporations and firms producing generic drugs in the South promise to make biomedical research safer and ethically acceptable and ensure greater accessibility of low-cost drugs. The urgency of these measures is indicated by the large number of HIV infections; the need to increase understanding of the efficacy of different ARV drugs and candidate vaccines in order to increase ART uptake, adherence, and optimum outcomes; and impending funding shortfalls. South–South collaboration in health biotech development is rapidly expanding in an increasingly favorable regional research and trade environment, an encouraging sign that Africa and other developing regions are beginning to assert their desire and capacity for greater self-sufficiency in the health field.

This volume indicates that moving forward in the current environment of stepped-up anti-HIV/AIDS efforts and emerging challenges presents many new needs and opportunities for social science and interdisciplinary research. In addition to the above-mentioned issues that need to be addressed, the spatial distribution of culture-specific high-risk environments and social HIV networks requires more attention. Research results may help to identify HIV-vulnerable communities; facilitate the evaluation of innovative, effective, and sustainable community-based prevention, treatment, care, and support programs; guide interventions; and identify constraints in achieving universal accessibility to treatment, care, and support. The continuing increase in the number of people living with HIV/AIDS makes the evaluation of care and support programs designed to meet their needs one of the most urgent tasks of HIV/AIDS governance. Notwithstanding the maturing of the epidemic and greater inroads made by prevention and control programs, the various challenges for further progress identified in this volume will increase the need for stepped-up social science input in interdisciplinary projects. Exchange of experiences and discussions by social, behavioral, and biomedical scientists across national boundaries has been energized by the biannual International AIDS Conferences, local conferences and workshops, and the First International HIV Social Science and Humanities Conference, held in June 2011 in Durban, South Africa.

References

Barnett, T. and Whiteside, A. 2008. *AIDS in the Twenty-First Century: Disease and Globalization.* 2nd ed. New York: Palgrave Macmillan.

Chin, C. 2007. *The AIDS Pandemic: The Collision of Epidemiology with Political Correctness.* Oxford: Radcliffe Publishing.

de Walque, D. and Kline, R. 2010. The relationship between HIV infection and education: An analysis of six African countries. In Sahn, D.E. (ed.), *The Socioeconomic Dimension of HIV/AIDS in Africa: Challenges, Opportunities and Misconceptions,* pp. 42–56. Ithaca, NY: Cornell University Press in collaboration with the United Nations University.

Epstein, H. 2007. *The Invisible Cure: Why We Are Losing the Fight against AIDS in Africa.* New York: Picador.

Glick, P. 2010. HIV prevention in Africa: What has been learned? In Sahn, D.E. (ed.), *The Socioeconomic Dimensions of HIV/AIDS in Africa: Challenges, Opportunities and Misconceptions,* pp. 231–267. Ithaca, NY: Cornell University Press in collaboration with the United Nations University.

Green, E.C. 2003. *Rethinking Prevention: Learning from Successes in Developing Countries.* Westport, CT: Praeger.

Haaker, M. 2010. HIV/AIDS, economic growth, inequality. In Sahn, D.E. (ed.), *The Socio-Economic Dimension of HIV/AIDS in Africa: Challenges, Opportunities and Misconceptions,* pp. 12–41. Ithaca, NY: Cornell University Press in collaboration with the United Nations University.

Kalipeni, E., Craddock, S. and Ghosh, J. 2004. Mapping the AIDS pandemic in Eastern and Southern Africa: A critical overview. In Kalipeni, E., Craddock, S., Oppong, J. and Ghosh, J. (eds.), *HIV/AIDS in Africa: Beyond Epidemiology,* pp. 58–69. Oxford: Blackwell.

Maughan-Brown, B. 2010. Stigma rises despite antiretroviral roll-out: A longitudinal analysis in South Africa. *Social Science and Medicine* 70:368–374.

Muchini, B., Benedikt, C., Gregson, S. et al. 2010. Local perceptions of the forms, timing and causes of behavior change in response to the AIDS epidemic in Zimbabwe. *AIDS and Behavior* 15:487–498.

Pisani, E. 2010. Treating ourselves to trouble? The impact of HIV treatment in Africa: Lessons from the industrialized world. In Sahn, D.E. (ed.), *The Socio-economic Dimensions of HIV/AIDS in Africa: Challenges: Opportunities and Misconceptions,* pp. 268–286. Ithaca, NY: Cornell University in collaboration with the United Nations University.

Shafer, L.A., Nsubuga, R.N., White, R. et al. 2011. Antiretroviral therapy and sexual behavior in Uganda: A cohort study. *AIDS* 25:671–678. doi.10.1097/QAD.06013e328341fb18

Skovdal, M., Campbell, C., Madanhire, C. et al. 2011. Masculinity as a barrier to men's use of HIV services in Zimbabwe. *Globalization and Health* 7:13.

Tallis, V. 2002. *Gender and HIV/AIDS: Overview Report.* Sussex: University of Sussex, Institute of Development Studies.

UNAIDS. 1999. *Acting Early to Prevent AIDS: The Case of Senegal.* Geneva: UNAIDS.

UNAIDS. 2000. *National AIDS Control Programmes: A Guide to Monitoring and Evaluation.* Geneva: UNAIDS.

UNAIDS. 2012. *AIDS Dependency Crisis: Sourcing African Solutions.* Geneva: UNAIDS.

Venkatesh, K.K., de Bruyn, G., Lurie, M.N. et al. 2010. Decreased sexual risk behavior in the era of HAART among HIV-infected urban and rural South Africans attending primary care clinics. *AIDS* 24:2687–2696. doi: 10.1097/QAD.0b013e32833e78d4

Wilhelm-Solomon, M. 2010. *Stigmatization, Disclosure and Social Space of the Camp: Reflections on ARV Provision to the Displaced in Northern Uganda.* Center for Social Science Research Working Paper No. 267. Cape Town: University of Cape Town.

Books, papers, websites, and other resources for further reading

Mills, E.J., Barninghausen, T. and Negrin, J. 2012. HIV and aging-preparing for the challenge ahead. *New England Journal of Medicine* 366:1271–1274.

UNAIDS. 2012.*UNAIDS Strategy 2011–2015.* Geneva: UNAIDS.

UNAIDS. 2012. *2012 Progress Reports Submitted by Countries.* Geneva: UNAIDS

Index

262